Discover the Amazing Healing Powers of Nature . . .

❧ PANSIES ARE PURPLE, VIOLETS ARE BLUE—and, believe it or not, they both can help treat glaucoma.

❧ WHAT'S AN "ANTI-ULCER COCKTAIL"? Find out Dr. Duke's secret recipe for ulcers—a delicious fruit smoothie to soothe the pain.

❧ SUSPICIOUS OF SILICONE IMPLANTS? Try fenugreek seeds or sprouts to increase breast size.

❧ DOES STINGING NETTLE HURT? No, but this versatile herb—a common weed that grows throughout the United States—is used to treat a multitude of ailments, from allergies to tendinitis.

❧ IS THERE A CURE FOR BALDNESS? An herb called saw palmetto may prevent the conversion of testosterone into a substance that kills off hair follicles.

READ ON TO FIND OUT MORE ABOUT
THOUSANDS OF OTHER HERBAL REMEDIES
AND THE HUNDREDS OF COMMON
CONDITIONS AND DISEASES THEY TREAT!

THE GREEN PHARMACY

The Ultimate Compendium of Natural Remedies from the World's Foremost Authority on Healing Herbs

JAMES A DUKE, Ph.D.

St. Martin's Paperbacks

The Green Pharmacy is meant to increase your knowledge of the latest developments in the use of plants for medicinal purposes. Because everyone is different, a physician must diagnose conditions and supervise the use of healing herbs to treat individual health problems. Herbs and other natural remedies are not substitutes for professional medical care. We urge you to seek the best medical resources available to help you make informed decisions.

Published by arrangement with Rodale Press Inc.

THE GREEN PHARMACY

Copyright © 1997 by James A. Duke.

Illustrations copyright © 1997 by Peggy K. Duke.

Library of Congress Catalog Card Number: 97-6175

ISBN: 0-312-96648-2

Printed in the United States of America

Rodale Press Inc. hardcover edition published 1997
St. Martin's Paperbacks edition/July 1998

St. Martin's Paperbacks are published by St. Martin's Press, 175 Fifth Avenue, New York, NY 10010.

10   9   8   7   6   5   4

Illustrations

The illustration of ginkgo on page 34 was previously published in *CRC Handbook of Nuts* by James A. Duke (Boca Raton, Fla.: CRC Press, 1989).

The illustrations of Asian ginseng on page 163 and American ginseng on page 233 were previously published in *Ginseng: A Concise Handbook* by James A. Duke (Algonac, Mich.: Reference Publications, 1989).

The illustration of goldenseal on page 249 was previously published in *Herb Companion Magazine* (Loveland, Colo.: Interweave Press, April/May 1994).

The illustrations of evening primrose on page 443 and red clover on page 483 were previously published in *CRC Handbook of Edible Weeds* by James A. Duke (Boca Raton, Fla.: CRC Press, 1992)

The illustration of cat's claw on page 508 was previously published in *Cat's Claw: Healing Vine of Peru* by K. Jones (Seattle, Wash.: Sylvan Press, 1996).

*T*his book is one more flower for Momma, Martha Truss Duke (deceased November 1995), who for at least 66 of her 98 years encouraged my love of forests and flowers. May her spirit merge with the pine forests of the red hills of Alabama.

Dedicated to four professors who most shaped my fascinating ecotour through life:

Dr. A. E. Radford of the University of North Carolina, now retired, who taught me the Carolina flora, aquatic and terrestrial

Dr. C. R. Bell of the University of North Carolina, now retired, who stretched me to Mexico, Guatemala and Costa Rica

Dr. R. E. Woodson of the Missouri Botanical Garden, deceased, who stretched me to Panama and Peru, at least in the herbarium

Dr. R. S. Davidson of the Battelle Memorial Institute, now retired, who moved me, Peggy, John and Celia to Panama, where my midlife conversion to ethnobotany and herbalism and my love for Latin America and its forests was entrenched

Contents

Part One

Your Guide to the Green Pharmacy

Part Two

Choosing the Herbs That Heal

-A-

-B-

-C-

-D-

-E-

-F-

-G-

-H-

-I-

-L-

-M-

-N-

-O-

-P-

-R-

-S-

-T-

-U-

-V-

-W-

-Y-

Acknowledgments

It takes a lot of good people to make a good book. If this proves to be a good book, and I hope it will, credits are due to many. First of all, I'd like to thank the staff at Rodale Press, especially my editor, Alice Feinstein. She was there all the way, all the time, to help and advise me as I plowed through new literary crossroads. She steered me to a writer and editor I have long admired, Michael Castleman, who was able to take my scientific jargon and translate it to the gentle language you'll read in this book. It's interesting for me to compare the stuffy stuff I wrote to the laymanese generated by Alice and Michael.

Closer to home, there's my incredible "right-hand man," Judi duCellier. For 20 years now, she has been an indispensable and patient helper—first as secretary, then as program assistant and co-author of one of my books. At home, there's my wife, Peggy, who's grown with me as we wheeled through a rich and interesting life. Peggy did the illustrations for this book.

As with so much in life, I'm indebted to so many people besides the four mentioned above for helping me solve my nitty-gritty problems. But I'm going to stop right here, lest I run the risk of making many people unhappy by failing to include them in what could easily be a list that goes on for pages.

There are more than a hundred diseases and hundreds of herbal remedies included in this book, and I've had conversations with hundreds of people from Maine to Peru as I've gathered this information through the years. I've especially appreciated all the participants in my field classes. I probably enjoy my classes more than the participants do, because they continually add to my store of anecdotes with all the interesting tidbits and stories they pass my way. I'll wager that more than a hundred readers recognize themselves in these pages, and I'd like to say thank you to all of them.

Finally, it seems appropriate to acknowledge my teachers. My grade school teacher, Miss Horne, and my high school teacher, Miss Beddingfield, encouraged and catalyzed my interest in the outdoors. My major professor at the University of North Carolina, Dr. A. E. Radford, taught me the flora of the Carolinas. C. Ritchie Bell took me to Mexico, Guatemala and Costa Rica and passed me on, as a post-doc, to the Missouri Botanical Garden. There, Dr. Edgar Anderson, Dr. Hugh Cutler, Dr. Fritz Went and Dr. R. E. Woodson, Jr., put some polish on me. Each of my teachers contributed in some way to this book, and I thank them for their patience and good work.

Introduction

Welcome to *The Green Pharmacy!*

This book is the culmination of many decades of work with medicinal plants throughout the world and many years of plant-hunting, from China to Costa Rica, from Peru to Pennsylvania, from the hills of Virginia to the upper reaches of the Amazon.

For most of my 30-year career, I've worked for the U.S. Department of Agriculture (USDA) as a botanist specializing in medicinal plants. Technically, I'm what is known as an ethnobotanist, which simply means that I've studied how plants are used as food and medicine in many different cultures. During that career, I've personally seen medicinal herbs successfully treat conditions that high-tech pharmaceuticals could scarcely touch.

I've also used many of these medicinal remedies myself and recommended them to friends and family when they seemed appropriate. Obviously, I wouldn't do this unless I had a high degree of confidence in the healing power of these plants as well as in their safety. In the next four chapters, and in the alphabetical entries throughout this book, you'll find my advice and cautions. These are based on my personal experiences as well as an extensive database of scientific information about the various chemicals and compounds found in plants.

In part Two, "Choosing the Herbs that Heal," I have applied a rating system of sorts to highlight the herbs and herbal remedies that I believe to be the most effective for each of the diseases and health problems. The most highly recommended herbs have a three-leaf ✺✺✺ rating. For alternate remedies, however, be sure to pay attention to herbs with two-leaf ✺✺ and one-leaf ✺ ratings. (I could have used stars, of course, but leaves seem a lot more appropriate in a book called *The Green Pharmacy*.)

You'll also find throughout this book that I give many subjective opinions as well as some personal anecdotes about my experiences with medicinal plants and natural healing. Since these experiences really come from a lifetime of interest, I hope you'll also read the personal postscript.

But first, let's have a look at the Green Pharmacy.

PART ONE

❦

Your Guide to the Green Pharmacy

Entering the Green Pharmacy

If you're reading this book, you probably know what an herb is . . . or do you? The term *herb* should be easy to define, but actually, it's surprisingly difficult.

The classic botanical definition is that an herb is a nonwoody plant that dies down to its roots each winter. Clearly, this definition was concocted by botanists in a cold climate, specifically that of northern Europe. According to this definition, there are no herbs in the Amazonian rain forest, one of the world's most botanically diverse, herb-rich habitats, because there is no winter.

The classic definition also excludes woody trees and shrubs, including ginkgo and hawthorn, two of the biggest-selling medicinal "herbs" in Europe. That's why some people prefer the term *botanicals* (and *botanical medicine*): It includes trees and shrubs as well as herbs.

Using a broader definition, some people consider an herb to be simply a useful plant. The big problem with this definition is that in one very important sense, all green plants are useful, even those that are not food and have no place in medicine or commerce. All green plants perform photosynthesis, combining sunlight, carbon dioxide and water and releasing the oxygen we all breathe. I'd say that's pretty useful.

For the purposes of *The Green Pharmacy*, I define an herb simply as a medicinal plant. It can be woody or nonwoody, from a cold climate or a tropical one. It can be a wild or tame food, a weed, a culinary spice or whatever. It doesn't even have to be green. Plenty of barks, roots and plant parts that are not green are medicinal and therefore part of the Green Pharmacy. And there are a lot of medicinal mushrooms out there that are not green and that do deserve more attention than they'll get in this book.

The Green Pharmacy Challenge

Most Americans believe that we have the best health-care system in the world—at least that's what all the doctors and government health experts keep trying to tell us. But anyone who has ever gotten the run-around from a doctor or had to deal with a health insurance company knows that if what we have is the best, then the best still leaves a lot to be desired.

Most Americans assume that the pharmaceuticals their doctors prescribe are unquestionably better than the herbal medicines that few doctors and relatively few Americans know much about. It delights me to no end that this picture is changing rapidly.

I've been a botanist specializing in medicinal plants for most of my 30-year career, and I've personally seen medicinal herbs successfully treat conditions that high-tech pharmaceuticals could not touch.

The reason herbs are not more popular in the United States is that the drug companies can't patent them. The drug companies make their money by pulling the medicinally active molecules out of herbs and then tinkering with them a little until they're chemically unique. The companies can then patent their new molecules, give them brand names and sell them back to us for a lot more money than their original herbal sources cost.

Herbs Are Good Medicine

Of course, the drug companies always say that their unique molecules are better, stronger, more targeted and safer than herbs. I'll readily agree that they are stronger. In fact, they're often too strong and have bad side effects that their herbal precursors might not have.

As for pharmaceuticals being better, that's sometimes hard to say. In some studies, herbal products clearly perform better. Ginger, for example, has been shown to be superior to pharmaceutical dimenhydrinate (Dramamine) as a preventive therapy for motion sickness.

I'm not saying that pharmaceuticals are bad. I am saying that we need more research that tests herbs against pharmaceutical drugs. Until that happens, we simply won't know which is better. That leads me to the rather shocking conclusion that Americans are not necessarily getting the best medicine. The Green Pharmacy with its herbal therapies may, in many cases, prove to be more economical, more effective and safer—all with fewer side effects—than the pharmaceuticals.

Our challenge is to transcend the assumptions that are made by doctors, the advertising and promotion of the drug companies and the narrow and restrictive drug approval process used by the U.S. government. Our challenge is to think green—not the mercenary, monetary green of the pharmaceutical firms but the cleansing, empowering green of chlorophyll, the green that feeds, fuels, oxygenates and medicates our planet.

Economics drives the pharmaceutical companies, but what drives the Green Pharmacy and the green lifestyle in general is ecology, the idea that we're connected to everything else on the planet and that we all thrive or fall together.

Putting Safety First

I'll be the first to admit that herbal medicine is not risk-free. To benefit from using herbs, you need to have some basic background information. Then you need to have confidence in the herbs you use and in any herbal practitioner you consult. This is no different from conventional medicine, where you need to have confidence in your physician and any pharmaceutical you take.

As a rule, however, rational herbal medicine is safer than conventional medicine because the medicines are more dilute and side effects tend to be less severe.

But you still have to exercise caution when using herbal medicines. You also need to understand that things can go wrong. There are a number of strategies that you can use to protect yourself.

First of all, get the right stuff. Unless you are absolutely sure of an herb's identity, don't take it. This rule applies mainly to people who are picking herbs in the wild, of course. People have been known to eat poisonous or dangerous plants simply because they misidentified an herb and took something other than what they thought they were taking. The classic killer is poison hemlock, which looks rather like wild parsley or wild parsnip.

The Universe of Herbs

While there are some 300,000 higher plant species that are all chemically distinct, fewer than 10 percent of them have been carefully screened for their medicinal and toxic constituents. A really good herbalist might know 1,000 to 2,000 species, rarely more.

This means that experienced as well as inexperienced herbalists can make mistakes. Not too long ago, while gathering herbs for a weekend class in the Blue Ridge Mountains, yours truly got all excited at the discovery of some "wild ginseng." Later, on closer examination, I was chagrined to discover that the supposed ginseng was Virginia creeper.

❧

Herbs to Shun while Pregnant

As a general rule, you shouldn't take herbs while you're pregnant unless you discuss your selections with your obstetrician.

There's a good reason for this. Quite a few herbs can increase the risk of miscarriage. Maine herbalist Deb Soule, author of the feminist herbal *The Roots of Healing*, advises pregnant women to avoid the following herbs: barberry root bark, cascara sagrada, feverfew, juniper berries, mugwort, pennyroyal, pokeroot, rue, senna, southernwood, tansy, thuja and wormwood. That sounds like good advice to me, and I would add a few more to this list: balsam pear, chervil, Chinese angelica, hernandia, hyptis, mayapple and mountain mint. Lately I've also seen caution flags about evening primrose and St.-John's-wort, but I haven't seen the rationale behind these caveats.

It's also a good idea not to binge on celery or parsley. Eating a little of these healthy vegetables won't do any harm, but eating a lot could conceivably cause a problem.

You should limit your consumption of caffeine as well. One study showed what the researchers called a "strong association of caffeine intake during pregnancy and fetal loss." As little as 163 milligrams of caffeine per day—the amount in one to two cups of brewed coffee—might double the risk of spontaneous abortion.

In addition, here are a few more "don'ts" during pregnancy: Don't smoke, don't drink alcohol, and again, don't take any drugs, including over-the-counter products, except on the advice of your physician.

❦

Of course, herbalists are not alone in making the occasional error. Physicians and pharmacists make them as well. And I personally feel safer consulting a well-informed herbalist than I do consulting most doctors. As for the perils of pharmaceuticals, read the fine print on labels or in the advertisements.

As for the identities of commercially packaged herbal products, especially those that are chemically standardized, you can usually trust the labels. But even with standardized extracts, as with pharmaceuticals, there is a very small but still real chance for error.

Watching Out for Problems

Whatever herb you're taking, I recommend that you learn as much as you can about what to expect from it. If anything unexpected happens, stop taking whatever it is and check with an expert you trust.

In addition, here's some further advice for anyone using herbal medicine.

Make sure of the diagnosis. Herbal devotees sometimes get the idea that they can diagnose illness as well as come up with herbs to treat it. But diagnosis is a separate art and one that is best left to physicians. I discourage self-diagnosis.

Diagnosing illness is not easy, and sometimes even good doctors make mistakes. But physicians' diagnostic batting average is usually better than that of anyone who has not had medical training. Once you're confident of a diagnosis, then you can discuss with your physician how to treat it: drugs, herbs, some combination of the two or any of the foregoing plus diet, exercise and lifestyle changes. Some holistic physicians will stress diet and lifestyle more than drugs for some ailments.

Watch out for side effects. I'm convinced that all medicines, natural or synthetic, have side effects. It's hard to imagine an active plant chemical (phytochemical)—or an herbal mixture containing thousands of them—having just one targeted chemical reaction in our body. Of course we have other reactions, unrelated to the illness, that could appropriately be termed side effects—some desirable and some undesirable. That's why you have to watch yourself when taking any new herb for the first time.

If you have an unpleasant reaction to an herb, such as dizziness, nausea or headache, cut back on your dosage or stop taking the herb. Listen to your body. If the herb doesn't feel right, don't take it.

Be alert for allergic reactions. People can be allergic to anything. Even if you have no known allergies, you might be allergic to a new herb that you try. Be careful. Again, listen to your body. If you develop any unusual symptoms, stop taking the herb and consult an allergist or physician.

If you experience any difficulty breathing within 30 minutes or so of trying a new herb, food or drug, call 911 immediately. You may be having an anaphylactic reaction, the most severe form of allergic reaction, which can prove rapidly fatal unless treated promptly.

Anaphylactic reactions to herbs are rare, and I'm not saying that you need to be unduly apprehensive about trying new things. Just be careful and understand the possible risks.

Beware of interactions. Pharmaceutical medicines sometimes interact badly with each other and with certain foods. The same goes for herbal medicines, although many herbal reference books neglect to mention this. Always be particularly careful when taking more than one drug or herb or a combination of a drug and an herb. Bad interactions are always possible. If you suspect a bad interaction, consult your physician or pharmacist.

Here's one interaction that you should be particularly aware of: Antidepressants known as monoamine oxidase (MAO) inhibitors interact badly with wine, cheese and many other foods. If you take a pharmaceutical MAO inhibitor, you shouldn't eat these foods.

The antidepressant herb St.-John's-wort is also an MAO inhibitor, so the same food restrictions apply. If you take St.-John's-wort regularly, consult a physician, pharmacist or consumer drug guide about which foods to avoid.

Open lines of communication. Too many people listen to both their physicians and their herbalists and do what both advise. Usually there's no problem with this, such as when a physician gives you sleeping pills for insomnia, for example, and an herbalist recommends a hot bath before bed with a blend of sedative aromatherapy oils.

But just as too many cooks can spoil the broth, too many health practitioners can also be too much of a good thing. Let's say your physician prescribes an MAO inhibitor for depression, and your herbalist recommends St.-John's-wort, also an MAO inhibitor. You may wind up taking too much. Or let's say your physician prescribes half an aspirin a day to prevent heart attack, and your herbalist tells you to drink a daily cup of tea made from willow bark or wintergreen. The teas contain the herbal equivalent of aspirin, and you might wind up taking more than you need, with more anti-clotting action than you want.

To avoid the too-many-cooks problem, be sure to tell your physician and your herbalist about *all* the medicines you're taking as well as any unusual foods you might be eating.

Shopping and Harvesting the Green Pharmacy

Are you interested in herbal medicines, but you're not quite sure how to get started? Never fear—the information in this book will help you, whether you're an herbal neophyte just taking the first steps or someone who already uses herbs on a regular basis.

The chapters in part 2 of this book will tell you which herbs you need to prevent and treat specific diseases. But before you ever use your first herb, you need to know how to obtain them.

There are, in fact, several ways to get the herbs that I discuss in *The Green Pharmacy*. Many you can buy, but there are some that you may want to plant, harvest and process yourself.

It's quicker, easier and sometimes safer and surer to simply buy herbal medicines, but in doing so, you forgo the exercise and miss the spiritual power of planting, nurturing, harvesting, processing and preparing your own green medicines. I'm an avid gardener. If you are, too, you know the joy it brings. But the important thing is to go green on any level that suits you.

Buying Standardized Medicinal Herbs

It is perfectly acceptable to buy what are known as standardized herbal products at a health food store or herb shop. In fact, these herbal preparations are gaining in popularity so rapidly that there's a good chance you'll even be able to find many of them at your local drugstore.

Standardized means that the herbal products have been processed a bit to guarantee a known minimum level of one or more of the major active ingredients. These products are the best quality you can purchase. Standardization largely compensates for the natural variability you find in bulk herbs—the kind available in bins or jars and measured out according to weight—and it takes the uncertainty out of herbal preparations. You know exactly how much of the active ingredients you're getting.

Unfortunately, standardization makes herbs more expensive than the bulk herb would be. Even so, these "expensive" standardized herbal extracts are still only about a tenth as costly, on average, as the pharmaceuticals that treat the same conditions, so you're still way ahead when you take the standardized green route.

Standardized extracts do vary somewhat, because the longer these herbal medicines are stored, the less potent they become. But then, pharmaceuticals are not perfect either.

You can usually find standardized herbal extracts quite easily wherever herbal products are sold. If you don't see them, ask for them. If an herbal product is standardized, it will say so on the label.

What the Labels Won't Tell You

Unfortunately, the labels of herbal preparations often don't say much else. That's because an herb must be approved as a "drug" in the eyes of the Food and Drug Administration (FDA) in order to specify its medical or therapeutic use. Herb marketers must spend on the order of $200 million proving to the agency's satisfaction that the herb in question is safe and effective enough to justify a medicinal claim. Of course, only the big drug companies have this kind of money, and who in his right mind would spend millions to prove the benefits of a plant no one can patent?

In the same way, manufacturers are prohibited from labeling herb products to specify possible side effects. That's because the FDA views this information as medicinal claims. Without clear labeling, consumers are left largely uninformed.

One purpose of this book, of course, is to provide you with the information that you need in order to use herbs safely and effectively. Nevertheless, I sincerely wish the FDA would allow good information to be included on herb labels. Anyone should have access to this information when they buy an herbal medicine. I hope that if enough of us pester the FDA long enough, perhaps one day we will be able to buy standardized herbs that are well-labeled for consumers.

Here are a dozen very important medicinal herbs that I'd suggest buying as standardized products. (If for any reason you can't buy the standardized products, it's certainly fine to use these—with the exception of ginkgo—as bulk herbs.)

Calendula. Buy it as a salve to treat bruises, cuts and scrapes.

Camomile. A tincture provides a reliable sedative and can be used to make a stomach-settling tea.

Echinacea. The flowers and roots stimulate the immune system to help fight disease.

Evening primrose. This flower produces a valuable seed oil that's too difficult to extract at home.

Ginkgo. This herb comes from a huge tree whose leaves must be processed into a concentrated extract to be medically useful.

Ginseng. The medicinal roots of this plant do not mature for at least five years. It is too complicated to grow and process this plant yourself. (At present, the deer are harvesting my own ginseng patch.)

Hawthorn. This slow-growing shrub is useful for treating heart problems. It's a powerful medicine that should be taken only under a doctor's supervision.

Kava kava. This herb is a safe, mild tranquilizer that grows only in tropical forests.

Licorice. Here's an anti-ulcer herb that is simply too hard to grow, at least where I come from. (This fact comes from someone who has tried several times to grow licorice but has never been successful.)

Milk thistle. The prickly leaves of this herb make it too painful to harvest yourself.

Red pepper. A plant that grows in tropical climates, red pepper contains a potent, pain-relieving compound—capsaicin—that often shows up in standardized products.

Teatree. A tropical plant that will not grow in most of the United States, teatree is an excellent, widely used antiseptic.

Buying Bulk Herbs

I use bulk herbs frequently, picking them by the handful in my six-acre Herbal Vineyard, my home of 25 years in Fulton, Maryland. Along with making teas, I also juice them, and I frequently add them to foods and beverages.

You don't have to be into gardening to get bulk herbs, however. Many health food stores and herb shops have rows of bins of dried bulk herbs that sell for a reasonable price.

There's a downside, however. Whether you buy herbs or grow them yourself, you can never be certain of the levels of active constituents in bulk plant material. This is the main shortcoming of bulk herbal medicines compared with standardized extracts and pharmaceuticals.

The payoff, to my way of thinking, is that using bulk herbs gives you the opportunity to experiment a little more and become more intimate with the plant. This produces a spiritual connection of the kind American Indians have long celebrated. I believe that this spiritual connection is therapeutic. It always has been for me.

But what about safety?

Not to worry. The vast majority of the medicinal herbs discussed in this book are safe even in large doses. And if you need to use special caution with a particular herb or when treating a particular health condition, I let you know in that chapter. So using bulk herbs doesn't really present much of a safety issue. The one concern is that with some batches you might not get enough potency—enough of the active compounds—to give you the therapeutic results you need.

The Variability Factor

Why can't you be sure of the potency of bulk herbs? There are many reasons.

Genetics. Different strains of an herb can have genetic differences in potency. For example, levels of sanguinarine, a biologically active compound found in the antiseptic bloodroot plant, *Sanguinaria*, may vary tenfold based on the genetics of different plants. And variations of a thousandfold or ten thousandfold may occur even within a given species of thyme.

Growing conditions. These affect the overall health and vigor of the plant. Plants grown in poor soil under stressful climate conditions may not have the same potency as plants grown in rich soil under ideal conditions. (Surprisingly, stressed plants often have higher levels of medicinal compounds.)

Timing and method of harvesting. Think of the difference in taste, texture and succulence between immature peaches and ripe peaches. Herbs don't ripen as fruits do, but the concentrations of active constituents vary considerably during their life cycles. For optimal potency, ginseng roots should not be harvested before they are at least five years old, but some growers harvest earlier to rush the roots to market. Those roots won't necessarily contain optimal levels of the active compounds.

Drying. Fresh herbs are most appealing. Just think of the difference between fresh mint and dried mint. Both smell and taste minty, but the fresh leaf is much more aromatic, meaning that it contains more of its medicinal oil. Whenever you smell an herb, it loses a tiny bit of its essence and power because its potency is contained in the aromatic molecules that land on the smell receptors in your nose. Once they leave the plant, they're gone.

Of course, herbs don't stay fresh for very long. That's why the convention among herbalists is to develop recipes using dried herbs, which can be stored fairly easily for many months. But the longer you store the herbs, the less potent they become. Light, oxygen and heat trigger chemical changes that make them lose potency—go stale—over time. That's why most herbalists recommend storing dried herbs in airtight, dark glass containers and keeping them cool. Careful storage greatly extends shelf life.

Packaging. In general, the best way to be sure of preserving an herbal medicine's potency is to buy an alcohol tincture or a glycerin extract. These can remain potent for a year or so. The same cannot be said for herbs in tea bags, powdered herbs or herbal capsules, unless they are guarded by added antioxidants. They are quicker to suffer damage from light, oxygen and heat.

Adding Some Spice

In addition to the many herbs that you can buy in bulk or standardized form, there are many spices that double as medicines. You probably already have some of them in your spice rack. With the exception of capsicum, garlic, ginger and turmeric, they are not available in the United States as standardized extracts and, again with the exception of garlic, most are tropical plants that don't grow well here. So you'll probably have to buy them in bulk or powdered form.

Allspice. This tropical herb has a complex aroma and is useful for indigestion.

Cardamom. An expensive spice, cardamom can be a mild stimulant.

Cinnamon. This common, tasty spice has potent antimicrobial action and can settle an upset stomach.

Cloves. Cloves have proven pain-relieving and antiseptic properties.

Garlic. Deservedly called Russian penicillin, this pungent bulb is useful in preventing our major killers—heart disease and cancer.

Ginger. The world's best nausea preventive, ginger is also useful in treating arthritis.

Red pepper. This native American spice works on pain by three different mechanisms.

Sesame. The seeds of this plant are a great source of antioxidants and other therapeutic chemicals.

Turmeric. This yellow spice shows great promise in treating arthritis and diabetes.

In Search of Wild Medicinals

Foraging for wild herbs is known in botanical lingo as wildcrafting. When you're wildcrafting, of course, you aren't dealing with standardized extracts. But in my humble opinion, the physical and mental exercise of wildcrafting, plus the spiritual connection to the plant and the forest where it grows, provides a therapeutic power that more than compensates for the loss of exactness.

As a botanist, wildcrafting is easy for me. I know my plants well and have been foraging in the wild for more than 60 years. Of course, picking wild medicinal herbs can be hazardous, and you don't want to try it unless you can positively identify the plants you're selecting. (I recall one elderly couple out West who mistook foxglove for comfrey. Unfortunately, foxglove is the source of the heart-stimulating drug digitalis, and it had fatal consequences.)

I advise anyone who is not really familiar with field botany to steer clear of the potential hazards of harvesting wild plants. But if you know what you're doing, in just about any part of the United States you can harvest a bounty of useful medicinal herbs just by stepping out your front door.

If you're not familiar with herbs at first, you can have a good deal of fun finding out more about them. Most metropolitan areas have botanical organizations—museum groups, scout groups, hiking clubs or university extension departments—that offer classes in the identification of local edible and medicinal plants. Take it from a long-time forager: Hiking is much more fun when you can munch your way along the trail.

Growing Your Own, Indoors

Like wildcrafting, growing your own herbs gives you non-standardized bulk plant material. But it also gives you an even deeper spiritual connection to your medicines than foraging, so I'm all for it.

No matter what you grow, gardening is a therapeutic, self-empowering hobby. And from what we know about mind-body medicine, I'm confident that self-grown herbal medicines should work better than anything store-bought or foraged.

I love my Herbal Vineyard, but you don't need an estate—or even a yard—to grow medicinal herbs. All you need is a kitchen windowsill where you can grow a potted aloe plant—your instant, herbal emergency kit in case of accidental burns. (Just snip off a leaf, slit it open and apply the yellow-green inner leaf gel to the burn.)

There are many other herbs that you can raise on a windowsill or on your back porch. If you're a city dweller, you can find space in a roof garden, courtyard, balcony or fire escape. Quite a few medicinal-culinary species that are native to semi-arid climates will also flourish on sunny kitchen windowsills. Here are some to consider.

Basil. This insect-repelling herb is recommended for treating bad breath and headache.

Chives. Along with their cousins garlic, leeks and onions, chives help prevent cancer and treat high blood pressure.

Dill. This herb is deservedly famous as a remedy for colic and gas.

Fennel. This herb is good for treating upset stomach and indigestion.

Hyssop. Mentioned in the Bible, hyssop contains several antiviral compounds and is useful in treating herpes. (It's also under review as an AIDS therapy.)

Lavender. Some varieties of this lovely herb are loaded with sedative compounds that can penetrate the skin. Toss a handful into your bathwater if you want a nice-smelling way to relax.

Parsley. Best known as a great source of chlorophyll for combating bad breath, parsley is rich in zinc, which is good for men's reproductive health. (Yet more than 90 percent of parsley served in restaurants is thrown away.)

Peppermint. This is a major source of cooling, soothing, stomach-settling menthol.

Rosemary. Rich in antioxidants, this tasty culinary spice may help prevent Alzheimer's disease.

Sage. Sage shares much of the medicinal potential of rosemary.

Savory. Europeans add this herb to bean dishes to reduce flatulence.

Thyme. This is one of the best sources of thymol, an antiseptic, stomach-soothing compound that helps prevent the blood clots that cause heart attack.

Growing an Outdoor Herb Garden

In my Herbal Vineyard, I have some 200 species of herbs, most of them medicinal. During the growing season, one of my great pleasures in life is to stroll the grounds and check on all the plants.

Almost hourly, when I'm spending the day at the computer, I take breaks and visit my herb garden. When I harvest a handful of this or that, I often select mints to make up one of my aromatic beverages, usually hot mint tea on a cool morning or iced mint tea on a hot afternoon.

Growing and loving these herbs is one of the most healthful activities I engage in, and I heartily recommend it.

It would take another book to tell you how to grow all the herbs I discuss in *The Green Pharmacy*. But if you do have garden space, here are the perennial medicinal herbs that I recommend. They flourish in my own garden, and I think they'll do well for anyone who gardens in a temperate climate more or less like Maryland's.

Chasteberry. A perennial flowering shrub, this is a great herb for treating women's problems.

Goldenseal. An antibiotic herb, goldenseal grows best when planted in a shady area.

Lemon balm. Also known as melissa, this weedy antiviral mint has sedative properties. Although it sometimes looks like it has died away, it always comes back.

Mountain mint. An insect-repelling herb that should be more popular among gardeners than it is.

Oregano. Another weedy mint—a great source of antioxidants.

Self-heal. The reputation of this mint as a panacea is only slightly exaggerated.

Spearmint. This herb is about as good as peppermint for settling the stomach.

St.-John's-wort. Simply the best herbal treatment for depression.

Tansy. This herb contains some of the same anti-migraine compounds as feverfew.

Valerian. The roots contain a great anxiety-relieving sedative. But be warned—the tea smells like dirty gym socks.

Wild yam. Many herbalists recommend this herb for women's reproductive health.

Willow. The willow tree's easy-peeling bark contains the herbal version of aspirin.

Harvesting and Storing Herbs

Okay, so you've got a big peppermint patch, or whatever, growing in your garden or on your windowsill. Now what?

First you must harvest your herbs. You can snip off leaves and use them as needed. Taking a cue from the American Indians, the romantics among us like to thank the herb for serving us and apologize for mutilating it.

Down in Panama and Peru, I listened as Indian shamans sang long chants to the herbs they were about to harvest, often while facing the East. When I'm not in a hurry, I remember that the plants, too, have lives, and that their lives sustain ours.

In fact, the more we clip the leaves of medicinal plants, the more medicinal they become. This makes sense botanically because herbs' medicinal constituents are basically part of the plant's self-protection system. Harvesting the leaves makes the plant respond as if it's under attack (which it is), so it produces more of what protects it. Studies have shown that infections, insect infestations and leaf-plucking, among other attacks on the plant, increase the levels of some of the same chemicals that we view as medicines.

Collection Times

Although some herbalists argue for harvesting herbs early in the morning while there is still dew on them, I disagree. That dilutes the herb with water, meaning that it has proportionately more water and less chemical until it's dried. In my view, you get the greatest concentration of plant chemicals and the least water when you collect leaves during a hot, dry day, but before the leaves have wilted.

Roots are best collected in spring or fall. Bark may be collected in spring, especially if the compounds you seek are in the living bark. If you're collecting seeds for food, I recommend that you get them before they have dried out and hardened. But if you're harvesting them to plant next year rather than to use immediately, you may want to wait until they've dried out.

Feel free to use herbs fresh, especially in cooking. Fresh culinary herbs and spices almost always taste best. You can also freeze them, dry them or use them to make tinctures. (When harvesting fresh culinary herbs, I generally use a plastic bag to help retain the moisture.)

Preserving the Goods

If you intend to preserve your herbs for future use, it's cheaper to dry them. Collect them in a brown paper bag rather than a plastic bag, and write the name of the plant and the collection date on the outside of the bag.

If you don't stuff it too tightly, many herbs can be dried right in the bag. I always make a run through my herb garden with paper bags before the last killing frost, collecting herbs for my winter medicines, soups and teas.

Check your brown-bagged herbs after about a week, and if they are not clearly drying—becoming papery and crumbly—spread them out on newspapers or clean wood or screen in a dry, shaded area so that they can dry before mildew attacks.

When it comes to success in drying, a great deal depends on your local weather conditions. In arid weather, herbs may dry too rapidly, especially in direct sunlight. In humid and especially in foggy weather, you may have to apply heat by baking the herbs in an oven to get the moisture out.

Once dried, herbs can be kept in paper bags or stuffed into plastic bags. You can also use glass jars with lids.

Light, heat and oxygen are the enemies of herb potency, so store your herbs in a cool, dark place, like a cellar or cupboard far from any heat source. To minimize the oxygen around stored herbs, fill your containers as full as possible and move the herbs to smaller containers as you use them.

Using the Green Pharmacy

There are many easy ways to use medicinal herbs. Whether you use them as foods, introduce them as seasonings or make teas, you'll get the benefit of their healing properties.

I have nothing against taking vitamin and mineral supplements. In fact, I suggest them for many of the conditions discussed in this book. But an ounce of fruit or vegetables has many more useful constituents than a pound of purified supplements.

My favorite way to use herbs is simply as foods or mixed into foods. In the United States, we make a distinction between foods and drugs, but in many cases there is no real difference. Is garlic, for example, a food or a drug? The correct answer is that it's both. The same goes for all of the culinary spices and many of the herbs discussed throughout this book.

Making Meals That Heal

When it comes to meals that heal, I think it's hard to beat a big mixed green salad, a bowl of vegetable soup (minestrone, which I often call Medi-strone) and a fruit salad topped with some herbs such as mint, basil or cinnamon.

In the early 1990s, I was involved with the Designer Food Program of the National Institutes of Health (NIH). The idea was to identify medicinal chemicals, such as plant estrogens (phytoestrogens), which appear to reduce the risk of breast cancer, in plants and to breed or augment these chemicals in food plants.

While the people I worked with in the Designer Food Program were all very bright, charming and well-intentioned, we had some differences of opinion. They wanted to pump plant chemicals (phytochemicals) into foods, while I kept saying that the beneficial chemicals were already there—if you knew where to look. For example, phytoestrogens abound in most beans. If you want to take a big step toward preventing breast cancer, eat bean soup or a bean salad a few times a week, try some Mexican food with refried beans or add tofu to just about anything.

The More Servings, the Better

Many of those in the Designer Food Program endorsed the Strive for Five program promoted by the NIH to encourage Americans to eat five servings a day of fruits and vegetables. An enormous amount of research shows that as fruit and vegetable consumption increases, risk of all the major cancers decreases. In fact, the risk of heart disease, diabetes and many other diseases declines as well. Based on this research, the NIH figured that it was prudent to recommend *at least* five servings a day of fruit and vegetables.

Unfortunately, few Americans get their five a day. And even that goal is shortsighted, in my opinion. I personally think people should strive for at least ten a day—five fruits and five veggies, seasoned with five different herbs and garnished with five different nuts.

As Hippocrates supposedly said, "Let your food be your medicine." Amen to that, especially if you add lots of medicinal spices.

To encourage as many servings of healing foods as possible, I've scattered several recipes throughout this book. But I would certainly never pretend to be a great cook: I rarely measure ingredients at home, and I almost never cook the same dish exactly the same way. I go with a little of this and a handful of that, trusting my taste buds and the wisdom of using as broad a range of fruits, vegetables and herbs as possible. My "recipes" may seem imprecise at times, but the objective is to get you to experiment as much as possible with these tasty herbs. What pleases your palate may not please mine, and vice versa.

How to Make a Healing Tea

You can make a good tea with dried herbs. You can even pop open capsules of powdered herbs and use the contents to make tea. But whenever possible, I use fresh herbs, at least in spring, summer and fall.

Why? Simply because fresh herbs are more fun and more flavorful.

The main difference between fresh herbs and dried herbs is their water content. Leaf for leaf, herbs retain their supply of medicinal phytochemicals even after they've been dried for a while. But phytochemicals are more concentrated in dried herbs because they contain less water. While fresh herbs are about 80 percent water, dried are only about 20 percent. So ounce for ounce, the dried herb is more potent, and when you add it to water, more of the phytochemicals are infused in the tea.

Herbal tea recipes usually assume that you're starting with dried herb material. If you have fresh herbs on hand, you'll need to use four times as much as the recipe calls for if you want to get the same potency.

To Infuse or Decoct?

There are really two types of teas—infusions and decoctions. An infusion is similar to what most people think of as tea. But there's a big difference between beverage teas and medicinal herb infusions. With a beverage tea, you might dunk a tea bag in hot water a few times and then drink it. If you're preparing an herb infusion, the tea should steep for 10 to 20 minutes to allow the therapeutic phytochemicals to pass out of the herb and into the water.

To make a good cup of medicinal tea, here's a good rule of thumb. Start with boiling water and steep your medicinal herbs until the water is cool. If you like to drink it hot, reheat the tea gently.

Decoctions, on the other hand, involve putting herbal material in the water, then boiling or simmering for 10 to 20 minutes. Infusions work best for leaf and flower material because they usually yield their phytochemicals more easily. The decoction method, on the other hand, is typically used for root and twig material because it can be difficult to extract medicinal phytochemicals from them.

Throughout this book, I include suggestions for amounts of herbs to be used in infusions and decoctions. But I must confess that I make my own herb teas the same way I cook—a little of this, a handful of that. In summer I cruise my garden, grabbing whichever aromatic herbs I pass—sometimes more than a dozen—taking bigger portions of the delicate-smelling herbs and smaller portions of the coarse-scented herbs like dittany, horsebalm and thyme. Like my soups and salads, no two of my herb teas are exactly the same.

Suggestions and Safety

What I'm leading up to is this: Use the suggestions in this book as just that—suggestions. I've concentrated mostly on herbs that are safe even in amounts considerably greater than those suggested in the recipes, so don't feel concerned if you use a bit more or less than the recipe suggests. (When exact dosages are extremely important, I note that. And whenever any precautions are needed, I note that as well.)

If there is no recipe for a specific herb, try making an infusion or decoction with one to two teaspoons of plant material. Then tinker with the amounts to suit your personal needs. You can't expect all medicinal teas to taste good; some of them are quite bitter. But if you like the taste and want a stronger tea, it's okay to use a little more of the herb next time around. I mask unpleasant tastes with powdered or real lemonade. The acidity may even extract more of certain medicinal chemicals.

At the same time, however, you must remember that these herbs are medicine. You have to pay attention to how your body responds to the herb and adjust your dose accordingly. If you're looking to relax and end up feeling overly sedated, for example, you'll want to make a weaker tea the next time you're using that particular herb. Our personal chemistries may be just as variable as the herbs'.

As for frequency, I typically suggest one to three cups of tea a day. Again, these are merely suggestions. In general, I wouldn't recommend much more than four cups of most herbal teas per day.

Tinctures and Vinegars

Classically, a tincture is made by steeping herb material in drinkable alcohol, such as ethyl alcohol (ethanol). My personal favorite when I'm creating my own tinctures is cheap vodka. It works just fine.

The alcohol extracts a great deal of the medicinal essence of the herb. Tinctures have longer shelf lives than dried herbs or capsules.

You can buy ready-made tinctures at most places that sell herbs. You can also make your own quite easily.

To make a tincture, you can use anything from 40-proof alcohol to almost 200-proof, which translates as anything from 20 percent alcohol to almost pure alcohol. Most herbalists suggest two ounces of dried herb (or a loose handful of fresh herb) per pint of alcohol. Allow your herb-alcohol mixture to stand for about a week, shaking it occasionally. Then strain it. Discard the plant material (preferably in the compost pile) and store the tincture in a bottle with a dropper lid.

Tincture dosages can run anywhere from 5 to 50 drops or from a fraction of a dropperful to several dropperfuls. Sometimes they're even measured in teaspoons or tablespoons. I usually add tinctures to beverage herbal teas or to juices.

One advantage of buying a tincture is that appropriate dosages are generally indicated on the label.

While alcohol is a great preservative, we want to pickle the herb, not the consumer. One nonalcoholic option that's often available these days is glycerides, tinctures that have been prepared using glycerin rather than alcohol. These are nice options for infants or for recovering alcoholics who wish to avoid alcohol in any form.

Herbal vinegars are another good option, and you can even make your own. To do this, simply steep your herbs in vinegar rather than alcohol. The same ratios might be used: one pint of vinegar for every one to two ounces of dried herb or loose handful of fresh herb.

You can use many herbal vinegars straight as salad dressings, which can be especially helpful for people who are overweight. Herbal vinegars can also be added to soups or cooked vegetables.

Using Poultices and Compresses

A poultice is a wad of chopped, fresh (or dried but remoistened) plant material that is applied directly to a wound or infection on the skin and usually held in place by a wet dressing that is covered by a bandage.

It's best to soften the herb first to coax out more of the medicinal phytochemicals. You can do this by boiling, steaming, chewing or pounding it. Then shape the material into a small, coin-size wad that can lie flat against the wound. Many herbalists recommend mixing one part herb with three parts water, alcohol or vinegar thickened with flour to make the poultice easier to handle and apply. In a pinch, you can simply ball up some whole leaf and use that.

Poultices work primarily at the application site, typically preventing infection and hastening the healing of wounds. But there are doubtless many compounds in poultice plants that pass through the skin and have internal benefits as well.

Compresses are clean cloths that have been dipped in an herbal solution—an infusion, decoction, tincture or vinegar. Compresses can be used in two ways. You might hold a poultice in place with a compress, in which case it doubles as a bandage. Or you might apply it directly to the skin. This type of compress is also known as a fomentation.

Soothing Salves

Many commercial salves contain herbs, and probably your best bet is to buy a salve rather than make it. Making your own salves is a pretty messy business, but you can certainly go that route if you choose. Making salves involves mixing medicinal herbs with water, beeswax, animal fat (lard or lanolin), vegetable fat (corn oil, Crisco, margarine or olive or safflower oil) and other ingredients to create spreadable lotions.

I confess that I've never had much luck mixing up salves.

Mine tend to be either too runny or too dry. But other herbalists are much better at it.

If you'd like to try making a salve, start with pulverized herb and cover it with water. Boil or simmer for 15 to 30 minutes, then let it cool. Add some oil, then gently heat the oily mixture until the water has evaporated, perhaps 15 to 30 minutes.

Finally, add beeswax and/or a fat to give your salve the proper consistency. Cool before using. A well-prepared salve can keep for up to a year. Salves can be used like poultices, except that you often don't need the bandage.

If you'd rather not make salves from scratch, you can also simply add pulverized, simmered herb material to any of the commercial skin ointments sold in drugstores.

Healing with Aromatherapy

Aromatherapy is the treatment of medical conditions with the aromatic essential oils of fragrant herbs. Aromatherapists often use essential oils from the mint family, which includes such aromatherapeutic superstars as lavender (a tranquilizer) and rosemary (a stimulant).

The essential oils used in aromatherapy, which come in little vials, are extremely concentrated. You can simply sniff directly from the vial, or you can use the oil for massage.

Since the oils are so concentrated, they can be irritating to the skin. If you're using an oil for massage, first dilute it by adding a few drops to vegetable oil or massage lotion. If you doubt that essential oils can pass through your skin, here's an experiment for you to try: Massage a few drops of diluted lavender oil into your skin. Within a short time, your friends may notice that you have lavender breath when you exhale.

Another nice way to use essential oils is to add a few drops to your bath. (You can also use a handful of fresh or dried herbs if you choose.) Since many of the fragrant compounds are readily absorbed through the skin, this is a particularly pleasant way to get your medicine. If you have insomnia, for example, I suggest adding sedative lavender and lemon balm (also known as melissa) to your bath. I bet you'll fall asleep more easily and sleep more soundly.

Whatever you do, though, do not ingest essential oils. Many are quite toxic, and as little as a half-teaspoon can kill you. (A few essential oils can be taken in diluted form, but this is not something that you can experiment with on your own. An experienced herbal practitioner may occasionally recommend ingesting diluted essential oils.)

PART TWO

Choosing the Herbs That Heal

Aging

As I write this, I'm entering the latter half of my sixties, and I confess that aging frightens me.

I watched uncomfortably as my 101-year-old grandmother languished almost immobilized in the last decade of her life. I went through the same anguish with my 98-year-old mother. I do not want to spend my last decade bedridden!

Age Factors

Being a botanist, I have a particular interest in herbs that can hold back the aging process. But I'm forced to admit that I think lifestyle changes are a whole lot more important than herbs—and even more important than hormone supplementation—in helping you stay youthful. So before I discuss the most helpful herbs, I want to be really specific about those lifestyle changes. They should form the foundation of any anti-aging herbal treatments that you decide to try.

Not being a doctor, I don't prescribe, but I would not hesitate to suggest the following to my 30-year-old daughter so she could hold on more tenaciously to her vibrant youth. Come to think of it, this is good advice for men and women of any age who are trying to hold back the clock.

Drink two antioxidant herb teas a day. Antioxidants are substances that neutralize free radicals, naturally occurring oxygen molecules that damage the body and are thought to play a significant role in the aging process. Most fruits and vegetables contain significant amounts of antioxidants, as do many herbs. If you're a heavy coffee drinker, you might consider replacing two cups of coffee a day with herb tea. Good research suggests that oregano, rosemary, bee balm, lemon balm (also known as melissa), peppermint, sage, spearmint, savory and thyme contain significant levels of antioxidants.

Eat at least one big salad a day. You can use both wild greens—things like purslane, if you have access to them—and a variety of domestic salad vegetables, such as spinach and chicory. Green leaves are chock-full of antioxidant nutrients that help protect you from heart disease, cancer and other degenerative diseases that tend to come on as we age. Usually, the greener the leaf, the more antioxidants it contains, so fill up on those dark, leafy greens.

Eat one or two Brazil nuts a day. The average Brazil nut contains more than the Daily Value of the antioxidant mineral selenium—70 micrograms.

Eat a handful of sunflower seeds a day, along with a sprinkling of other nuts. Among nuts and seeds, sunflower seeds are one of the better sources of vitamin E. They're also cheap.

One caution, however: If you're watching your waistline, don't eat more than an ounce of nuts a day. Nuts are high in fat.

Eat at least one broccoli spear, carrot and celery stalk a day. They're all high in fiber. Broccoli and carrots are also high in beta-carotene, the powerful antioxidant that the body transforms into vitamin A. Celery is high in apigenin, a chemical that expands (dilates) the blood vessels and may help prevent high blood pressure.

Drink a fruit smoothie every day. Take any fruits that appeal to you—apples, oranges, bananas, grapefruit, melons or berries—and run them through a blender. Don't use a juicer, which extracts just the juice by separating it from the fiber. Leave the fiber in there; it's great for the digestive tract. If you like, add some nonfat yogurt and cinnamon. Or make my Strive-for-Fiveade by blending one diced apple, two diced carrots and diced sections of one lime and one grapefruit with some water and a little stevia. (Stevia is available in many health food stores. You can open a tea bag and use a pinch of the herb in place of artificial sweetener.)

Replace one meat course a day with a vegetarian dish. One of my favorites is guacamole—mashed avocado. You can lace your guacamole with onion, hot chili peppers, garlic and lemon juice and sprinkle it with chopped nuts such as hazelnuts, macadamias, pistachios, cashews, peanuts or Brazil nuts. All of these nuts are rich in monounsaturated fatty acids, beneficial fats that are good for your heart, among other things. (Anyone who is carrying extra pounds, however, should forgo the nuts, which are high in calories.)

Use olive oil. Corn oil and other vegetable oils are polyunsaturated oils. Olive oil is a monounsaturated oil. There is a complex chemical explanation for how these differ, but all you really need to know is that there's good reason to believe that monounsaturated oils are a lot better for you. In salad dressings, replace polyunsaturated oils with olive oil.

Eat a wide variety of fruits and vegetables. Also eat a good selection of herbs, legumes, nuts and spices. These are the foods that our ancestors consumed back in the days before the invention of burgers, hot dogs, pizza, ice cream and all the junk we eat today. They ate more nutritiously than we do.

Make love regularly with someone you love. There's no explanation needed here except that it's good for you.

Go for a walk every day. Weather permitting, get outdoors and take a vigorous half-hour walk, well-protected from sunlight (ultraviolet radiation). Use the time to unwind and commune with the natural world. Contemplate the miraculous ecosystem around you and consider what it is that makes you—and it—tick. Respect, don't fear, the mystery of it all.

I also recommend some lifestyle don'ts to go with the do's.

Don't smoke. This goes without saying.

Don't drink alcohol. If you do imbibe, don't have more than two drinks a day, and don't drink every day. Give your liver a sabbatical every now and then. A few weeks out of every year, don't drink any alcohol or take any medications (other than those your doctor tells you are absolutely necessary). Your liver has to work hard to clear alcohol, medications and environmental pollutants from your body; it will appreciate getting a breather.

Don't sunbathe—ever. You probably get enough sun to produce a healthy amount of vitamin D with moderate outdoor activities that don't involve actively seeking the sun.

Don't take life or death too seriously. That can age or kill you.

Don't be a dietary faddist. It's never a good idea to base your diet on just a couple of foods, even fruits or carrots. Vary your diet, your food sources, your mode of preparation and even the company you keep when you dine.

Don't let industry outvote the environmentalists. If you do, we'll all pay the price eventually.

Green Pharmacy for Aging

I think that all of these lifestyle changes are a lot more important than herbs. There are, however, several herbs that you should know about for holding back the ravages of age.

✻✻✻ **Ginkgo** (*Ginkgo biloba*). This is the most intriguing herb for counteracting the neurological slings and arrows of aging. There's good European research showing that it helps improve blood flow to the brain. Some studies suggest that ginkgo helps people with Alzheimer's disease and other forms of dementia become more alert and sociable, think more clearly, feel better and remember more. In Europe, many older people regularly take a standardized extract of this herb to help keep them mentally fit.

Ginkgo's ability to increase blood flow to the brain has been shown to offer a number of benefits to people who are aging. It improves alertness, memory and the ability to concentrate, it elevates mood, and it relieves tinnitus (ringing in the ears), dizziness and anxiety.

Huge, stately ginkgo trees grow all over the United States, but it takes barrels of leaves to produce a few days' worth of usable extract. The best way to use this herb is to buy a standardized extract or capsules at a health food store or herb outlet. Still, I confess to blending a few leaves into my fruit smoothies with no obvious ill effects. You can try 60 to 240 milligrams of standardized extracts a day, but don't go any higher than that. In large amounts, ginkgo may cause diarrhea, irritability and restlessness.

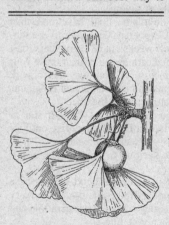

Ginkgo

For medicinal purposes, the leaves of the ginkgo tree are made into standardized extracts.

✻✻ **American ginseng** (*Panax quinquefolius*) **and Asian ginseng** (*P. ginseng*). The Chinese and Koreans revere ginseng as the Fountain of Youth. They regard this herb as a tonic for the elderly because it tones the skin and muscles, helps improve appetite and digestion and restores depleted sexual energy.

While on a trip to China in 1978 for the express purpose

of investigating ginseng, I had one elderly Chinese man tell me not to waste this herb on young people. He said I should save it for old age, when it would make me feel young again. I'm almost ready. The house is paid off, and I have five species of ginseng growing on my six-acre farmette.

Ginseng is slowly gaining supporters among American physicians. One big booster is Andrew Weil, M.D., herb advocate, professor at the University of Arizona College of Medicine in Tucson and author of *Natural Health, Natural Medicine*. He frequently recommends ginseng to help strengthen people who are weakened by old age or chronic illness.

❧❧ Echinacea (*Echinacea*, various species). This herb is native to our own Great Plains, and it's America's best herbal immune booster. I've been very impressed with German research showing that its antimicrobial action helps prevent and treat colds, flu and all sorts of other viral, bacterial and fungal infections.

❧❧ Evening primrose (*Oenothera biennis*). The seeds of this lovely night-flowering blossom contain an oil rich in gamma-linolenic acid (GLA), a substance that has excited a great deal of research interest in the past few years. GLA seems to help alleviate several conditions: premenstrual syndrome (PMS); eczema, a chronic skin condition that causes itchy, red, scaly patches; diabetic polyneuropathy, a type of nerve damage associated with diabetes; and perhaps even alcoholism and obesity. It also shows promise against America's biggest killers, heart disease and cancer.

❧❧ Garlic (*Allium sativum*). Besides being a potent antibiotic and antiviral herb, garlic reduces high cholesterol levels and lowers high blood pressure.

I also read a fascinating Japanese study suggesting that garlic helped slow physiological aging and age-related memory loss in experimental animals. I don't hang my hat on a single study—especially not an animal study—but since I'm recommending garlic anyway, I thought I'd mention this one.

❧❧ Gotu kola (*Centella asiatica*). Gotu kola is widely used in India to improve memory and extend longevity. If you want to use it, add a fresh leaf or two or a teaspoon or so of dried herb to beverage teas. You can also add a few fresh leaves to salads.

❧❧ Milk thistle (*Silybum marianum*). This is my favorite liver protector. The liver processes drugs and environmental toxins, so it's under constant assault in the modern world. Anyone who drinks alcohol, takes drugs (legal or illicit) or comes in contact with any pollutants might benefit from this herb.

❧❧ Peppermint (Mentha piperita). Thank goodness for peppermint's ability to relieve indigestion and gastrointestinal distress. It also contains antioxidants that help prevent cancer, heart disease and other diseases associated with aging.

❧❧ Purslane (Portulaca oleracea). Exceptionally rich in antioxidants, purslane is the top herb that pops up in my database when I'm looking for combinations of the antioxidant vitamins A, C and E. It's also rich in the compound glutathione, which is both a powerful antioxidant and an immune system booster.

Speaking of glutathione, other vegetables rich in this anti-aging compound include asparagus, broccoli, cabbage, cauliflower, potatoes and tomatoes. Fruits with this antioxidant include avocados, grapefruit, oranges, peaches and watermelon.

❧❧ Thyme (Thymus vulgaris). Thyme is another good source of beneficial anti-aging chemicals. You can even benefit from soaking in it. I would regularly add a handful of the dried herb to hot baths if I were a tub type instead of a shower type. Thyme's aromatic oil helps soothe my back spasms.

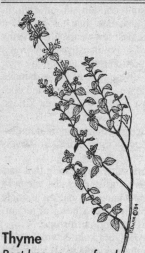

Thyme
Best known as a food flavoring, thyme contains chemicals with healing properties.

❧❧ Willow (Salix, various species). The bark of this tree was the original source of aspirin. It can be made into a tea that relieves headache, toothache, arthritis and other painful conditions. It also helps prevent heart attack, stroke and colorectal cancer.

❧ Camomile (Matricaria recutita). This popular herb is a mild tranquilizer with anti-inflammatory constituents that might help relieve arthritis.

❧ Horsetail (Equisetum arvense). With age and declining hormonal activity, levels of the mineral silicon decrease in the arteries and skin. Silicon also plays a role in the repair of bone, cartilage and connective tissues. Horsetail, a good herbal source of silicon, is a longtime folk remedy for fractures, torn ligaments and related injuries. I'm intrigued by this herb, but since I'm not yet convinced that it has all the anti-aging value that some sources suggest, I take it only rarely. If you want to try it, you can do so in consultation with a holistic practitioner.

Allergies

If you've ever had a sneezing fit in the midst of house-cleaning, you probably blamed it on all that stirred-up dust. But an allergist or immunologist would disagree. It's not the dust that causes the sneezing, they've found. It's your body's *reaction*, and the chemicals it releases, that prompt your sneezing. It's true that some people are more sensitive than others to the dust, dust mites and mold spores that float through the air. But that just means that their bodies go a little overboard in the process of reacting to the free-floating invaders.

Stress, Dust and Annoyance

Allergies are abnormal reactions to everyday substances. They are caused by the immune system's overreaction to histamine, a chemical that the body releases to fight microbial invaders. But in allergies, the invaders are not viruses or bacteria. They are harmless substances: pollens, dust, mold spores or harmless microscopic bugs called dust mites that live in carpets, clothing and bedding.

Hay fever, one of the most common allergies, is triggered by pollens. Ragweed pollen reportedly accounts for about 75 percent of cases of hay fever in the United States. Some 25 to 30 million Americans suffer from hay fever every year. Another 12 million are allergic to things other than pollen (bee stings or certain foods or drugs).

Allergy Emergency

Writing about herbal treatments for allergies reminds me of a woman I met in the early 1970s. She was an attractive, energetic young lady from the Smithsonian Institution in Washington, D.C. She came out to my office in Beltsville, Maryland, one December to borrow a lengthy report that I'd prepared on the poppy plant. We discussed collaborating on a revised version of the report and then parted, assuming that we'd talk again after Christmas. But I never saw her again.

This woman, I later learned, died from a very rare allergic reaction to peanuts. (On average, two people each year are known to die from this allergy.) Knowing that she was deathly allergic to peanuts, the woman had always shunned them. But, I was told, she inadvertently ate one Christmas cookie that contained powdered peanuts, and that was enough to kill her.

Such fatal reactions are not what most of us refer to when we say "allergy." More often, allergic reactions are merely annoying. They involve things like sneezing, itching, watery eyes and hives.

Allergic reactions that are life-threatening, on the other hand, are in a class by themselves. The medical name for this kind of allergic reaction is anaphylaxis.

If an allergic reaction is a firecracker, then anaphylaxis is a stick of dynamite. Everyone should be aware of what an anaphylatic allergic reaction is, because a person who is having this kind of reaction must receive medical treatment within about a half-hour.

Anaphylaxis develops suddenly shortly after ingestion of a substance that a person is extremely allergic to. Symptoms include difficulty breathing, collapse and convulsions. If these develop, call 911 immediately, and say "Suspected anaphylaxis." In fact, if you know that you're severely allergic, you might want to discuss injectable epinephrine with your doctor. She might agree that it would be a good idea for you to have this emergency treatment on hand.

❦

Standard medical treatment for allergies involves taking decongestants and antihistamines. Decongestants open clogged nasal passages and have drying action. Antihistamines suppress the body's release of histamine.

In severe cases, doctors prescribe immunotherapy, popularly known as allergy shots. The shots contain tiny quantities of the substances (allergens) to which the person is sensitive. Over time, with exposure to slowly increasing amounts of allergen, the body becomes desensitized and stops reacting with allergy symptoms.

Decongestants, antihistamines and allergy shots work well for some people, but I'm not a big fan of them. These approaches treat only the symptoms of allergies, not the cause, which is a confused immune system.

Decongestants can cause insomnia and raise blood pressure. Antihistamines may cause drowsiness. Both may lose effectiveness after a while. They also interfere with—and according to some experts, weaken—the immune system. Allergy shots don't work for everyone, and when they do, they often involve years of treatment.

Green Pharmacy for Allergies

You won't be surprised to learn that I prefer "greener," more natural approaches. Some of these approaches help with allergy symptoms. Here are the helpful herbs.

❦❦ **Garlic (*Allium sativum*) and onion (*A. cepa*).** These may be beneficial because of the high concentrations of compounds such as quercetin found in these plants. These compounds retard inflammatory reactions. If you have allergies, I'd suggest adding generous amounts of these foods to your menu.

❦❦ **Ginkgo (*Ginkgo biloba*).** The leaf extract of the stately ginkgo tree contains several unique substances (ginkgolides) that interfere with the action of a chemical that the body produces—platelet-activating factor, or PAF. PAF plays a key role in triggering allergies, asthma and inflammation. My own allergies have never been severe enough to make me reach for ginkgo, but if they got bad, I would probably try it. You can try 60 to 240 milligrams of standardized extract a day, but don't go any higher than that. In large amounts, ginkgo may cause diarrhea, irritability and restlessness.

❦❦ Stinging nettle *(Urtica dioica).* Some good research shows that nettle preparations may effectively treat allergic nasal symptoms. Every spring, visitors to my herb garden dig up roots from my nettle patch to treat their hay fever. We shouldn't be surprised that nettle does, in fact, help relieve allergy symptoms. For centuries, cultures around the world have used this herb to treat nasal and respiratory troubles: coughs, runny nose, chest congestion, asthma, whooping cough and even tuberculosis. At a Columbia University Workshop on Botanical Medicine for Physicians, herb advocate Andrew Weil, M.D., professor at the University of Arizona College of Medicine in Tucson and author of *Natural Health, Natural Medicine,* said that he knew of nothing so dramatic as the allergy (hay fever) relief afforded by freeze-dried nettle leaves.

❦ Camomile *(Matricaria recutita).* Aromatherapists, especially in Europe, recommend massaging with camomile preparations to treat skin allergies such as hives and itching. That sounds reasonable to me. There are compounds in this herb that have significant anti-inflammatory and anti-allergic properties. You can buy camomile essential oil and creams containing camomile at many natural food stores.

If you have hay fever, you should use camomile oil and herbal products cautiously, however. Camomile is a member of the ragweed family, and in some people, it might trigger allergic reactions. (Documented cases are extremely rare.) The first time you use camomile, watch your reaction. If it seems to help, go ahead and use it. But if it seems to make the itching worse, simply discontinue use. (For other herbs that can help relieve the itch associated with skin allergies, see Hives on page 318.)

❦ Feverfew *(Tanacetum parthenium).* Feverfew is best known these days for its proven effectiveness in treating migraine headaches. But this herb may also help relieve allergies. If you use it, take capsules or some other commercial preparation. I've tasted the leaves, and the experience is not pleasant. If I developed sufficiently annoying allergy symptoms and had no other medication, I would likely use feverfew.

Pregnant women should not take feverfew because of a remote possibility that it might trigger miscarriage. And women who are nursing should not use it because of the possibility of passing the herb to infants via milk. Finally, long-term users often report a mild tranquilizing or sedative effect, which may be welcome or unwelcome, depending on your temperament.

❧ **Horseradish (*Amoracia rusticana*).** There's nothing like a bite of fresh horseradish (or a spoonful of prepared horseradish dressing) to clear the sinuses. Or if you like Japanese food, try Japanese horseradish, called wasabi. This recommendation comes from the good book, *Natural Health Secrets from around the World* by Glenn W. Geelhoed, M.D., professor of surgery at George Washington University in Washington, D.C., and Robert D. Willix, M.D., a cardiac surgeon and sports medicine specialist in Boca Raton, Florida. They report that "a daily dosage is necessary only until the symptoms of your allergy subside. Thereafter, you need only a few teaspoons of horseradish each month to prevent another allergy attack."

I enjoy horseradish as a spice, so I would not hesitate to try it for allergy relief. You should be aware that while horseradish is hot, wasabi is even hotter. If you don't enjoy hot, spicy food, you'd best opt for a different treatment.

❧ **Vitamin C.** Not too long ago, C. Leigh Broadhurst, Ph.D., stopped by my office to talk about allergies. Dr. Broadhurst is a geochemist with expertise in nutritional medicine. At the time of our conversation, he was working for the U.S. Department of Agriculture.

To prevent and treat allergies, Dr. Broadhurst recommends taking 1,000 milligrams of vitamin C with bioflavonoids three times a day. This sounds fine to me. One review of some 40 vitamin C studies showed that people who took vitamin C regularly had fewer allergy problems, respiratory infections and asthma attacks. Vitamin C is a powerful natural antihistamine with no known side effects, except diarrhea. Some people develop diarrhea after taking as little as 1,200 milligrams of vitamin C a day, but this is rare. If you'd like to try this therapy, cut back on the amount of vitamin C if you develop diarrhea.

Don't confine yourself to supplements, either. Plants that are rich in vitamin C include Chinese bitter melon, bell peppers, cayenne pepper, pokeweed shoots, guava and watercress.

Altitude Sickness

I celebrated my 65th birthday climbing Machu Picchu, the famous 9,000-foot mountain in Peru. And just the day before that, I had climbed its steeper sister peak, Huainu Picchu. Two days of tough climbing nearly two miles above sea level and I could have suffered a bad bout of altitude sickness, what people in the Andes call *soroche*.

But before both climbs I knew that I might develop the symptoms of altitude sickness—headache, thirst, dizziness, weakness, heart palpitations and shortness of breath. So I did what Peruvian mountain hikers have done for thousands of years: I had a cup of *mate de coca*, or coca tea.

This tea is perfectly legal in Peru and Bolivia but not in the United States, because the coca leaf (*Erythroxylum coca*) is the source of cocaine. Cocaine is a highly processed derivative of coca, and coca tea contains only a little bit of it. But there's enough to act as a stimulant, which is why many Peruvians drink coca tea the way many of us drink coffee. In fact, hotels in Cusco and La Paz offer mate de coca as a reinvigorating refreshment to new arrivals from the lowlands. And they're well-aware that coca tea helps relieve altitude sickness.

For native Andeans, the straight, unbrewed coca leaf is the classical Andean energizer. On one ecotour to Peru, 27 of our 35 participants, myself included, experimented with chewing coca leaves. Some of us truly seemed to be energized. Several people commented that I climbed those mountains like a mountain goat.

Of course, I wouldn't recommend trying to get coca here in the United States. The association with cocaine has permanently tainted its legality and reputation, and getting relief from altitude sickness is not worth the prison sentence. But anywhere that coca is legal, it would be my top three-star recommendation for relief of soroche. I've never suffered any ill effects from coca tea, nor have I seen Peruvians become gangsters from chewing coca leaves.

In the United States, you might consider sipping Coca-Cola or Pepsi-Cola to relieve altitude sickness. The cocaine came out of these beverages many years ago, and they now contain decocainized coca leaves. Coca leaves still contain more than a dozen compounds that are closely related to cocaine but are completely legal, some of which help produce similar effects.

Why Going High Flattens You

Altitude sickness doesn't really have to do with the change in altitude but with the change in oxygen levels. The higher you go, the less oxygen there is. At 8,000 feet the atmosphere contains half the oxygen of the air at sea level. If you ascend slowly, a few thousand feet a day, your body will probably adjust to decreased oxygen with few ill effects. But rapid ascents—as in vigorous mountain climbing—leave your body deprived of oxygen availability, and the result is altitude sickness.

A key component of altitude sickness is dehydration. At high elevations, fluid moves out of the blood and into body tissues. As the blood thickens, dehydration interferes with efficient distribution of nutrients and oxygen and impedes the elimination of toxic wastes. The result is the headache, fatigue and malaise of altitude sickness, as well as extreme thirst.

One thing you can do to minimize or avoid altitude sickness is to drink plenty of nonalcoholic fluids before you start your ascent and continue taking in liquids as you climb. Plain water or juice works well. In the Andes, I eat a great deal of vegetable soup to get fluid as well as cooked vegetables (raw vegetables can cause problems). I also drink herb teas.

Green Pharmacy for Altitude Sickness

Since using coca leaf won't be an option in most of your travels, here are some other herbs that can help prevent altitude sickness.

❧❧ **Clove (*Syzygium aromaticum*).** Clove oil is rich in eugenol, a compound that is a potent blood thinner (anti-aggregant). Other high-eugenol herbs in my database, in descending order of potency, include allspice, bayrum leaf, galangal, carrot seed, shrubby basil, cinnamon, bayleaf and marjoram.

Mix several of the anti-aggregant herbs together, and you get my Altitude Adjustment Tea: In a pot of boiling water, steep cloves, allspice, bayleaf, celery seed, cinnamon and marjoram as available and to taste. Mix in, as available, any or all of these mints: basil, mountain dittany, savory and thyme.

☘☘ Garlic (*Allium sativum*). Garlic contains at least nine compounds that help thin the blood. Its anti-aggregant effect is valued as a heart attack preventive, but it also helps soroche sufferers. According to my database, other plants that have anti-aggregant activity include tomatoes, dill and fennel with seven blood-thinning compounds; onions, hot peppers and soybeans with six; and celery, carrots and parsley, each with five. You can cook them all in a big pot of water, and you will get what I call my Anti-aggregant Soup. Enjoying these foods in a vegetable soup before a mountain hike really can help prevent altitude sickness.

☘☘ Horsebalm (*Monarda*, various species). Many mints contain thymol, menthol or menthone, all compounds that have anti-aggregant activity. In my database, horsebalm wins as the herb with the most. Here are several more herbs, in descending order of potency, that contain these helpful ingredients: thyme, nude mountain mint, wild bergamot, winter savory, mountain dittany, lemon mint, basil and California bay.

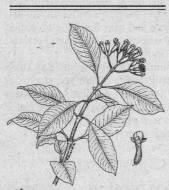

Clove

Cloves are the dried flower buds of a tropical evergreen tree.

☘☘ Reishi (*Ganoderma lucidum*). People in the mountains of Asia use this mushroom the way Peruvians use coca leaf. According to scientific reports, reishi significantly reduced altitude sickness symptoms in Chinese workers who climbed to over 15,000 feet over three days in Tibet. The theory is that reishi increases the body's oxygen consumption.

☘ Ginkgo (*Ginkgo biloba*). This herb increases blood flow throughout the body, especially to the brain. In animal studies, rats fed a ginkgo

extract show definite increases in cerebral blood flow and toler-
ance to low-oxygen effects. This sounds to me like a potential preventive and treatment for altitude sickness. You can try 60 to 240
milligrams of standardized extract a day, but don't go any higher
than that. In large amounts, ginkgo may cause diarrhea, irritability and restlessness.

Alzheimer's Disease

Nearly a decade ago, four different people approached me
independently in rapid succession, asking if I could find
them some Chinese club moss. They had all heard that
huperzine, a compound derived from this herb, might help slow
the progression of Alzheimer's disease. Each of these people
had a parent who had this disease, and they were desperate to
find anything that might help.

I'd never heard of using Chinese club moss (*Huperzia ser-
rata*) for Alzheimer's, so I did a little digging—in my database,
not in my garden—and learned that *Huperzia* is an alternate
name for some of the *Lycopodium* club mosses, including one
that grows around my Herbal Vineyard in Maryland.

Moss Compounds for the Brain

I dimly recalled that an Indian tribe had eaten *Lycopodium*,
and sure enough, after a little more research I found that it was
the Chippewa tribe of the eastern United States. I sampled some
of the club moss growing in my garden and found it rather
unappetizing. But as my research continued, I came across
some interesting information: The two species of club moss
sought by the Chippewa contained huperzine.

Researchers have found that huperzine inhibits the breakdown of acetylcholine, a brain chemical (neurotransmitter) that
plays a key role in cognition and reasoning. People with
Alzheimer's often have an acetylcholine deficiency. It's still not
clear whether this deficiency causes the disease or results from
it. But Alzheimer's researchers are actively pursuing treatments

that either prevent the chemical breakdown of acetylcholine or add its precursor, choline, to brain tissues. It would seem that anything that boosts acetylcholine in the brain, including a number of herbs, is currently our best approach to dealing with this disease.

The Brain Drain

Alzheimer's is the leading cause of mental deterioration as people age. The National Institute on Aging estimates that Alzheimer's affects four million Americans. It strikes about 10 percent of people over 65 and about half of those who live beyond 85.

Until a couple of years ago, there was no way to treat Alzheimer's. Then the Food and Drug Administration (FDA) approved tacrine hydrochloride (Cognex), a medication that reportedly slows progression of the disease by preserving acetylcholine in the brain. The problem with this drug is that it is toxic to the liver, with a high potential for causing liver damage.

Other drugs are in the pipeline. As usual, they are synthetics. And as usual, the drug companies and the FDA seem to be overlooking some promising herbal alternatives, namely all of the herbs containing compounds that prevent the breakdown of acetylcholine.

Green Pharmacy for Alzheimer's Disease

Fortunately, along with club moss, there are a number of other herbs that show promise in preventing and treating this devastating disease.

❦❦❦ **Horsebalm (*Monarda*, various species).** Horsebalm contains the beneficial compound carvacrol, which Austrian scientists have discovered helps prevent the breakdown of acetylcholine. Horsebalm also contains thymol, which also prevents the breakdown of acetylcholine.

Some compounds in horsebalm apparently can cross the blood-brain barrier. Normally your body's protective blood-brain barrier helps prevent harmful substances in the blood from reaching the tissues of the brain. But because this blood-brain barrier sometimes works too well, it can also prevent helpful medicines from reaching the brain. The horsebalm compounds seem to cross that great divide, which means it might have some positive effects even if you use it as a shampoo or skin lotion.

That being so, I'd be willing to wager my head of hair, if not my brain, that a horsebalm shampoo might work nearly as well as FDA-approved tacrine hydrochloride. It would probably be safer, easier on the liver and a whole lot cheaper.

You won't be able to buy shampoo that contains horsebalm, but it's easy to make your own. Simply add several dropperfuls of horsebalm tincture to your favorite herbal shampoo.

🌿🌿🌿 Rosemary (*Rosmarinus officinalis*). Some evidence suggests that oxidative damage caused by highly reactive (free radical) oxygen molecules in the body plays a role in Alzheimer's. If that's so, rosemary should help. It contains a couple of dozen antioxidants—that is, compounds that help mop up free radicals. Among the antioxidants is a particularly potent one, rosmarinic acid.

Rosemary also contains a half-dozen compounds that are reported to prevent the breakdown of acetylcholine. Interestingly enough, aromatherapists suggest using rosemary oil for treating Alzheimer's disease. (They also recommend oils of balm, fennel and sage.)

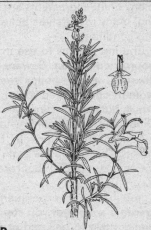

Rosemary has a long history as a memory-enhancing herb, so much so that it's known as the herb of remembrance. I think rosemary shampoo, rosemary tea and rosemary in the bathwater would have anti-Alzheimer's activity similar to that of tacrine or huperzine.

The good thing about this recommendation is that it's safe and pleasant to use rosemary in all of these forms. If I'm wrong, there's little or no harm done. And if I'm right, it's all to the good.

Rosemary

Originally used to preserve meats, rosemary is said to improve memory.

Of the rosemary compounds that retard the breakdown of acetylcholine, several if not all can be absorbed through the skin, and some probably cross the blood-brain barrier. Thus, using rosemary shampoo regularly could conceivably help preserve acetylcholine in the brain just as tacrine does. You can buy commercial herbal shampoo that contains rosemary, or you can make your own by adding rosemary tincture to your favorite herbal shampoo.

❧

Biblical Brainfood Soup

This soup, made entirely from plants mentioned in the Bible, is a good bet for anyone with Alzheimer's disease. Many of the ingredients are rich in choline, a compound that many researchers believe is helpful for people with this condition.

The ingredients to use in the soup are barley, bottle gourd, dandelion flowers and greens, fava beans, flaxseed, lentils, poppy seeds, stinging nettle, ground walnuts and cracked wheat. (You'll need to wear gloves when harvesting stinging nettle leaves, but the fuzzy stingers lose their sting when the leaves are cooked.)

Season the soup with balm, rosemary, sage and savory. These help the brain hold on to its acetylcholine, another compound that researchers believe to be helpful.

You'll have to experiment with these ingredients to create a soup that you can enjoy. Not all of the ingredients have to be used at once. In fact, you probably won't have access to them all at once. You could simply keep the list handy and add as many of these ingredients as possible to other soups you might be making.

❧

✷✷ Brazil nut (*Bertholettia excelsa*). In addition to looking into treatments focused on preventing the breakdown of acetylcholine, researchers have also been studying possible treatments that will supplement people's supply of choline, a building block for acetylcholine.

Lecithin contains choline, and according to my database, Brazil nuts are the richest food sources of lecithin (up to 10 percent on a dry-weight basis). Many other plant foods and herbs also contain generous amounts of lecithin. They include, in descending order of potency, dandelion flowers, poppy seeds, soybeans and mung beans.

There are also a number of plants, including fenugreek leaves and shepherd's purse, that contain choline itself. Other plant foods and herbs that contain small amounts of choline include horehound, ginseng, cowpea, English pea, mung beans, sponge gourd, lentils and Chinese angelica, also known as *dang-quai*.

Researchers have tried feeding high-choline and high-lecithin foods to people with Alzheimer's. Preliminary results were encouraging, but more recent studies have failed to find significant memory improvement. I remain cautiously optimistic that eating foods containing choline and lecithin might help.

✷✷ Dandelion (*Taraxacum officinale*). These flowers are one of our better sources of lecithin, and they're also a reasonable source of choline (the two often show up in the same foods). Lecithin increases concentrations of acetylcholine in the brain and improves memory in laboratory mice. There's no proof yet that this treatment works in people, but I'm optimistic about the possibility. Besides, dandelions are very nutritious.

✷✷ Fava beans (*Vicia faba*). These beans are quite rich in lecithin. Fava beans are a key ingredient in my Biblical Brainfood Soup. In fact, many beans are rich in lecithin and choline and should be included in any diet, not just those for people concerned about preventing and treating Alzheimer's.

✷✷ Fenugreek (*Trigonella foenum-graecum*). Little did I know when I had *alu methi* at an Indian restaurant that I was indulging in steamed fenugreek leaves. These are among the better dietary sources of choline (up to 1.3 percent on a dry-weight basis). As we have seen, dietary choline could conceivably help prevent and treat Alzheimer's.

Fenugreek greens are also a good source of beta-carotene, an antioxidant that might also help prevent or slow the progression of Alzheimer's.

❧❧ Ginkgo (*Ginkgo biloba*). Hundreds of European studies have confirmed the use of standardized ginkgo leaf extract for a wide variety of conditions associated with aging, including memory loss and poor circulation. There's not much data on using ginkgo to treat Alzheimer's, but I wouldn't be surprised if it helped. It's probably worth trying. You can take 60 to 240 milligrams of standardized extract a day, but don't go any higher than that. In large amounts, ginkgo may cause diarrhea, irritability and restlessness.

❧❧ Sage (*Salvia officinalis*). Seventeenth-century herbalist John Gerard said that sage "helpeth a weake braine or memory and restoreth them . . . in a short time." British researchers have confirmed that sage inhibits the enzyme that breaks down acetylcholine, thus preserving the compound that seems to help prevent and treat Alzheimer's. Like rosemary, sage is also well-endowed with antioxidants. Just be judicious: Sage contains a fair amount of thujone, a compound that in very high doses may cause convulsions.

❧❧ Stinging nettle (*Urtica dioica*). This herb contains considerable amounts of the mineral boron, which can double levels of the hormone estrogen circulating in the body. And estrogen, tested in several studies, helped improve short-term memory and also helped elevate the moods of some people with Alzheimer's.

❧❧ Willow (*Salix*, various species). Some studies have shown a lower incidence of Alzheimer's in those who have taken a lot of anti-inflammatory drugs for arthritis. If these medicines help prevent Alzheimer's, then willow bark, the herbal source of aspirin, should help as well. Remember, though, that if you're allergic to aspirin, you probably shouldn't take aspirin-like herbs, either.

❧ Gotu kola (*Centella asiatica*). This herb has a centuries-old folk reputation as a memory herb that helps maintain strong mental vigor. I doubt that it would have maintained this reputation if there weren't something to it.

❧ Herb gardening. If you have a family history of Alzheimer's or are otherwise concerned about this disease, you might want to consider starting an herb garden. This would give you an ongoing source of the herbs that show promise against Alzheimer's. All of them can be grown, at least as annuals, in the lower 48 states. Not only that but also gardening requires thought, creativity and physical activity, all of which I believe help to preserve brain function. (For more detailed instructions on how to grow herbs, see pages 17 and 18.)

Amenorrhea

S he was under 40, not pregnant, and she hadn't had a period in six months. The doctors had checked her for everything—including endometriosis and cancer—and found nothing.

Amenorrhea—the medical term for lack of menstruation in women who should be having regular periods—is a sign that something in the body has gone wrong. The cause could be anything from a stress reaction or a hormone imbalance to something more serious, and it sometimes takes a while to pinpoint the problem.

In desperation, this woman called me after being referred by Washington's Mind-Body Institute. She thought that maybe her problem was caused by a medication that she was taking, which was possibly altering the levels of the female hormone estrogen in her body.

I told her that she might normalize her estrogen levels with the help of the estrogen-like substances called phytoestrogens that are found in many plants, including soybeans and wild yams. I also mentioned chasteberry, an herb with a well-deserved reputation for restoring menstrual flow. She said she'd try chasteberry and phytoestrogens. Months later, she called again to say she was quite satisfied with the results.

Green Pharmacy for Amenorrhea

Herbs that bring on menstrual flow—for whatever reason—are known as emmenagogues. Back in the days before modern medicine, women often used emmenagogues for two reasons. Some used the herbs as a kind of morning-after contraception, because not much else was available. Others used them to treat amenorrhea.

Emmenagogues are no longer necessary for contraception,

but they might still help with amenorrhea. There are dozens, if not hundreds, of emmenagogue herbs and plant chemicals (phytochemicals) in my various databases.

You should see your doctor for a diagnosis if you have amenorrhea. The standard medical treatment is hormone therapy, but hormone treatments are tricky, require sophisticated monitoring and in many cases, fail to get results. In my experience, emmenagogues often restore normal menstrual flow and provide considerable emotional relief. You might ask your doctor about trying these safe and gentle herbs before resorting to hormones.

From the longer list in my database, here are some of my favorites.

❦❦❦ **Chasteberry (*Vitex agnuscastus*).** In one small study, 20 women with amenorrhea were given 40 drops daily of a *Vitex* extract, then were monitored for six months. Fifteen completed the study, and 10 of them had their menstrual cycles restored.

Amenorrhea is often associated with elevated blood levels of

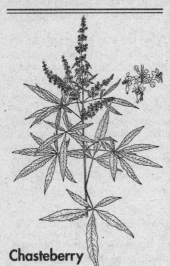

Chasteberry

An extract of these berries helps restore the menstrual cycle to normal.

the hormone prolactin, and drugs that reduce prolactin usually restore the menstrual cycle to normal. Chasteberry acts just like these drugs.

The typical dose is 20 milligrams per day of a tincture made from the fruits. In Germany, herbal medicines are widely used and often recommended by doctors. One popular German ' amenorrhea preparation (Femisana) is a tincture of chasteberry fruits, along with greater celandine, black cohosh and pasqueflower (*Pulsatilla vulgaris*).

❦❦ **Black cohosh (*Cimicifuga racemosa*) and blue cohosh (*Caulophyllum thalictroides*).** These were the American Indians' two favorite herbs for gynecological complaints. It turns out that black cohosh has potent estrogen-like activity, and blue cohosh stimulates uterine contractions.

❧ **Carrot (*Daucus carota*).** Many Pennsylvania Dutch have used wild carrot (Queen Anne's lace) seed, which is apparently effective as both an emmenagogue and a morning-after contraceptive. Indian researchers have confirmed that carrot seed has anti-implantation activity in laboratory animals.

❧ **Celery (*Apium graveolens*).** Celery seed contains butylidenephthalide, a chemical that helps trigger menstrual flow.

❧ **Dill (*Anethum graveolens*).** The compound apiole in dill is such a powerful emmenagogue that most herbalists I respect warn pregnant women not to use it in medicinal concentrations. (Don't panic, though—eating a dill pickle is okay.) If you want to encourage menstrual flow, you can brew a tea using two teaspoons of mashed seeds.

❧ **Marsh mallow (*Althaea officinalis*).** This herb contains up to 4 percent betaine, a phytoestrogen and emmenagogue that is also found in beets, carrots, chard, chicory, oats, oranges and yarrow.

You might try marsh mallow and yarrow tea. For a tasty vegetable dish that delivers a good dose of betaine, try steamed carrots and chard with beets.

❧ **Turmeric (*Curcuma longa*).** Traditional Chinese and Indian physicians recommend turmeric to treat amenorrhea. I have no reason to doubt its safety, but I cannot vouch for its efficacy. It's probably worth a try. For a medicinal dose, you can make a curry, heavy on the turmeric, or simply brew a strong tea.

❧ **Assorted herbs.** Other herbs that help amenorrhea are so plentiful and widely available that I'd feel as if I weren't doing my job if I didn't list some of them. You could combine dashes of whichever of these herbs you have on hand, pour boiling water over them and steep for 15 minutes. They are agrimony, angelica, betony, calaminth, caraway, catnip, coriander, cilantro, cumin, Chinese angelica (also known as *dang-quai*), fennel, feverfew, ginger, horehound, hyssop, juniper, lavender, lemon balm (also known as melissa), lovage, marigold, marjoram, motherwort, nutsedge, oregano, parsley, pennyroyal, roselle, rosemary, rue, saffron, tansy, tarragon, thyme, wild chervil, wintergreen, wormseed (also known as *epazote*), yarrow and ylang-ylang.

I should also note that fruits and roots with enzymes that

break down protein (proteolytics) are folkloric emmenagogues. These include figs, ginger, papaya and pineapple.

Angina

It's amazing how much herbal information you can pick up wandering the halls of the U.S. Department of Agriculture (USDA). Many of my colleagues there used to ask me for herbal advice and for solutions to assorted health problems.

One of my more conservative colleagues—not the kind of person who gravitated toward herbal medicine—surprised me one day by asking me what sort of herbal concoction I might recommend for angina. This problem had been bothering him for several months.

I mentioned a couple of the herbs in this chapter—hawthorn and garlic—and he thanked me. Then he told me that he'd been taking ginger for about a week, and he felt considerably better.

That was a new one on me. I knew that ginger helped lower cholesterol and blood pressure, which benefits the heart, but I didn't know that it had anti-angina benefits as well. It turned out that he was right—it does.

Angina, technically angina pectoris, is a form of heart disease that causes moderate to severe chest pain. In stable angina, the pain develops after some form of physical exertion, anything from a brisk jog to a leisurely stroll. In unstable angina, the pain strikes while a person is at rest.

Angina is caused by atherosclerosis, a disease in which cholesterol-rich deposits called plaque cause the coronary arteries to narrow. Atherosclerosis limits blood flow into the heart, and the resulting lack of nourishment and oxygen triggers angina pain. Both kinds of angina (but particularly unstable angina) indicate that a person has major risk of heart attack.

Green Pharmacy for Angina

Anyone with angina should be under a physician's care, and it's extremely important to follow your doctor's recommendations. Typical recommendations involve taking nitroglycerin, aspirin and frequently other medications that lower cholesterol and blood pressure.

In addition to these measures, there are a number of medicinal herbs that can help. Before you take any of these herbs, however, you should discuss it with your doctor.

❧❧❧ Hawthorn (*Crataegus*, various species). In Europe, hawthorn berry preparations are widely used to treat mild angina.

Extensive research has demonstrated that hawthorn extracts improve heart function by opening up the coronary arteries. This in turn improves the blood and oxygen supply to the heart. Hawthorn also decreases blood cholesterol levels, another heart-healthy benefit, and it is safe to use for extended periods of time, according to European clinical experience.

In his excellent book *Herbs of Choice*, Varro Tyler, Ph.D., dean and professor emeritus of pharmacognosy (natural product pharmacy) at Purdue University in West Lafayette, Indiana, explains that hawthorn's heart benefits are due to special compounds in the plant—oligomeric procyanidins (OPCs). People get additional beneficial effects from several other compounds known as flavonoids, which open (dilate) the smooth vessels of the coronary arteries.

Commission E, the German expert panel that evaluates medicinal herbs for the German government, approves hawthorn for a number of heart problems. Naturopaths recommend a daily dosage of 240 to 480 milligrams of standardized extract. Hawthorn is a powerful heart medicine, so do not take it without discussing it with your doctor.

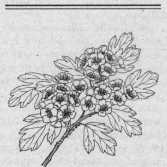

Hawthorn

The flowers, leaves and fruits of this plant are all used for medicinal purposes.

❧❧ Angelica (*Angelica archangelica*) and other herbs of the carrot family. Calcium channel blockers are a standard class of antiangina drugs, and angelica contains 15 compounds that act much like these channel blockers. Similar compounds appear in other plants in the carrot family: carrots, celery, fennel, parsley and parsnips.

If I had angina, I'd combine them all in a drink that consists of juiced angelica, carrots, celery, fennel, parsley and parsnips, with some water and spices added.

It's well-known that vegetarians have a low incidence of heart disease. Usually, their lower-fat diet gets the credit. But I'd be willing to bet that part of the reason is that they eat lots of plants from the carrot family.

≈≈ Bilberry (*Vaccinium myrtillus*) and other fruits. Bilberry contains compounds known as anthocyanins that have a cholesterol-lowering effect. This herb is also a vasodilator that opens blood vessels and lowers blood pressure. Anthocyanins help prevent formation of the blood clots that trigger heart attack.

Until pharmaceutical firms start studying anthocyanins, we won't know how effectively these compounds help to prevent coronary problems. But one thing is clear. Bilberries are not the only fruit that contains them. Other good sources include blackberries, black chokeberries, boysenberries, black currants, blueberries, cherries, cranberries, red grapes and red raspberries. I suspect that all of these fruits might help prevent and treat angina.

≈≈ Garlic (*Allium sativum*) and onion (*A. cepa*). Both of these spicy herbs help treat heart disease by lowering cholesterol and blood pressure and by preventing formation of the blood clots that trigger heart attack.

According to one study, munching one clove of garlic daily cuts cholesterol by 9 percent. Every 1 percent decrease in cholesterol translates to a 2 percent decrease in heart attack risk, so a clove a day reduces risk of heart attack by 18 percent. Onions have similar benefits, although not as pronounced.

≈≈ Ginger (*Zingiber officinale*). After my USDA colleague persuaded me to explore ginger's anti-angina benefits, I read that it was endorsed for heart attack prevention in *Ginger: Common Spice and Wonder Drug* by New England herbalist Paul Schulick. He notes that an Israeli cardiology clinic now recommends a daily half-teaspoon of powdered ginger.

It seems that ginger is an antioxidant that offers the blood vessels some protection against the damage caused by cholesterol. Ginger also boosts the strength of heart muscle tissue, as does the medication digitalis. If I had angina, I would take ginger regularly and use it liberally in cooking.

Khella (*Ammi majus*). A 1951 article published in the *New England Journal of Medicine* touted the anti-angina benefits of khellin, a compound in khella that increases blood flow into the heart. The article called khellin "a safe and effective drug for the treatment of angina pectoris."

As little as 30 milligrams of khellin a day can help, but noted naturopath Michael Murray, N.D., co-author of *Encyclopedia of Natural Medicine* and several other scholarly books on nutritional and naturopathic healing, recommends taking 250 to 300 milligrams daily of khella extracts that are standardized for khellin content (typically 12 percent). If you buy khella in standardized extract form, that information will be on the label.

Kudzu (*Pueraria lobata*). Chinese clinical studies attest to the anti-angina benefits of kudzu. In one study, 71 people took 10 to 15 grams of a root extract a day for 4 to 22 weeks. During this time, 29 were much improved, 20 showed some improvement, and 22 showed little or no improvement.

Kudzu extracts dilate coronary arteries, increasing blood flow and decreasing blood pressure. They also help stabilize heart rhythm. Kudzu root preparations have produced no adverse effects in human trials.

Purslane (*Portulaca oleracea*). Antioxidants are substances that protect cells from damage caused by free radicals, highly reactive oxygen molecules in the body. And they appear to play a key role in preventing heart disease. I recommend purslane because it's extremely well endowed with antioxidants, and in addition, it's our best leafy source of omega-3 fatty acids, beneficial oils that also help prevent heart disease.

Willow (*Salix*, various species). Studies have shown that low-dose aspirin—anywhere from 30 milligrams to a standard 325-milligram tablet a day—helps prevent heart attack by preventing the formation of blood clots. This is a major concern for people with angina.

Willow bark is herbal aspirin. A daily cup or two of willow bark tea would probably provide the equivalent of the low aspirin dose recommended for heart attack prevention. (Incidentally, the latest studies show that aspirin, and presumably willow bark as well, also help prevent colon cancer. So there's more than one reason to adopt it.) Remember, though, that if you're allergic to aspirin, you probably shouldn't take aspirin-like herbs, either.

❧ **Evening primrose (*Oenothera biennis*).** Primrose is an excellent source of gamma-linolenic acid (GLA), a compound that lowers both cholesterol and blood pressure. GLA also has an anti-clotting effect. My friend C. Leigh Broadhurst, Ph.D., a geochemist with expertise in nutritional medicine, suggests that evening primrose and flaxseed, which is discussed below, should be taken together.

❧ **Flax (*Linum usitatissimum*).** Flaxseed contains an abundant amount of alpha-linolenic acid, a compound that many claim has heart-protective ability.

❧ **Sichuan lovage (*Ligusticum chuanxiong*).** This Asian herb helps prevent the formation of heart attack–triggering blood clots, according to pharmacognosist (natural product pharmacist) Albert Leung, Ph.D., and noted Arkansas herbalist and photographer Steven Foster. In their book, *The Encyclopedia of Common Natural Ingredients*, they note that this herb contains compounds similar to those in angelica. These compounds dilate the coronary arteries, increasing blood flow to the heart. Small wonder that Sichuan lovage is used in China to treat angina and other heart conditions.

Ankylosing Spondylitis

I have ankylosing spondylitis (AS), a form of arthritis most people have never even heard of. AS causes inflammation along the spinal column, resulting in back pain and stiffness. (*Ankylosing* means "rigid," *spondy-* is "spine," and *-itis* means "inflammation").

Men develop AS 2.5 times more often than women. Current estimates are that it affects about 318,000 men and 127,000 women. Ninety percent of cases develop between the ages of 20 and 40, but I wasn't diagnosed until I was 60, after my slipped disk operation in 1991.

While no one knows what causes AS, there's been some

suggestion that it may be an autoimmune disease, a description that also fits rheumatoid arthritis, another kind of joint disease. Normally, the immune system attacks only invading microbes, which keeps you from succumbing to infection. Sometimes, however, the immune system gets confused about what it's supposed to be attacking and turns its lethal power against the body itself. Depending upon what part of the body it attacks, any number of so-called autoimmune diseases can result.

Pain Gets a Grip

In my case, AS has affected the vertebrae in my neck, the disks between the vertebrae and the surrounding ligaments and connective tissue. They're stiff and painful, and occasionally pressure on the nerve roots causes pain to radiate down my arms. AS has also made me lean forward a bit.

It often takes years for AS to be diagnosed, because many people assume that it's ordinary low back pain, which is very common. (AS often makes its appearance in the low back.) If AS remains untreated, the risk is lifelong back disability. The chronic inflammation can destroy the cartilage between the vertebrae. AS can also lead to bony growths that fuse the vertebrae and cause permanent spinal rigidity.

When I slipped a disk and had surgery, my expensive neurosurgeon dismissed exercise, saying that it wouldn't help me because of my AS. If I ever happen to run into him again, I'll be sure to tell him that exercise has worked quite well to help relieve the pain these last five years. I'll also be sure to tell him that the kind of operation that he performed on me is now regarded as medically useless.

While he was deep inside my neck, my neurosurgeon performed a cervical fusion, meaning that he fused two of the vertebrae. That's exactly what Nature was doing all along, just going about it a little more slowly. Fused disks are exactly what happens eventually with ankylosing spondylitis. Maybe I just should have waited for Nature to take its course. Maybe not. I'll never know.

❧

Socorro's Secret

Socorro Guerra and her husband, Cesar, live in eastern Peru at the junction of the Yanomono Creek and the Amazon River. That's some 15 minutes on foot from the Explorama Lodge that houses the ecotourists who attend my tropical herb workshops. Cesar runs a sugar cane distillery that turns out aguardiente, or cachasas, an Amazonian rum used by the locals both medicinally and for social drinking.

Socorro is quite the Amazonian herbalist. Back in her kitchen, she proudly shows off her remedio para reumatismo—her rheumatism remedy. I call it Socorro's Secret, having concluded that it might be as useful as anything out there for rheumatoid arthritis and possibly for ankylosing spondylitis (AS) as well.

The significant ingredients are the herb dragon's blood, fig latex (a milky substance that oozes from the fig tree), ginger, port wine and, of course, her husband's rum. Ginger and fig latex contain protein-digesting (proteolytic) enzymes that are useful in alleviating the inflammatory symptoms of rheumatoid arthritis and possibly AS. As for the dragon's blood and port wine, they both contain generous amounts of compounds known as oligomeric procyanidins (OPCs). OPCs are antioxidants—substances that mop up free radicals, highly reactive oxygen molecules that damage the body's cells.

Of course, Socorro doesn't know about proteolytic enzymes or OPCs. She simply uses her fiery formula to obtain relief from her reumatismo. I've taken the liberty of adding pineapple to Socorro's Secret, making a very tasty herbal punch that's loaded with proteolytic enzymes.

Here's the modified recipe: Add one tablespoon of

dragon's blood and one tablespoon of fig latex to one pint of red wine and one pint of pineapple juice. (Both dragon's blood and fig latex are imported into the United States but are not widely available, and they are not approved by the Food and Drug Administration. You may have to do some searching.) Stir in one cup of shredded ginger root. Sit back and enjoy, without worrying about your back.

❦❧

Green Pharmacy for Ankylosing Spondylitis

My neurosurgeon also said that there are no herbal approaches to back problems. What he should have said was that there were none that he knew of. In fact, several herbs can help. I should be clear right here that herbs won't cure your AS. If you have it, get yourself a good rheumatologist and follow his advice. But herbs can definitely help. They've helped me.

✿✿✿ **Ginger** (*Zingiber officinale*). Ginger contains zingibain, a special kind of proteolytic enzyme that has the ability to chemically break down protein. Adolph's meat tenderizer works because it contains this kind of enzyme.

Clinical studies have shown that proteolytic enzymes have antiinflammatory properties, according to noted naturopath Michael Murray, N.D., co-author of *Encyclopedia of Natural Medicine* and several other scholarly books on nutritional and naturopathic healing. That means that they should help relieve AS.

Proteolytic enzymes, of which there are several besides zingibain, also play an additional role in controlling autoimmune diseases. They help reduce blood levels of compounds known as immune complexes, high levels of which activate the immune system to attack the body itself, ultimately leading to tissue damage.

At least one researcher, Paul Schulick, New England herbalist and author of *Ginger: Common Spice and Wonder Drug*, suggests that zingibain, which comprises as much as 2 percent of fresh ginger root, is as powerful an enzyme as the bromelain in pineapple or the papain in papaya. He insists that ginger is one of nature's richest sources of proteolytic enzymes, containing approximately 180 times more than the papaya plant.

❧

Help from the Animal Kingdom

Cartilage. I realize that it is not green, but the bottom-line advice is going to translate into the suggestion to toss a soup bone into your vegetable soup. So bear with me for a moment.

Over the past few years, health food publications have been promoting shark cartilage for preventing cancer. It seems that sharks, whose nonbony skeletons are all cartilage, don't get cancer. I can't say much of a positive nature about taking shark cartilage for cancer, but there is some intriguing research suggesting that chicken and cattle cartilage may help those of us with ankylosing spondylitis (AS).

Harvard researcher David Trentham, M.D., has discovered that eating type II collagen, a connective tissue and component of cartilage, may significantly reduce the symptoms of autoimmune forms of arthritis, specifically rheumatoid arthritis and, quite possibly, AS. The work of immunologist Rachel E. Caspi, Ph.D., at the National Eye Institute supports the use of collagen therapy for other autoimmune diseases.

Now AutoImmune, a biotech company in Lexington, Massachusetts, is collaborating with Dr. Trentham on collagen studies involving 280 people. Preliminary results suggest that the lowest dose of collagen was the most effective, prompting researchers to consider even lower dosages in the future. Dr. Trentham does not yet say that eating animal cartilage will alleviate rheumatoid arthritis or AS, but the studies reported to date just might make a cartilage eater out of me.

Some people go in for chicken gristle, but I prefer to

get my collagen from soup bones, which contain a good deal of it. So tossing a soup bone or two into your vegetable soup as it simmers is probably a good idea if you have AS.

❧❧

Ginger is also well-known for its anti-inflammatory properties. Indian and Scandinavian studies have consistently shown that ginger (and closely related turmeric) is useful for treating most kinds of arthritis.

Ginger also contains more than 12 antioxidants, which help neutralize the highly reactive molecules—free radicals—that play a role in causing inflammation.

Finally, Schulick also notes that ginger offers a big advantage over mainstream medicine's treatment of choice for AS, which is nonsteroidal anti-inflammatory drugs (NSAIDs). Aspirin and other NSAIDs are hard on the stomach, and long-term use can lead to ulcers. Ginger does not cause stomach problems.

I enjoy ginger, and I hope it's helping to postpone any serious complications of AS for me. You can take ginger as an herb in tea, tincture or capsules. It's also a tasty spice that you can use generously in the kitchen. A dish prepared with ginger will actually give you a medicinal dose of the herb.

❧❧❧ **Pineapple (*Ananas comosus*).** Like ginger, pineapple contains a proteolytic enzyme, called bromelain.

Dr. Murray recommends taking 400 to 600 milligrams of bromelain three times daily on an empty stomach. You can buy pure bromelain in natural food stores.

Liking pineapple as I do, I prefer to get my bromelain from the natural source, so I eat lots of pineapple. In addition to zingibain and bromelain, there are several other potent proteolytic enzymes that should have similar effects. You can get these enzymes by eating the fruits and herbs that contain them. The best sources include breadfruit, ginger, kiwifruit, papaya and figs.

❧❧ **Corn (*Zea mays*).** How well I remember my first trip to Amazonian Peru back in 1991. I was suffering the indignity of one of those neck (cervical) collars. It helped correct that forward-leaning head posture that so many old men are prone to exhibit, especially those with AS. But in the Amazonian humidity, the collar really chafed, and it seemed to hurt my neck more than it helped my spine.

Back home, I would have rubbed on some soothing talcum powder. But I didn't have any until one nice ecotouring lady, with an Alabama accent like mine, gave me some of her "tropical talcum powder"—finely pulverized cornstarch. She had wisely brought this along to avoid just such chafing problems herself. When she applied the first sprinkling to my aching neck, relief was almost immediate. Then she gave me a plastic bag with my own stash of finely powdered cornstarch. I'm not suggesting cornstarch to alleviate AS itself, just to help relieve the dermatitis you might have if you happen to be strapped into a cervical collar as a result of having this condition.

🌿🌿 **Pigweed (*Amaranthus*, various species).** There's no doubt that getting enough calcium helps prevent osteoporosis. I believe it's useful for preventing AS as well.

In my database, pigweed is the best plant source of calcium. Other plants that are also good sources of the essential mineral include lamb's-quarters, stinging nettle, broadbeans, watercress, licorice, marjoram, savory, red clover shoots, thyme, Chinese cabbage, basil, celery seed, chaya, dandelion and purslane.

I recommend eating green leafy vegetables often as a regular part of your meals. It's also good practice to drink broths or pot-likkers made from these plants between meals.

🌿 **Vegetarianism.** Several studies and a good deal of anecdotal evidence suggest that a low-calorie vegetarian diet helps alleviate the pain and inflammation of rheumatoid arthritis. Research has shown that this type of diet helps relieve the symptoms of a broad range of autoimmune diseases. If AS is, in fact, a form of autoimmune arthritis, then a calorie-restricted vegetarian diet should help relieve this condition as well.

This type of diet is good for health and longevity in general, even if you don't have an autoimmune condition. And if you do have AS, at the very least, this diet can help you lose weight, which takes pressure off arthritic joints. Considering our evolutionary past, I can't recommend strict vegetarianism. I prefer Jeffersonian vegetarianism, letting meat be a "spice" rather than a major meal constituent.

Arthritis

I'm the bass fiddle player in a five-member band called Durham Station. In recent years three of our band members or their relatives have been using an herb known as stinging nettle to relieve their arthritis pain. Although stinging nettle does cook up into a tasty vegetable, these musicians aren't eating it. Rather, they're stinging themselves with it by grasping the plant in a gloved hand and then swatting their stiff, swollen joints.

This practice, called urtication—from nettle's botanical name, *Urtica dioica*—dates back at least 2,000 years to biblical times. Although it's an odd-sounding practice, there's no escaping the fact that it's been around so long precisely because it helps so many people.

Not only does our banjo player keep a plant in his kitchen so that he can self-urticate when his arthritis flares up, but he and the other arthritis-afflicted band members are convincing nonmembers to try the remedy. The guitar player's mother-in-law was unable to write because of arthritis in her hands, but the sting of the nettle improved that. The fiddle player's mother now has stinging nettle taking over her garden, and she says her arthritis is "much improved."

And just so you don't think that urtication is something that only crazy musicians indulge in, my former secretary at the U.S. Department of Agriculture (USDA) kept a nettle plant in the office. She would remove the nettles and discreetly sting herself any time arthritis stiffened her fingers.

Urtication often provides considerable relief. Sometimes the stuff works pretty fast; I have seen arthritic swelling subside within minutes after the stings were administered.

The Case for the Sting

I'm open to the notion that stinging nettle's anti-arthritic action is based on distraction, meaning that the irritation of the sting simply takes people's minds off their arthritis pain. That's an explanation you might hear from doctors. But as a botanist,

I have to say that I think what's going on is more chemical than psychological.

❧

The Gin-and-Raisins Cure

Some years ago, the newsman Paul Harvey recommended raisins soaked in gin for all manner of aches and pains, including arthritis. Here's a letter I received on this subject from a correspondent in Mesa, Arizona: "After reading a Paul Harvey commentary on gin-soaked raisins, a group of friends and I decided to give it a try. It really works. We have all enjoyed great relief from arthritic aches and pains. After 15 years of pain, I'm almost totally pain-free. I've been taking pain pills for years with only minimal relief. Some kinds of pain that have been relieved or eliminated after taking the gin-soaked raisin formula include migraine headaches, gout and arthritic pain in joints. Several people reported a decrease in pains that awakened them at night, enabling them to have an uninterrupted sleep. In your research, have you discovered why it works so well?"

I replied: "No, but I am going home to a gin Collins with grape juice, since I prefer grapes to raisins."

If you benefit from gin-steeped raisins, the raisins probably do you more good than the gin. Grapes and raisins contain many pain relieving, anti-arthritic and anti-inflammatory chemicals. Looking over the long list of compounds that occur naturally in grapes, I see such pain relievers as ferulic acid, gentisic acid, kaempferol-glucosides and aspirin-like salicylic acid. Grapes and raisins also contain several anti-inflammatory compounds: ascorbic acid, cinnamic acid, coumarin, myricetin, quercetin and quercitrin. And in 1997, there was a flurry of interest in resveratrol, yet another anti-inflammatory compound of which grapes are the best source. Ounce for ounce, raisins contain more of all of these compounds than grapes because they contain less water.

All of these pain relievers occur at low levels in raisins, so I doubt that the mere seven gin-soaked raisins that Harvey touted would contain significant doses. My correspondent might have benefited from a placebo effect: Believing enough in a remedy really can help it work. But a large quantity of raisins might well provide significant pain-relieving and anti-inflammatory benefits. Personally, I'd be tempted to try raisins before depending on nonsteroidal anti-inflammatory drugs.

The raisins are surely less likely to do you any harm than the gin they're soaked in, especially if you're prone to gout. Alcohol is a major trigger of excruciating gout attacks. I can guarantee that my big toe will swell if I drink a six-pack of beer and don't take my allopurinol. But if you don't have gout (and are not an alcoholic), modest consumption of alcohol may help relieve arthritis pain.

✺

The tiny stingers of the nettle plant actually provide microinjections of several chemicals that are responsible for the stinging sensation that the plant causes. One M.D. told me that many of these chemicals might also trigger anti-inflammatory action that would help relieve arthritis.

And there's strong folkloric evidence that stinging nettle has some specific anti-arthritic properties. On every continent where it grows, stinging nettle has developed a reputation as a treatment for arthritis. That might be a coincidence, but I don't think so.

If you'd like to give urtication a try, you shouldn't have much problem locating a plant. It's a common weed throughout most of the country. (See the illustration on page 118.) If you're not sure how to identify it, you'll need to ask someone in the know; someone who works at a plant nursery or your local county agricultural extension agent should be able to help.

Joints in Trouble

Arthritis literally means "joint inflammation." According to the Arthritis Foundation, there are more than 100 different diseases that produce joint pain and inflammation—everything from the flu to certain cancers. But when people say "arthritis," they usually mean osteoarthritis.

Also known as degenerative joint disease, osteoarthritis is the most prevalent of more than a dozen different kinds of arthritis. Some 16 million Americans have it. The hips, knees, spine and the tiny joints of the hands and feet are most frequently affected. Osteoarthritis usually develops gradually, beginning with minor aches that eventually lead to extended pain, stiffness, swelling and limited range of motion. Symptoms sometimes subside with gentle physical activity, but not always.

Another common form of arthritis is the rheumatoid variety. Rheumatoid arthritis (RA) has a nasty reputation because it can cause crippling joint deformity. But many of the 2.1 million Americans with RA—approximately 75 percent of whom are women—have milder, noncrippling cases that flare up and subside mysteriously.

※·※

Arthritis Soup

Here's one for people who like quantitative recipes. Start by combining the main ingredients, then season them with dashes of any of the seasonings that appeal to you. You don't need all of these, and you can play with the proportions and flavors, if you like. If an ingredient doesn't appeal to you or is unavailable, simply leave it out.

3–4	quarts water
2	cups chopped cabbage
1	cup sliced string beans (1" pieces)
1	cup chopped celery
1	cup stinging nettle leaves

½   cup diced carrots
½   cup chopped asparagus
½   cup dandelion leaves
½   cup finely chopped dandelion root
¼   cup chopped spinach
¼   cup cubed eggplant
¼   cup chopped chicory
2   tablespoons minced garlic
2   tablespoons turmeric
2   tablespoons licorice
2   tablespoons evening primrose seeds
     Ground red pepper
     Ground black pepper
     White mustard
     Flaxseed
     Sarsaparilla
     Fenugreek
     Lemon juice

Place the water in a large soup pot. Add the cabbage, beans, celery, nettle, carrots, asparagus, dandelion leaves, dandelion root, spinach, eggplant, chicory, garlic, turmeric, licorice and evening primrose seeds. Season with the red pepper, black pepper, mustard, flaxseed, sarsaparilla, fenugreek and lemon juice. Bring to a boil over high heat. Reduce the heat, cover and simmer for 20 to 30 minutes, or until the vegetables are tender.

Makes 4 servings

Frequently, both hands are affected, but RA can strike other joints as well. In addition to joint pain, swelling and warmth, possible symptoms include fatigue, fever, loss of appetite, enlarged lymph nodes, lumps under the skin and muscle stiffness after sleep or inactivity. Stiffness usually subsides with moderate activity.

Green Pharmacy for Arthritis

Fortunately, along with stinging nettle, there are a number of other herbs that can help.

❧ ❧ ❧ **Ginger (*Zingiber officinale*) and turmeric (*Curcuma longa*).** In one study, Indian researchers gave three to seven grams (1½ to 3½ teaspoons) of ginger a day to 18 people with osteoarthritis and 28 with rheumatoid arthritis. More than 75 percent of those participating in the study reported at least some relief from pain and swelling. Even after more than two years of taking these high doses of ginger, none of the people reported side effects. This study is one reason that Jean Carper, author of *Food: Your Miracle Medicine*, drinks ginger tea for her osteoarthritis.

The curcumin in turmeric is a close chemical relative of some compounds found in ginger, so I'm not surprised that this herb also has a major reputation as an arthritis treatment.

You can enjoy both herbs in a wide variety of spicy dishes as well as use them to make teas.

❧ ❧ ❧ **Pineapple (*Ananas comosus*).** Some intriguing research suggests that bromelain, a chemical in pineapple, helps prevent inflammation. For some time now, athletic trainers have been recommending pineapple to athletes to prevent and treat sports injuries. I think it's also a good bet for people with arthritis. Bromelain can help the body get rid of immune antigen complex, compounds that are impli-

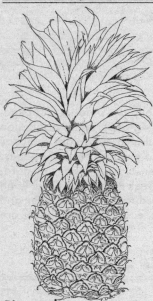

Pineapple

This tasty fruit is rich in vitamin C and immune-boosting minerals.

cated in some arthritic conditions. It also helps digest fibrin, another compound suspected of being involved in some types of arthritis. If you need an excuse to indulge yourself with fresh, ripe pineapple, this is it.

❧❧❧ **Red pepper (*Capsicum*, various species).** Red pepper causes some pain on the tongue, but ironically, it interferes with pain perception elsewhere around the body. The pain-relieving chemical in red pepper, capsaicin, triggers the body to release endorphins, nature's own opiates. Red pepper also contains aspirin-like compounds known as salicylates.

You can make a tea by mixing red pepper into water, but it would be a whole lot more pleasurable to have your red pepper cooked in a variety of spicy dishes. For a quick hit, try a splash of hot-pepper sauce in tomato juice.

Compounds in red pepper can also help relieve arthritis when you apply the herb to the skin. Researchers have discovered that you'll get significant pain relief if you apply capsaicin cream directly to painful arthritic joints four times daily. In one study of this treatment, the capsaicin cream reduced RA pain by more than half. Osteoarthritis pain was reduced by about one-third.

Capsaicin creams are generally believed safe and effective for arthritis. Look for capsaicin in the ingredient list of over-the-counter pain creams such as Zostrix or Capzasin-P or ask your doctor for a prescription capsaicin product. If you use a capsaicin cream, be sure to wash your hands thoroughly afterward: You don't want to get it in your eyes. Also, since some people are quite sensitive to this compound, you should test it on a small area of skin to make sure that it's okay for you to use before using it on a larger area. If it seems to irritate your skin, discontinue use.

❧❧❧ **Stinging nettle (*Urtica dioica*).** Beyond stinging painful joints, there's another method of using this herb to treat arthritis—steaming the fresh leaves and enjoying them as a vegetable. You'll be relieved to know that although you do have to wear gloves to harvest the leaves, the fuzzy stingers lose their sting when the leaves are cooked.

The Rheumatoid Disease Foundation suggests that three milligrams of boron, taken daily, may be helpful in treating osteoarthritis and RA. An analysis of stinging nettle provided to me by USDA scientists shows that this herb contains 47 parts per million of the mineral boron, figured on a dry-weight basis. That means that a 100-gram serving of stinging nettle, easily prepared by steaming several ounces of young, tender leaves, could easily contain more than the recommended three milligrams of boron. (You can also get a good portion of nettle in my Arthritis Soup; see page 68.)

⋘·⋙

Multi-mint Antioxidant Arthritis Tea

Rosemary and oregano are both antioxidant mints. Add several more antioxidant herbs to these two, and you get my Multi-Mint Antioxidant Tea. The mints are basil, bee balm, horehound, hyssop, lemon balm (also known as melissa), marjoram, oregano, peppermint, rosemary, sage, savory, spearmint and thyme. It makes sense to top it off with a dash of ginger and turmeric.

I checked my database to see if, in addition to their antioxidant value, any of these herbs contain proven anti-arthritic compounds. Sure enough, basil had five, while marjoram, oregano and rosemary weighed in with a few each.

How much of each herb should you use to make this tea? People always ask me that, and I never know what to say. My teas are never the same; I use a little of this and a little of that. But to satisfy people who need recipes, I'll say to use two parts of the ingredients you like and one part of those you find less appealing. Pour boiling water over the herbs and let them steep for 10 to 20 minutes before drinking.

⋘·⋙

According to the Rheumatoid Disease Foundation, boron is effective because it plays a role in helping bones retain calcium.

It also has a beneficial influence on the body's endocrine (hormonal) system, and hormones play a role in helping the body maintain healthy bones and joints.

✿✿ **Oregano (*Origanum vulgare*).** Studies are accumulating that the "pizza herb," oregano, is a powerful antioxidant. Like other antioxidants contained in fruits and vegetables, the compounds in oregano may help prevent the cell damage caused by free radicals—highly unstable oxygen molecules that steal electrons from other molecules they encounter. Free radical reactions are probably involved in inflammation, degenerative arthritis and the aging process in general. And evidence is accumulating that antioxidants may help relieve osteoarthritis and RA.

In a test of nearly 100 plants in the mint family, of which oregano is a member, the pizza herb was the one that had the greatest total antioxidant activity. Research has shown that the antioxidant activity of oregano and other medicinal mints is due in large part to rosmarinic acid, a compound with antibacterial, anti-inflammatory, antioxidant and antiviral properties. Considering how highly it ranks for this kind of protection, oregano is definitely worth adding to your pizza, or any other food, if you have arthritis. You could also try my Multi-Mint Antioxidant Arthritis Tea.

✿✿ **Willow (*Salix*, various species), garlic (*Allium sativum*) and licorice (*Glycyrrhiza glabra*).** Willow bark was the original herbal aspirin. It contains a chemical called salicin, which the Bayer Company eventually transformed into little white tablets of acetylsalicylic acid—the painkilling drug called aspirin that so many people with arthritis take daily.

Willow bark tea has pain-relieving and anti-inflammatory effects similar to those of aspirin. But because the irritation-causing ingredient in aspirin tablets is diluted in tea, you'll have less risk of stomach upset, ulcer and overdose if you take the tea instead of the pills.

Still, willow bark might upset your stomach. That's why I've included licorice in this formula. Not only does licorice have anti-inflammatory effects, it may also help treat any gastrointestinal problems caused by the willow.

But the formula is not quite complete without garlic. While long-term use or ingestion of large amounts of licorice can raise some people's blood pressure and lead to other problems (headache, lethargy, sodium and water retention, excessive loss of potassium), garlic helps reduce blood pressure. So here's the formula for a well-balanced Anti-Arthritis Tea: approximately three parts dried willow bark, two parts dried licorice root and one part minced garlic. Pour boiling water over the mixture and steep for about 15 minutes. If you don't like the taste, add lemon and/or honey, plus ginger and turmeric to taste.

❧·❦

Arthritis Broth

To make this broth, begin with a couple of cups of water and add red pepper, burdock, black pepper, celery seed, dandelion, garlic, ginger, horseradish, juniper, lemongrass, oregano, parsley, sarsaparilla, thyme, turmeric, valerian, watercress, white mustard and willow bark. Bring to a boil, then turn down the heat and simmer for a few minutes.

I confess that I have never made this broth in its entirety. I just opportunistically seize any of these ingredients that are near at hand. If you press me for a recipe, I'd say use four dashes each of burdock, dandelion, parsley, turmeric and watercress; two dashes of celery seed, garlic, ginger and oregano; and one dash each of the others, as available. This might be too spicy for your taste, but if so, you have my permission to alter the recipe to suit your own taste.

❧·❦

❧ **Brazil nut** (*Bertholettia excelsa*) **and sunflower** (*Helianthus annuus*)**.** SAM is shorthand for S-adenosyl-methionine, a chemical shown to have pain-relieving and anti-inflammatory properties similar to those found in the over-the-counter medication ibuprofen.

SAM can be found in high-methionine seeds and nuts, particularly sunflower seeds and Brazil nuts. It would take 250 grams of sunflower seeds (about 9 ounces) or 500 grams of Brazil nuts (18 ounces) to provide a dose of SAM that's more effective than a standard dose of ibuprofen. It's not feasible to eat that many nuts and seeds, but I believe that every little bit helps, especially if you use the other natural approaches this chapter recommends.

So go ahead and sprinkle some sunflower seeds on your salad. And when you're nibbling mixed nuts in company, don't apologize for monopolizing the Brazil nuts.

❧ **Broccoli (*Brassica oleracea*) and other herbs containing glutathione.** Studies indicate that people who are low in the antioxidant compound glutathione are more likely to have arthritis than those who have higher amounts.

Vegetables rich in glutathione include asparagus, cabbage, cauliflower, potatoes, tomatoes and purslane. Fruits with healthy amounts include avocados, grapefruit, oranges, peaches and watermelon.

❧ **Rosemary (*Rosmarinus officinalis*).** Rosemary was known in antiquity as the herb of remembrance. I find that quite fitting, since rosemary has antioxidants that help prevent aging in cells, and the aging process is certainly associated with memory loss. One Greek-American herb grower tells how her fishing relatives set out to sea with fish dishes heavily covered with rosemary. Even when it was unrefrigerated, this food lasted for days, thanks in part to the antioxidant activity of the rosemary.

Can an herb that keeps fish from spoiling help preserve your youth? The jury is still out on that one, but rosemary has preservative powers comparable to the commercial preservatives BHA and BHT. And since we know that antioxidants do help treat arthritis, it makes sense that this antioxidant-rich herb would help thwart this disease.

❧ **Vitamin C.** Vitamin C inhibits the progression of osteoarthritis in guinea pigs. Does it work in humans? There's no proof yet that it does, but it certainly can't hurt to get more vitamin C. Red pepper and many of the other herbs and vegetables mentioned in this chapter contain good amounts.

Asthma

M artha was one of my favorite people—a tall, pretty, free-spirited woman in her thirties who worked as a technician with me in the Medicinal Plants Research Laboratory of the U.S. Department of Agriculture (USDA). We were both involved with the joint USDA/National Cancer Institute plant-screening program, looking for plants with anti-cancer potential.

Martha loved to hike in the woods, and we occasionally hiked together. I can see her now, working happily in my ginseng patch in big, tall cowboy boots. I would never have imagined that she would become one of the thousands of Americans who die each year of asthma.

Asthma Takes Your Breath Away

Asthma is a chronic respiratory ailment that causes wheezing, coughing, chest congestion, shortness of breath and often tremendous anxiety about being unable to breathe.

More than 4,000 people die each year from complications of serious asthma attacks, a number that's increased over 30 percent since 1980. For reasons that remain unexplained, children are more likely to die in summer, while people over 65 are more likely to die in winter.

Many people consider asthma a childhood illness, and there's certainly no shortage of kids with this disease. In 1995, some 3.7 million children and adolescents had it, up sharply from 2.4 million in 1980. But asthma can develop at any age, and the fact is, most people with asthma are adults. About 14 million Americans now have asthma. The disease costs us more than $6 billion a year in medical care and lost productivity.

Doctors say that they don't know what causes asthma or why the number of people who have it keeps rising. Neither do I. But it seems that the closer we get to chemical pollution and the farther we stray from natural foods, the more asthma we see. I believe that outdoor air pollution and "sick buildings" with indoor pollution are a big part of the growing asthma. problem.

❧⋆❧

The Coltsfoot Controversy

Coltsfoot (Tussilago farfara) has been a folk favorite for asthma and coughs for centuries. Its generic name, Tussilago, comes from the Latin for "cough," and this herb does indeed contain some compounds proven effective against cough and asthma.

Coltsfoot has expectorant activity. In other words, it stimulates the microscopic hairs that move mucus out of the air passages. And like garlic and ginkgo, it suppresses the body's production of platelet-activating factor, a protein in the blood that plays a role in triggering bronchospasms, the narrowing of the air passages that causes asthma symptoms.

But in recent years, coltsfoot has become controversial. This herb contains pyrrolizidine alkaloids (PAs), chemicals that are toxic and/or carcinogenic to the liver. Many herbalists, and more botanists, wanting to err on the side of caution, recommend against taking herbs that contain PAs. The primary herbs to be concerned about are coltsfoot and comfrey.

On the other hand, data published in the journal Science by noted biochemist Bruce Ames, Ph.D., of the University of California at Berkeley, would indicate that comfrey leaf tea is less carcinogenic than an equivalent amount of beer. Officially, I'd have to say don't ingest coltsfoot or comfrey. But privately, I'll confess that I take an occasional cup of comfrey or coltsfoot tea, just as I drink an occasional beer.

❧⋆❧

The symptoms of asthma are caused by bronchial spasms (bronchospasms), a sudden narrowing of the branching tubes that lead into the lungs. While asthma and hay fever–type allergies are distinct conditions, they overlap, especially among those under age 15. Ninety percent of children with asthma also have allergies, and these allergies can trigger asthma attacks.

The reason that bronchospasms can be triggered by allergies is that histamine, the chemical most responsible for allergy symptoms, seems to play a role in asthma attacks as well. But many other things besides histamine can trigger an attack: strenuous exercise, cigarette smoke, respiratory infections, industrial chemicals, aspirin, pet dander, indoor pollution and the sulfites added to many foods.

Stress also plays a role in asthma. Severe anxiety can trigger attacks, and stress generally aggravates asthma symptoms.

Green Pharmacy for Asthma

Doctors treat asthma with a variety of drugs—among them, theophylline (Aerolate, Theo-Dur)—that open up the bronchial tubes. These drugs, known as bronchodilators, are often taken with an inhaler.

If I had asthma, I'd certainly follow a physician's recommendations. This is a potentially fatal illness. But for my treatment, if my doctor suggested theophylline, I'd prefer to get it from its many natural sources, chief among them the plants containing caffeine.

✖✖✖ **Coffee, tea, caffeinated cola drinks, cocoa and chocolate.** All of these popular beverages, as well as chocolate candy, are derived from plants and count as herbal products. And all contain caffeine as well as other compounds that may help fend off asthma.

Joe Graedon, the pharmacist and syndicated newspaper columnist, once wrote in his column that in a pinch, if caught without their medication, people with asthma could drink a few cups of coffee, which is a potent bronchodilator. Some months later he received a thank-you note from a newlywed woman with asthma who forgot her medication on her Hawaiian honeymoon. At one point she started wheezing, realized she'd forgotten her drugs and became panicky, which made her wheezing worse. Then she remembered the column advocating coffee as a workable substitute. She quickly drank three cups.

Her wheezing subsided, saving her honeymoon and possibly her life.

Actually, coffee, tea, caffeinated cola drinks, cocoa and chocolate have more than caffeine. All reportedly contain two other major natural anti-asthmatic compounds, theobromine and theophylline, which, along with caffeine, belong to a family of chemicals called xanthines. These chemicals help stop bronchospasms and open constricted bronchial passages.

Levels of these anti-asthmatic compounds vary, depending on the strength of the brew and other factors. But in general, a cup of coffee has the highest levels (about 100 milligrams of caffeine per cup), while a cup of tea or cocoa or a 12-ounce can of cola has about half that amount. A 1½-ounce chocolate bar has a little less than a can of cola.

Of course, caffeine and the other anti-asthmatic xanthines are not entirely risk-free. As any java junkie knows, caffeine can cause insomnia and the jitters. But in their natural state, the anti-asthmatic compounds actually cause fewer side effects than pharmaceutical theophylline.

In one survey, 81 percent of pediatricians said that parents had expressed concerns about the side effects of their children's asthma medication, particularly the restlessness and difficulty concentrating that many children experience. At high doses, pharmaceutical asthma medications may also cause headache, insomnia, irritability, nausea, poor appetite, stomachache and even seizures.

At this point, though, I'd like to make myself crystal clear: If I were plagued by life-threatening asthma, I'd listen to my physician and take pharmaceuticals, and I'd use natural approaches only as supplemental treatments.

✿ ✿ ✿ **Ephedra (*Ephedra sinica*).** Many medical botanists say that ephedra is one of the world's oldest medicines. The Chinese, who call it *ma huang*, have used this herb for thousands of years to treat asthma and other respiratory ailments.

Scientists isolated its active chemical constituents, ephedrine and pseudoephedrine, in 1887. It wasn't until after World War I, however, that American doctors started prescribing these substances. At that time, doctors became aware of the chemicals' effects as bronchodilators, nasal decongestants and central nervous system stimulants. Pseudoephedrine has since become a common over-the-counter decongestant. The chemical inspired the brand name Sudafed.

Whole ephedra—as well as its chemical components ephedrine and pseudoephedrine—has side effects such as insomnia, anxiety, restlessness and possibly aggravation of high blood pressure. So you have to be careful with this herb. In fact, if you take really high doses, very strange things can happen. The medical literature contains 20 case reports of ephedrine psychosis, and the Food and Drug Administration has taken steps to curb the distribution and sale of ephedrine supplements.

Still, if you are careful, this herb is very useful in managing asthma. You might consider making a tea with the dried herb instead of taking the over-the-counter drugs that contain the active compounds. To make a tea, use a level teaspoon of ephedra or a half-teaspoon to one teaspoon of tincture from a health food store or pharmacy.

Because of ephedra's stimulant effect, some ephedra/ma huang products are sold as "energy formulas." In fact, over the last few years, several people have died as a result of abusing this herb. Because it does have stimulant properties, I would advise against using ephedra to treat asthma in children unless you first discuss it with the child's pediatrician.

🌿🌿🌿 **Stinging nettle (*Urtica dioica*).** Four hundred years ago, the British herbalist Nicholas Culpeper claimed that nettle roots or leaves, used in juice or tea, were "safe and sure medicines to open the pipes and passages of the lungs."

For many years, Australians have viewed nettle as a good treatment for asthma. Aussies drink the juice of the roots and leaves mixed with honey or sugar, and they firmly believe that it relieves bronchial troubles. But Americans didn't catch on until a little more than five years ago, when a scientific study was published showing that nettle is a potent antihistamine. Now nettle is increasingly recommended for hay fever and asthma. Friends with allergies and asthma visit my garden regularly to dig up my nettle patch. (You'll need to wear gloves when harvesting stinging nettle leaves, but the stinging hairs lose their sting when the leaves are cooked.)

🌿🌿 **Anise (*Pimpinella anisum*) and fennel (*Foeniculum vulgare*).** The Greeks use teas made from these herbs for asthma and other respiratory ailments. They both contain helpful chemicals—creosol and alpha-pinene—that help loosen bronchial secretions. Fennel seeds (actually fruits) can contain as much as 8,800 parts per million (ppm) of alpha-pinene. Ironically, despite its traditional use for respiratory problems, anise is no superstar. It has only 360 ppm of alpha-pinene.

Many other plants are good sources and could be expected to provide asthma relief. In descending order, they are parsley seed, coriander, juniper berries, sweet Annie, cardamom, sassafras, horsebalm, ginger, Chinese angelica (also known as *dang-quai*), dill, tarragon and yarrow. You could mix up a pretty good Asthma Tea with any or several of these, especially if you added a little licorice.

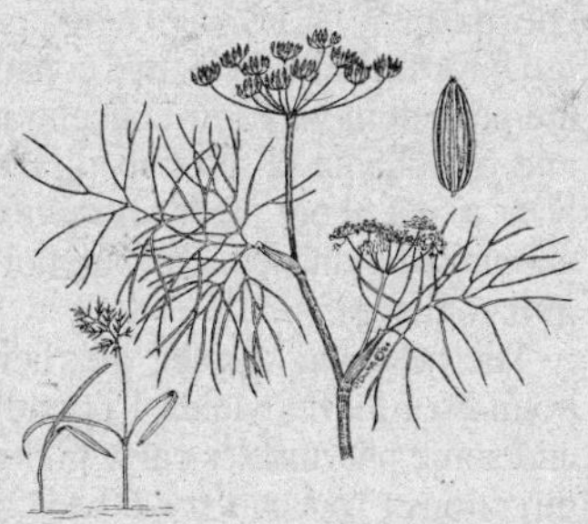

Fennel

Also known as finocchio, this herb is in the same plant family as carrots and parsley.

❦❦ **Licorice (*Glycyrrhiza glabra*).** Licorice tea soothes the throat and is often recommended for sore throat, cough and asthma. Licorice and its extracts are safe for normal use in moderate amounts—up to about three cups a day. However, long-term use or ingestion of excessive amounts can produce headache, lethargy, sodium and water retention, excessive loss of potassium and high blood pressure.

If you decide to use licorice steadily to manage asthma, opt for deglycyrrhizinated licorice extracts (DGLE), which cause fewer problems. There are many over-the-counter preparations of DGLE, especially overseas. You can find them in America, however. I use licorice (modestly), especially during severe episodes of stress, by using a piece of dried root to stir my herb teas.

❦ **Ginkgo (*Ginkgo biloba*).** Asian healers have used extracts of ginkgo leaves for thousands of years to treat asthma, allergies, bronchitis and coughs. Ginkgo has become popular in the West because of its benefits for the elderly: increased blood flow to the brain and treatment of stroke and other infirmities of old age. But in China, it's still widely used for asthma.

Ginkgo works because it interferes with platelet-activating

factor, a protein in the blood that plays a role in triggering bronchospasms.

Unfortunately, the active constituents in ginkgo ginkgolides—are present in very low concentrations in the tree's leaves. To get one reasonable dose of medicine, a person with asthma would have to eat about 50 fresh leaves. I eat a lot of plants that most people wouldn't touch, but not even I would eat that many ginkgo leaves.

The best way to take this herb is to buy a 50:1 extract (50 pounds of leaves yields 1 pound of extract). Health food stores and some pharmacies carry ginkgo extracts. Follow the package directions. You can try 60 to 240 milligrams of standardized extract a day, but don't go any higher than that. In large amounts, ginkgo may cause diarrhea, irritability and restlessness.

❧ **Tomato (*Lycopersicon lycopersicum*), citrus fruits and other foods containing vitamin C.** A review of some 40 good studies revealed that vitamin C—about 1,000 milligrams a day—helps prevent asthma attacks, bronchospasms, wheezing, respiratory infections, nasal congestion, watery eyes and other allergy symptoms. Why? Vitamin C inhibits the release of histamine.

I advise eating more plants that are high in vitamin C—not just citrus fruits and tomatoes but also bell peppers and strawberries. You can also take a supplement. The beauty of eating citrus fruits, however, is that in addition to vitamin C, they also contain flavonoids. These are substances that also block the release of histamine, in turn curbing allergy symptoms and allergy-related asthma.

❧ **Assorted herbs.** I searched my database for anti-asthmatic compounds and came up with quite a few herbs worth mentioning. I found at least six anti-asthmatic substances in tea, fennel and cayenne. Onion, coriander and bell pepper had five. And a large group contained four: cabbage, cacao, carrot, cranberry, currant, eggplant, grapefruit, orange, oregano, sage and tomato.

Looking for herbs with the largest amounts of anti-asthma compounds, I found that licorice and tea were the big winners. Cacao, cardamom, coffee, cola, onion and purslane looked relatively rich.

You could whip up some interesting anti-asthma dishes with these herbs. How about orange-grapefruit-cranberry fruit salad with fennel? Or eggplant with onion, tomato and sage?

Finally, Japanese wasabi is worth a try. The Japanese enjoy wasabi just as Americans and Europeans enjoy horseradish. It certainly clears the sinuses. There's some research suggesting that a spoonful a day can relieve allergies, especially hay fever. This tells me that it should be good for managing asthma as well.

If I had asthma, I'd try wasabi. You can buy it at any grocery store that carries a specialty line of Oriental products. You can use it just as you would horseradish. Try spreading it on crackers or mixing it in a dip, or have it with sushi, as the Japanese do.

You should be aware, however, that wasabi is *extremely* hot. If you don't enjoy hot foods, don't even consider using this as an asthma treatment.

❧ **Vitamin B_6.** Melvyn Werbach, M.D., assistant clinical professor of psychiatry at the University of California, Los Angeles, School of Medicine and author of several books on alternative medicine, cites cases of children with asthma who reduced their dosages of anti-asthma medications—bronchodilators and steroids—by taking a daily dose of 200 milligrams of vitamin B_6 in addition to their medication. Adults have experienced decreased frequency and intensity of asthma attacks by taking 50 milligrams of vitamin B_6 twice daily.

The Daily Value for B_6 is only 2 milligrams, and unusually large doses may damage the nervous system. If I had asthma, I'd probably try B_6, but if you want to take B_6 supplements or give them to your child, discuss it with your doctor.

Athlete's Foot

You might not think going barefoot is a healing remedy, but it is. To prevent and treat athlete's foot, doctors often recommend keeping the feet dry by going sockless and wearing open-toed shoes. I have an even better approach: I suggest a barefoot weekend at a salt-water beach.

I personally practice this particular form of therapy as often as possible. In fact, strange as this may sound, I even go barefoot in the jungles of Amazonian Peru. And I manage to stay free of the fungal skin infection known as athlete's foot.

Athlete's foot, medically known as tinea pedis, is a superficial fungal infection. The fungi (any of several species) can infect not only the feet but also other parts of the body in the form of tinea corporis, commonly called ringworm. And when the fungus gets to the groin or thigh, it's called tinea cruris, or jock itch (which women can get even though they don't wear jocks).

Athlete's foot fungus needs moisture and darkness to grow. That's why both conventional doctors and alternative practitioners recommend keeping the feet dry. And of course, your feet are drier if you go around barefoot rather than keeping your toes all trapped and humid in dark, closed shoes.

Green Pharmacy for Athlete's Foot

If my main form of prevention—going barefoot—ever stops working for me and I experience burning, itching and cracking skin between my toes, I'm ready: My Herbal Vineyard in Maryland is loaded with powerful antifungal herbs. Here are the ones I recommend for athlete's foot.

❧❧❧ **Garlic (*Allium sativum*).** This is my first-choice treatment. It's one of the most widely recommended antifungal antiseptics, and for good reason. Many scientifically rigorous studies show that it's effective in treating athlete's foot and other fungal infections, notably vaginal yeast infections.

A garlic footbath might be malodorous, but it usually relieves itching and burning between the toes. I suggest putting several crushed garlic cloves in a basin with warm water and a little rubbing alcohol.

If this approach doesn't appeal to you, consider the traditional Chinese approach: Crush several cloves of garlic and steep them in olive oil for one to three days. Strain out the plant material and use a cotton ball or clean cloth to apply the garlic oil between your toes once or twice a day.

Some herbalists I respect even suggest taping a sliver of garlic onto bad patches of athlete's foot. This might work better than many of the commercial treatments, but I see a problem here, as walking around with garlic between your toes could raise some eyebrows—and alert some nostrils. You could always try this approach just for the duration of the afternoon ball game on TV, provided you're not expecting any company.

One note of caution: If you try this whole-garlic approach and it seems to irritate your skin, discontinue use and switch back to using either a garlic footbath or garlic oil.

❦❦❦ **Ginger (*Zingiber officinale*).** According to my database, ginger ranks second among all herbs in the number of antifungal compounds with a total of 23. One compound—caprylic acid—is so potent that a chemist I know suggests taking three capsules a day for all manner of fungal infections. Of course, unless you're a chemist, you probably can't get pure caprylic acid, which is why I recommend using ginger instead. I'm still skeptical of isolated plant chemicals (phytochemicals) taken out of their evolutionary context.

You can prepare a strong decoction by adding an ounce of chopped ginger root to a cup of boiling water. Simmer for 20 minutes and apply it directly to the problem areas twice a day with a cotton ball or clean cloth.

❦❦❦ **Licorice (*Glycyrrhiza glabra*).** Garlic may be my numero uno treatment for athlete's foot, but ironically, in my database, it is nowhere near the top of the list of herbs containing the largest number of antifungal compounds. That distinction belongs to licorice, which has 25 reportedly fungicidal compounds. (Garlic has only 10, but they are quite potent.)

Licorice's clear antifungal action lends credence to the Chinese practice of using it to treat ringworm. I'd add some chopped licorice sticks to the garlic footbath mentioned above.

You could also simply brew a strong decoction using about five to seven teaspoons of dried herb per cup of water. Bring it to a boil, simmer for 20 minutes, then let it cool. Apply the decoction directly to the affected areas using a cotton ball or clean cloth.

❦❦❦ **Teatree (*Melaleuca*, various species).** Teatree oil is a powerful antiseptic that's very useful against athlete's foot. Dilute the oil with an equal amount of water or vegetable oil and apply it directly to the affected area three times a day using a cotton ball or clean cloth. Just don't ingest it. Like so many other essential plant oils, small amounts of teatree oil, on the order of a few teaspoons, can be fatal.

❦❦ **Camomile (*Matricaria recutita*).** Camomile oil is also fungicidal. In Europe it's incorporated into many over-the-counter antiseptics. I would suggest using camomile oil in the same way as teatree oil. Or you can mix the two.

If you have hay fever, however, you should use camomile

products cautiously. Camomile is a member of the ragweed family, and in some people, it might trigger allergic reactions. The first time you try it, watch your reaction. If it seems to help, go ahead and use it. But if it seems to cause or aggravate itching or irritation, discontinue use.

✿✿ Echinacea (*Echinacea*, various species). The immune-stimulating action of this herb is particularly beneficial for treating yeast infections, but I'd also recommend it for athlete's foot. To boost your immune system, you could buy a tincture at a health food store and add the recommended amount to juice three times a day to enhance the effectiveness of the other herbal approaches to athlete's foot. (Although echinacea can cause your tongue to tingle or go numb temporarily, this effect is harmless.)

✿✿ Goldenseal (*Hydrastis canadensis*). This herb contains berberine, a powerful antifungal and antibacterial compound, which makes it an excellent antibiotic. But it's not the only source of berberine. Barberry, goldthread, Oregon grape and yellowroot all contain it, and all have been used traditionally to treat yeast and other fungal infections.

You might buy a goldenseal tincture and follow the package directions. Usually, the guidelines suggest adding it to juice three times a day. If you want to use it externally, you can make a strong decoction with the dried herb. Add five to seven teaspoons to a cup of water, bring it to a boil and let it simmer for 20 minutes. After the liquid cools to a tolerable temperature, use a cotton ball or clean cloth to apply it to the affected area. You'll probably want to repeat the application up to three times a day.

✿✿ Lemongrass (*Cymbopogon*, various species). Scientists have demonstrated significant fungicidal activity for lemongrass oil against several common infection-causing fungi.

Enjoy drinking lemongrass tea one to four times a day. And for additional antifungal benefit, use the spent tea bags as compresses directly on the affected area.

✿ Arrowroot (*Maranta arundinacea*) and other herb powders. Since moisture and darkness help the growth of foot fungus, you're more likely to prevent it if you put some drying powder inside your socks and even your shoes. You can get a number of powders made from the dried leaves, stems or roots of herbs, including arrowroot, comfrey and goldenseal.

❧ **Cinnamon (*Cinnamomum*, various species) and other fungicidal herb teas.** While you're applying herbal oils and teas externally, there are also a number of beverage teas made with herbs that have fungicidal properties that could prove helpful. I went into my database and asked it to print a list of all the plants containing more than ten fungicidal chemicals. It didn't take the computer long to come up with 38 species, including cinnamon, fennel, peppermint, dill, tarragon, basil, tea, orange, black currant, sage, thyme, red clover, lemon and spearmint. Just brew them up in any combination that appeals to you for a little antifungal boost to whatever other treatment you happen to be using.

❧ **Turmeric (*Curcuma longa*).** Pakistani studies show that oil of turmeric inhibits many common problem fungi, even at very low concentrations. I'd go with commercial oil of turmeric, diluting it with water (one part oil to two parts water) and apply it directly to the affected area using a cotton ball or clean cloth.

❧ **Tomato-and-herb sauce.** Here's another way to take advantage of some other herbs that have fungicidal properties. Make a tomato sauce and go very heavy on the basil, celery, carrot, dill, fennel, sage and thyme. In one quick meal, you'll get a dish with dozens of fungicides: Just heat it up and pour over pasta. (I almost hesitate to say this, but if you're willing to put up with the mess, you could also spread a bit of this sauce between your toes for a couple of hours. It sounds like that tomato festival in Spain, where everybody gets splattered with tomatoes.)

Backache

Both my wife and I share a propensity for back problems. Peggy is a good example of how back problems often run in families. She and her two sisters (like their late mother) all have a peculiar kink in the same area of their backs that causes them grief, especially following extended kitchen work at sink height.

As for me, Scrooge that I am, I blame my most serious back problem on Christmas. It was December 23, 1991, when

Peggy and I went to a nearby Christmas tree farm to select a living tree. Wanting to replant the tree, I dug a big ball of earth with it and managed to heave it into the wheelbarrow the owner had lent me. I successfully wheeled that 100-pound load 100 yards up the hill to my station wagon, but when I attempted to lift it from the wheelbarrow to the wagon's trunk, something snapped.

❧

Moving toward a Cure

One of the worst things you can do for an aching back is to stop exercising, according to Leon Root, M.D., orthopedic surgeon and author of *Oh, My Aching Back*. In fact, exercise experts claim that 80 to 90 percent of back problems are caused by weak muscles. Doctors have also come around to this view and now recommend exercise instead of rest.

I can attest to the effectiveness of this approach. I do back exercises religiously every morning before my shower and also before and after activities that I know can trigger back pain—cutting my lawn (more than an acre), standing in long lines or at cocktail parties, and moving heavy objects. I swim when the opportunity arises, ride a stationary bike and walk a mile or two a day.

The YMCA has developed a popular nationwide back exercise program that combines strength training, flexibility exercises and relaxation. About 80 percent of enrollees report improvement, and 31 percent become pain-free. You might want to contact your local Y and ask about this program. Think about it: About one-third of bad backs can be cured with no medicine at all.

❧

Agony ensued. It grew worse as we drove home. Santa's
back was ruined. I could not lie, sit or stand comfortably. I
slept terribly, sideways on a couch with three pillows under my
left side. The only help we could find the following day,
Christmas Eve, was a chiropractor. He took a $95 x-ray,
declined to do major manipulations and said that I should see
an orthopedist.

A week later, the orthopedist said I should consult a neurosurgeon. Not surprisingly, he said I needed surgery. He insisted
this was my only option, given my x-rays. So ultimately (two
months later), I had surgery followed by physical therapy. I also
used healing herbs and had acupuncture treatments. I think the
alternative treatments gave me more relief than the physicians.

Backaches Abound

It seems that everywhere I look, people have back problems.
That's not surprising, because aching backs are one of America's most prevalent health problems. Estimates vary, but the
experts generally agree that somewhere between two and five
million Americans suffer serious back pain each year.

At some point in life, about four out of five Americans experience back pain severe enough to require medical interven-
tion—anything from taking aspirin to major surgery. And at any
given moment, something like one-quarter of the country is
dealing with previous back trouble by taking medication, doing
exercises or making other lifestyle adjustments to convalesce
and keep from reinjuring their backs.

Bad backs also cost the country a fortune—$16 billion a year
in medical treatment and $80 billion in lost wages and produc-
tivity.

Be Wary of Surgery

Doctors used to treat back pain with rest, long-term medication and surgery. Now they will generally recommend short-
term medication, exercise and, increasingly, chiropractic, yoga
or some other formerly scorned alternative therapy.

I'm glad surgery has fallen out of favor. My own back
surgery was useless. I did not seek a second opinion, even

though friends advised me to. Why? Because I'm a lazy cheap-skate who goes with the flow of an HMO, and I wanted so desperately to put my back pain behind me.

I'll go to my grave not knowing whether the surgery did me any good. I have since learned that cervical fusion—the operation I endured—is another of those overperformed operations. I found out that bad x-rays don't always mean bad backs and that good x-rays don't always mean good backs. I learned that 80 percent of people in the kind of distress I had recover in four months *without* surgery.

But unrelenting pain makes people desperate. We Americans undergo a lot less back surgery than we used to, but there are still about 20 times more back operations per capita in the United States than in Canada and Europe. So here's my advice: If a doctor says you need back surgery, get several other opinions before going under the knife. I should have, but now that's water over the dam.

In the meantime, what can you do about the pain? Immediately after a back injury or a flare-up of back pain, doctors recommend pain-relieving and anti-inflammatory medications such as aspirin and other nonsteroidal anti-inflammatory drugs. For really bad pain, stronger medications might be necessary, including codeine or other narcotics. If you're in serious pain, I'd suggest taking whatever the doctor orders. Recently, physicians are more inclined to give slow-release morphine, which actually comes from an herbal source—the opium poppy.

Green Pharmacy for Backache

For lesser pain or lingering pain, there are a number of herbal alternatives that can prove helpful.

🌶️🌶️🌶️ **Red pepper (*Capsicum*, various species).** Red pepper contains a marvelous pain-relieving chemical—capsaicin—that is so potent that a tiny amount provides the active ingredient in some powerful pharmaceutical topical analgesics. One product, Zostrix, contains only 0.025 percent capsaicin.

At this point, I don't know (or care) whether red pepper's effectiveness is due to capsaicin's ability to interfere with pain perception, to its ability to trigger release of the body's own pain-relieving endorphins, to its salicylates, or to all three. All I know is that it works.

You can buy a commercial cream containing capsaicin and use that. Outside the United States, however, people simply use red pepper. You can, too, at considerable savings. A hot pepper costs a few cents, while capsaicin drugs cost a few dollars.

You can mash a red pepper and rub it directly on the painful area. You can also take any white skin cream that you have on hand—cold cream will do—and mix in enough red pepper to turn it pink.

Whether you use a cream or a hot pepper, be sure to wash your hands thoroughly afterward: You don't want to get it in your eyes. Also, since some people are quite sensitive to this compound, you should test it on a small area of skin to make sure that it's okay for you to use before using it on a larger area. If it seems to irritate your skin, discontinue use.

☙☙☙ **Willow (*Salix*, various species) and other forms of natural aspirin.** I have no problem with taking aspirin, since it was originally derived from an herbal source. It originally came from compounds known as salicylates that occur naturally in willow bark, meadowsweet and wintergreen. Any of these herbs can be made into pain-relieving teas.

Many salicylate-rich plants also contain methyl-salicylate, an aspirin-like compound with a particularly pleasing smell. One is wintergreen. Another is birch bark, once used by American Indians to make a tea that they drank or applied externally to treat lower back pain. On occasion I have made such teas by throwing roughly a handful of birch bark or wintergreen into a cup or two of boiling water and letting it steep for about ten minutes. (Remember, though, that if you're allergic to aspirin, you probably shouldn't use aspirin-like herbs, either.)

Oil of wintergreen, which is high in methyl-salicylate, also serves as a good pain

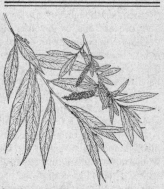

White Willow

The salicin in willow is "herbal aspirin" and has been used to relieve pain since 500 B.C.

reliever for external use. It may be applied during massage. (Please make sure you keep oil of wintergreen out of children's reach. It has a tempting aroma, but ingesting even a little can prove fatal.)

·· **Peppermint (*Mentha piperita*) and other mints.** You will find the compounds menthol and camphor in many over-the-counter backache medications. They are chemicals that can help ease the muscle tightness that contributes to many bad backs. Menthol is a natural constituent of plants in the mint family, particularly peppermint and spearmint, although the aromatic oils of all the other mints contain it as well. Camphor occurs in spike lavender, hyssop and coriander.

· **Assorted essential oils.** Treatment with essential oils can often help relieve the painful muscle spasms that contribute to back pain. Several of these—sage, rosemary, thyme, horsebalm and mountain dittany—are rich in thymol and carvacrol, compounds that help muscles relax.

To use any of these oils, add a few drops to a couple of table-spoons of any vegetable oil and massage the oil mixture directly into the affected area. You might also add a few drops of the oil to a hot bath and soak for a while, inhaling the steamy vapors. (Remember, though, never to ingest an essential oil, as small quantities of some oils, on the order of a single teaspoon, can be fatal.)

Other compounds with potent muscle-relaxing action that can relieve back spasms are borneol and bornyl-acetate. Plants rich in these chemicals include cardamom, sage and rosemary. My database tells me that borneol is an effective antispasmodic compound at a very dilute concentration, making it even more potent than menthol, camphor, thymol and carvacrol.

There are also a few other oils that you should know about. Aromatherapists often suggest using the oils of birch, lavender, black pepper, clary, ginger and marjoram to alleviate backache. I would not hesitate to use any of these, as all have a folkloric history for relieving cramps or backaches, and all contain pain-relieving and muscle-relaxing compounds.

Why use the plant oil if you can obtain chemically isolated menthol or some other muscle-relaxing chemical? Because, in my opinion, the whole aromatic herb oil is likely to work better. These oils evolved to protect the plants from pests and other environmental stresses. The fact that aromatic herb oils evolved into a chemically complex mixture suggests that all the chemicals in them work together.

Bad Breath

Herbalist Tom Wolfe, owner of the Smile Herb Shop in College Park, Maryland, and a friend of mine for more than two decades, is a student of Persian literature and an admirer of Persian culture. He once told me about a high-class Persian dinner he attended in the Washington, D.C., area, in part for the food and in part to brush up his Farsi language skills.

On a large round board in the center of the table stood four large bowls filled with fresh coriander, parsley, spearmint and tarragon; the guests rolled the herbs in pita bread and munched them between courses to cleanse the palate. Not coincidentally, all of these herbs also have a long history of use as breath fresheners. In fact, the ancient custom of ending a meal with a sprig of stomach-soothing, breath-freshening mint evolved into our use of after-dinner mints.

By the time the meal was over, Wolfe told me, nearly a pound of fresh herbs had been consumed in these Persian Phytochemical Pita Sandwiches. Which brings me to my first herbal tip in this chapter—for a quick breath cleanup at a restaurant, save the decorative parsley sprig and eat it last.

Bad Breath Basics

I've always said that bad breath is better than no breath at all. But when it comes to halitosis, I'm a hypochondriac. I'm by no means alone. Convene a convention of everyone who's certain their breath is always sweet-smelling, and you'd have an empty auditorium. It's no wonder that Americans spend more than $200 million a year on breath-freshening products.

Most bad breath is caused by bacteria in the mouth. Bacteria produce wastes that smell, well, bad. During the day, oxygen-rich saliva acts as a natural mouthwash, keeping oral bacteria largely at bay. But at night, salivation slows, and the chemical environment of the mouth shifts from mildly acidic to mildly alkaline, which encourages the growth of odor-causing bacteria. By morning, you have what those commercials call "morning mouth." An herbal mouthwash can help as much as, or more than, any of the store-bought products. The recipe appears on the opposite page.

In at least one-third of people with halitosis, the cause is gum (periodontal) disease. Bacteria worm their way down into the gums below the tooth line, where not even the fanciest toothbrush can reach. As they grow, they destroy gum tissue. If not treated, this gum damage eventually causes tooth loss. At the same time, the bacteria release the wastes that cause bad breath.

Flossing can help control gum disease. So can a mouthwash containing the right herbs. But chronic halitosis may also be a sign of several other conditions, according to Israel Kleinberg, M.D., chairman of the Department of Oral Biology and Pathology at the State University of New York at Stony Brook. Some are quite serious: cirrhosis of the liver, diabetes, kidney failure and cancer in the upper respiratory tract, among others. If your bad breath just won't quit, it's a good idea to discuss it with your doctor.

Green Pharmacy for Bad Breath

Most bad breath is just a passing inconvenience, and there are a number of herbs that can help erase it.

🌸🌸🌸 **Cardamom (*Elettaria cardamomum*).** In my database, cardamom is the richest source of the compound cineole, a potent antiseptic that also kills bad breath bacteria. And it may have more than just a breath-freshening benefit if you use it during a romantic date. Arab cultures consider it an aphrodisiac. If you're not partial to my Halitosisade, try chewing cardamom fruits (seeds). I chew them for a while and then spit them out. I also add them to herbal teas and liqueurs.

🌸🌸🌸 **Eucalyptus (*Eucalyptus globulus*).** Many commercial mouthwashes contain alcohol, which helps kill odor-causing bacteria, and eucalyptol, a compound that is derived from eucalyptus oil and is rich in cineole.

Instead of buying expensive mouthwashes, you can simply mix up some of my own unique Halitosisade using crushed eucalyptus leaves. No access to eucalyptus? No problem.

Many other herbs are also rich in cineole. While none of them except cardamom come close to eucalyptus's cineole content, any of these herbs would help freshen the breath:

spearmint, rosemary, sweet Annie, ginger, nutmeg, lavender, bee balm, peppermint, tansy, yarrow, cinnamon, basil, turmeric, lemon leaf, hyssop, tarragon, lemon verbena or fennel.

❧❧

Halitosisade

To make Halitosisade, my breath-freshening herbal alternative to commercial mouthwashes, steep any combination of the herbs in this chapter in vodka. You can put up to several ounces of herbs per pint of vodka in a wide-mouthed jar with a screw-on lid.

Personally, I favor eucalyptus, rosemary and spearmint, plus whatever else I have on hand. I don't usually use cardamom because it's so expensive. It does have a nice flavor, however.

For personal use, I just leave the herbs in the vodka and let it steep indefinitely. When making mouthwash for someone else, I might be elegant enough to strain out the herbs after several days so it looks nice and clear. The choice is yours, but I kind of like the look of all those herbs floating in my bottle of mouthwash.

❧❧

❧❧❧ **Parsley (*Petroselinum crispum*) and other plants rich in chlorophyll.** My cousin Suzie, who has high blood pressure, called recently to ask what I might recommend. I advised her to take garlic to lower her blood pressure, plus parsley to minimize the halitosis caused by the garlic. Bright green parsley is a rich source of the green plant pigment, chlorophyll, which is a powerful breath freshener. Munch some parsley after meals, after drinking coffee or after eating or drinking anything that might cause malodorous breath.

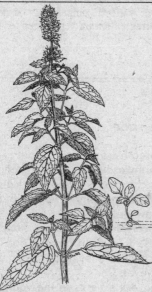

Peppermint

This mint has long been grown commercially to flavor everything from candies and liqueurs to toothpastes.

In fact, it's a good idea to refrigerate fresh sprigs of parsley and other plants rich in chlorophyll, notably basil and cilantro, and nibble as needed.

❧❧ **Anise** (*Pimpinella anisum*). The seeds of this licorice-flavored herb have been used for thousands of years to freshen the breath. I'm not surprised, because it works. Boil a few teaspoons of seeds in a cup of water for a few minutes. Strain, then drink or use as a mouthwash.

❧❧ **Coriander** (*Coriandrum sativum*). Coriander is a Cantonese folk remedy for bad breath. To use this herb, add a few ounces of fresh coriander (also known as cilantro), to two cups of water and boil for a few minutes. Strain, then drink or use as a mouthwash.

❧❧ **Dill** (*Anethum graveolens*). Like parsley, dill is rich in chlorophyll. Try dill tea after meals; use one to two teaspoons of leaves or mashed seeds per cup of boiling water. Or simply chew on a few dill seeds to freshen your breath. (If you are pregnant, using dill in medicinal amounts could cause problems. You should reserve it for occasional, moderate use.)

❧❧ **Peppermint** (*Mentha piperita*). Peppermint tea is highly recommended for halitosis, with good reason. Aromatic peppermint oil is a potent antiseptic, but it is toxic and should never be ingested.

❧❧ **Sage** (*Salvia officinalis*). An herbalist I respect recommends gargling several times a day with warm sage tea for mouth sores and bad breath. Sage has breath-freshening properties similar to parsley and peppermint, so I agree with him.

❧❧ Wild bergamot (*Monarda fistulosa*). If you like thyme, you'll like wild bergamot, either by itself or mixed into other herb teas. It contains some of the same antiseptic compounds used in commercial breath fresheners. Use two teaspoons per cup of boiling water and steep for ten minutes.

❧ Clove (*Syzygium aromaticum*). Before the people in some ancient Asian cultures were permitted to see their king, they had to chew cloves to freshen their breath. This herb's powerfully aromatic oil is antibacterial. Add several tablespoons to about a pint of vodka and steep for a few days to make a pleasant-tasting mouthwash. Or brew a tea using a teaspoon or two of dried herb.

Baldness

A nother phone call, another desperate voice, this one from far-off California. I'm always getting calls for help from people who are looking for herbal advice on how to deal with their health problems. Even though I never discovered how this man found me, I still remember how upset he was about losing his hair.

We talked, and I wound up faxing him information about saw palmetto. This herb works by preventing the conversion of the male sex hormone testosterone into dihydrotestosterone (DHT), a substance that plays a role in prostate enlargement. DHT is also the hormone that may kill off hair follicles and can lead to male-pattern baldness. I suggested to my caller that saw palmetto might help slow his hair loss.

Hair loss is genetically influenced but hard to predict. Sometimes all the men in a family go bald, and sometimes only a few do. But more than half of American men suffer significant hair loss by age 45. Many women also suffer hair loss, but it's almost always much less severe.

Green Pharmacy for Baldness

While I can't promise that my herbal approaches will cover your dome with a thick mat of hair, these natural alternatives might be worth a try.

❦❦❦ **Saw palmetto (*Serenoa repens*).** This remains my top choice, although you might want to use a combination of approaches that includes an anti-baldness medication such as minoxidil (Rogaine) or finasteride (Proscar). Biochemistry supports saw palmetto. We know that DHT kills off the hair follicles, and this herb blocks the formation of DHT. If it turns out that saw palmetto helps prevent hair loss, it would be *the* herb for men, since studies have shown that it also helps prevent prostate enlargement.

❦❦ **Licorice (*Glycyrrhiza glabra*).** Licorice contains one compound that prevents the conversion of testosterone to DHT. You could prepare a baldness-prevention shampoo by adding licorice to your favorite shampoo when you shower.

❦❦ **Rosemary (*Rosmarinus officinalis*).** For centuries, if not millennia, both men and women have massaged their scalps with rosemary in olive oil to keep their hair lush and healthy. Is there anything to really recommend this practice, besides wishful thinking? Massaging the scalp certainly stimulates circulation and encourages hair growth, according to Wilma F. Bergfeld, M.D., of the Cleveland Clinic Foundation in Ohio. Naturopaths often suggest nightly scalp massage with one part rosemary oil and two parts almond oil.

❦ **Danshen (*Salvia miltiorrhiza*) and sage (*Salvia officinalis*).** Danshen is actually Asian red sage. In folklore, both danshen and native sage have long-standing reputations as hair preservers.

In this country, people frequently used sage extracts in hair rinses and shampoos. The herb allegedly had the ability to prevent hair loss and maintain hair color. This folk use of herbs is unlikely to cause any harm, so I suggest that you try adding a few teaspoons of sage tincture to your favorite shampoo.

❦ **Horsetail (*Equisetum*, various species).** The minerals selenium and silicon both help promote circulation to the scalp, and as a result, they help maintain hair, according to naturopathic physicians. Both minerals abound in horsetail. I'd try adding a teaspoon or so of dried horsetail to herbal teas, but you should check with a holistic practitioner before using this herb.

❦ **Safflower (*Carthamus tinctorius*).** In Chinese herbal medicine, safflower is considered a vasodilator, a substance that causes blood vessels to open up. Apparently, it also helps open the blood vessels in the scalp, and Chinese physicians believe that safflower helps nutrients get to the hair follicles. You can massage your scalp with safflower oil or grind up a few table-spoons of whole seeds and add the powder to an herbal shampoo.

☙ Sesame (*Sesamum indicum*). Sesame seeds are also a Chinese treatment for hair loss, according to pharmacognosist (natural product pharmacist) Albert Leung, Ph.D. Just for taste, you can add toasted sesame seeds to all kinds of dishes, and if the additional sesame helps you keep your hair, so much the better.

☙ Stinging nettle (*Urtica dioica*). Tincture of nettle leaf can help prevent balding in those with thinning hair, according to Rudolf Fritz Weiss, M.D., the dean of German herbal physicians and author of *Herbal Medicine*. I don't know of any studies supporting this, but I respect Dr. Weiss.

Perhaps his endorsement of nettle is a remnant of the Doctrine of Signatures, which was the idea that a plant's appearance announces its medicinal value. Nettle is a hairy plant, so the doctrine would endorse its use for hair problems.

On the other hand, maybe there will be some other evidence to recommend this herb for balding. The more researchers look at nettle, the more uses they seem to find. Taking a teaspoon or two of tincture a day—or one or two cups of nettle tea—certainly shouldn't hurt.

Bladder Infections

Y ou're probably going to want to know right off the bat whether cranberry juice really helps prevent bladder infections. This one is easy: Yes, there is reason to believe that it does. And there are several other herbal treatments that can help as well.

Bladder infection, also called cystitis and urinary tract infection (UTI), is a bacterial infection that causes painful urination and a feeling that the bladder never completely empties. It can also cause fever and low back pain. Urine from an infected bladder may smell strong and contain tinges of blood. (If you develop any of these symptoms, you should see your doctor for treatment.)

Some 80 percent of bladder infections are caused by bacteria from the anal area, notably *Escherichia coli*, a microorganism that lives in the digestive tract.

Men can develop bladder infections, especially if they have an enlarged prostate gland, but this problem strikes mostly women. Women have a much shorter urethra (the tube through which urine exits the body) than men, so the *E. coli* can travel more easily into women's bladders.

Bladder infections occur in about 20 percent of women, many of whom suffer chronic, recurring infections. More than 20 percent of women who develop bladder infections have three or more a year.

Green Pharmacy for Bladder Infections

Doctors treat UTIs with antibiotics. But quite often, natural approaches—foods and herbs—work just as well.

❧ ❧ ❧ **Blueberry (*Vaccinium*, various species) and cranberry (*V. macrocarpon*).** I'm enthusiastic about these two fruits. Folk practitioners have claimed for a long time that they help. A study published in the *Journal of the American Medical Association* showed that certain compounds in cranberry and blueberry juice prevent bacteria from adhering to the bladder walls. And if they can't stick to the bladder walls, they won't cause infection there.

Both cranberry and blueberry also contain arbutin, a chemical compound that is both an antibiotic and a diuretic that helps relieve excess water retention. In another study of seven juices, cranberry and blueberry lowered *E. coli* adhesion, while grapefruit, guava, mango, orange and pineapple did not.

The only problem with the cranberry juice prescription is that you have to drink a lot of it. Naturopaths suggest drinking 17 ounces a day to treat UTIs. The juice is naturally tart and must be sweetened to be palatable, meaning that this prescription is rather high in calories. If you try this, make sure you adjust the rest of your diet accordingly.

❧ ❧ ❧ **Yogurt.** While this isn't an herb, I won't hold that against it. It's too good a natural healer to exclude from this chapter. Studies show that the active bacterial cultures in yogurt help prevent both bladder infections and yeast infections. The trick, of course, is to eat yogurt with live cultures. If it has live cultures, the label will say so.

How about yogurt with blueberries and cranberry juice for an infection-fighting breakfast?

✿✿ Parsley (*Petroselinum crispum*) and other vegetables. After cranberry and blueberry, juices that are often recommended for bladder infections include carrot, celery, cucumber and parsley. Parsley in particular has a long history of use for bladder problems, and no wonder. Good research shows that it's a diuretic that helps empty the bladder.

✿ Bearberry (*Arctostaphylos uva ursi*). For my other herbal recommendations to prevent and treat bladder infection, I'll turn to my friend Varro Tyler, Ph.D., dean and professor emeritus of pharmacognosy (natural product pharmacy) at Purdue University in West Lafayette, Indiana.

In his excellent book *Herbs of Choice*, Dr. Tyler relies on the recommendations of Germany's Commission E, the body of natural medicine experts that advises Germany's counterpart of the Food and Drug Administration.

Dr. Tyler's list leads off with bearberry, a close relative of cranberry and blueberry that contains a good amount of arbutin, a natural diuretic and antibiotic.

Calling bearberry the "most effective antibacterial herb for urinary tract infections," Dr. Tyler quotes the Commission E prescription: Take ten grams a day (about a half-ounce) to treat bladder infections. This much bearberry contains anywhere from 400 to 700 milligrams of arbutin. Maximum antibacterial activity occurs three to four hours after taking this herb.

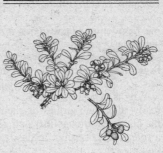

✿ Birch (*Betula*, various species). Commission E endorses birch leaves as a diuretic of value in treating both kidney and urinary tract infections. Chemicals called flavonoids (mostly hyperoside and quercetin) apparently account for the diuretic effect.

Bearberry

Dried leaves of this common, attractive ground cover are used to make a diuretic tea.

If you can find birch leaf tincture, Commission E suggests taking two to three grams (about a teaspoon) several times a day. If you have a birch tree, you can make your own tincture by putting two teaspoons of bark in a cup of vodka and letting it steep for a couple of days.

I prefer a tea made from cherry birch bark, which you can make by adding a handful of bark to a cup or two of boiling water.

❧ **Buchu (*Agathosma betulina*).** Buchu has long been a folk favorite as a diuretic and treatment for inflammation and infection of the kidneys and urinary tract. Oddly, Commission E did not endorse it. Other sources that I trust have been a bit more positive, saying that buchu can be used as an antiseptic and diuretic in mild cases of UTI. I'm inclined to consider buchu helpful. It contains diosphenol, which may have an antibacterial effect.

❧ **Couchgrass (*Agropyron repens* or *Elymus repens*).** The recommendation to use couchgrass, also known as quackgrass, for the treatment of urinary tract inflammation also comes from Commission E. I like the name quackgrass so much that I feel as if I have to endorse it, especially since I know that this herb is a diuretic with a long folk history of use for bladder and kidney stones. This common weedy grass occurs in almost all 50 states.

❧ **Dandelion (*Taraxacum officinale*).** Dandelion root is a particularly potent diuretic. Diuretics don't cure bladder infections, but they help flush urine out of the bladder, and some bacteria along with it. Long clinical experience suggests that this action is helpful in treating bladder infections.

Why is dandelion such a powerful diuretic? Scientists aren't really sure. Two groups of chemicals that have been found in the plant, eudesmanolides and germacranolides, appear to play a role. The potassium in dandelion may also contribute to its diuretic effect.

❧ **Echinacea (*Echinacea*, various species) and goldenseal (*Hydrastis canadensis*).** Echinacea, also known as coneflower, is an immune system booster. Taking echinacea along with antibiotics can be a good treatment for UTIs. If you'd like to use a natural antibiotic as well, try goldenseal.

You can use tinctures of echinacea and goldenseal alone or in combination. Take one to two dropperfuls (about a teaspoon) of each two to three times a day. (Although echinacea can cause your tongue to tingle or go numb temporarily, this effect is harmless.)

❧❧

Banishing Bladder Infections

Herbs are fine for treating bladder infections, but I'd be remiss if I didn't include the standard natural guidelines for preventing this condition. All women, whether they're prone to bladder infections or not, should:

- Drink eight glasses of water a day.
- Urinate whenever they feel the urge (a full bladder is more prone to infection).
- Not douche.
- Wipe from front to back to prevent anal-area bacteria from being introduced into the urethra.

Women with recurrent bladder infections should:

- Take showers instead of baths.
- Drink a glass of water before and after sexual intercourse.
- Urinate within 15 minutes after intercourse.

❧❧

❧ **Goldenrod (*Solidago virgaurea*).** Europeans praise goldenrod as one of the safest and most effective diuretic-antiseptic herbs. There is good clinical evidence of its diuretic activity. There is also clear scientific evidence that it is beneficial in treating kidney inflammation (nephritis). All of this suggests to me that this herb would also be of some benefit in treating bladder infections.

Several species of goldenrod are used widely in Europe to

alleviate urinary tract inflammations and to prevent the formation of and facilitate the elimination of kidney stones. Commission E suggests taking goldenrod for prevention and treatment of various types of bladder and kidney problems.

❧ Lovage (*Levisticum officinale*). Lovage looks and smells just like celery, and it is also an effective diuretic for treatment of urinary tract inflammations, according to Commission E reports.

❧ Marsh mallow (*Althaea officinalis*). You can use a cold-water infusion to soothe the burning of a bladder infection, according to Christopher Hobbs, a distinguished fourth-generation California herbalist, botanist and author of about a dozen books. Make the infusion by soaking about four teaspoons of dried marsh mallow in a quart of cold water overnight. Sip the resulting tea throughout the day.

❧ Stinging nettle (*Urtica dioica*). Commission E recommends taking stinging nettle for the prevention and treatment of kidney stones. Because nettle acts as a diuretic, this tells me that it should help with bladder infection as well. In one study, treatment over 14 days with fresh nettle sap significantly increased urine volume in people taking the herb.

Body Odor

The chemistry of armpits is rather interesting. Much of our body odor comes from emanations of the apocrine sweat glands, most of which are located in the underarm area. We're all born with these specialized glands, but they don't do much until puberty, when they start secreting a milky ooze that has no aroma. If we don't wash it off regularly—every six hours or so—bacteria begin to colonize these apocrine secretions. And a while later we develop . . . guess what?

Men have more and bigger apocrine glands than women, so they have more body odor, although I bet women spend more on deodorants.

In addition to poor hygiene, body odor may be caused by a zinc deficiency, diabetes or liver disease, chronic constipation

❧

The Amazing Amazonian Turn-On Shrub

Some years ago, the tropical shrub the Amazonians call *picho huayo* came up in a conversation I had with Alwyn Gentry, Ph.D., the late tropical botanist and senior curator at the Missouri Botanical Garden in St. Louis. He said that hunters in the Amazon rub the fruit of this shrub all over themselves in the belief that it prevents their quarry from smelling them. In other words, picho huayo masks their body odor. It's not a true deodorant, however, but just an aromatic mask.

Since that chat, I've asked several Amazonian guides about picho huayo. They use it not only when hunting wild game, they said, but also when courting women. It makes men smell more attractive to the opposite sex, the guides claim.

One noted Amazonian taxonomist (a specialist in classifying plants) swore to me that he had tried it with remarkable success, saying slyly, "I have good empirical evidence that it works." Picho huayo could be a gold mine for some enterprising entrepreneur with a flair for romance.

For those who would like to try picho huayo to attract members of the opposite sex, I'm sorry, but it's not available in the United States—at least not yet.

❧

and certain parasites. Vegetarians claim that meat-eaters have more body odor.

Bathing is probably the best way to control body odor, but if you don't feel socially at ease without a deodorant, there's no need to use commercial roll-ons or sprays.

Green Pharmacy for Body Odor

Herbs have a long and illustrious history of use as deodorants. Not surprisingly, the herbs most widely used all have antibacterial action against the microorganisms that make our apocrine secretions smell unpleasant. Here are some to try.

✿✿✿ **Coriander (*Coriandrum sativum*), licorice (*Glycyrrhiza glabra*) and other herbs.** My trusty database shows that coriander and licorice both contain 20 chemicals with antibacterial action. Oregano and rosemary have 19; ginger, 17; nutmeg, 15; cinnamon and cumin, 11; and bay, 10. (Black pepper has 14 and garlic 13, but I can't see rubbing them under my arms.)

✿✿

The Positive Side of BO

Body odor is really a two-way street.

Socially and cosmetically, we consider BO "bad." We bathe frequently to get rid of it and spend lots of money trying to cover it up. But it turns out that body odor also contains pheromones, mysterious chemicals that attract the opposite sex with their subtle aromas.

Scientists have known for a long time that pheromones play a principal role in animal mating. But until fairly recently, conventional scientific wisdom held that these chemicals had no amorous effect on us humans. Now studies have demonstrated that pheromones do indeed play a subtle but very real role in human attraction.

My wife is more apt to tell me to take a shower than to snuggle up to my armpits, but who knows? Maybe our aromas were part of what attracted us to each other in the first place. I'm inclined to believe that this is true.

✿✿

Looking at the quantity of bactericidal compounds in various herbs—as opposed to the number of compounds—we find that licorice contains up to 33 percent bactericidal compounds (on a dry-weight basis); thyme, up to 21.3 percent; oregano, up to 8.8 percent; rosemary, up to 4.8 percent; coriander, up to 2.2 percent; and fennel, up to 1.5 percent.

All of the herbs mentioned so far should have some impact against the bacteria that cause body odor. One way to use these deodorant herbs is to powder them and rub them into your underarms. It's an effective approach, but it might also stain clothing. So instead, I would suggest making a strong tea of the herb or herbs of your choice, soaking a cloth in it and applying the moist cloth as a compress for a few minutes.

Add plenty of sage, and if various reasonably well-informed sources are correct, your tea might also provide antiperspirant benefit.

You might also use these herbs in a bath. Scoop them into a cloth bag and run hot bathwater over it.

Another approach is to buy the essential oils of these herbs, dilute them in vegetable oil (try a drop or two of essential oil per tablespoon of vegetable oil) and use the resulting mixture as an underarm massage lotion. Just remember that you shouldn't ingest the oil, as even a small amount can be toxic.

Medical anthropologist John Heinerman, Ph.D., in *Heinerman's Encyclopedia of Fruits, Vegetables and Herbs*, suggests making an antiperspirant sage tincture by steeping ½ cup dried, powdered sage in 1¼ cup vodka. Age the mixture for two weeks, shaking it twice a day, then strain the sage out and store the liquid in a clean bottle. Try applying it three or four times a day. Alcohol can dry the skin, so discontinue use if it becomes irritating. (You can also sip it as sage liqueur.)

❧ **Baking soda and cornstarch.** Apply a mixture of these powders in malodorous areas. The drying action of both powders helps, and as anyone who has ever used an open box of baking soda to control odors in the refrigerator knows, baking soda has deodorant action. I know that baking soda is not an herb, but it's such a natural approach to this problem that I thought I'd include it.

❧ **Turnip juice.** Here is a personal anecdote from Dr. Heinerman that I find interesting: After a Japanese colleague told him about using turnip or daikon radish juice to control body odor, Dr. Heinerman juiced up some turnips and briskly rubbed one teaspoon under each arm. His conclusion: "Turnip juice won't prevent sweating, but it keeps body odor from occurring for up to ten hours." It sounds too good to be true, but I intend to try it if I'm home alone for about three days and have a good supply of turnips on hand.

❧ Vegetables containing zinc. Zinc deficiency may contribute to body odor. It's not easy to get zinc from processed foods, because it's often removed during processing, but whole foods contain good amounts. Good food sources of zinc include spinach, parsley, collard greens, brussels sprouts, cucumbers, string beans, endive, asparagus and prunes. Spinach has the most, and the rest of the foods are listed in descending order according to how much zinc they contain. If you'd like to make a deodorant cocktail, consider juicing any or all of these vegetables. (I'd leave out the prunes.)

❧ Vinegar. Dr. Heinerman recommends using cider vinegar in place of commercial deodorants. It makes sense to me, because vinegar is an antiseptic. I also steep some of the aromatic herbs, such as sage, in the vinegar.

Breast Enlargement

A few years ago, I wrote an article for *HerbalGram*, the excellent publication of the American Botanical Council in Austin, Texas, of which my friend Mark Blumenthal is executive director. I summarized the research showing that fenugreek, a tasty, vaguely maple-flavored herb, helps control blood sugar in people who have diabetes and that its sprouts just might enlarge women's breasts.

Some time later, I was invited to a meeting of herbalists in Arkansas. When I was picked up at the airport in Little Rock, the woman who drove me to the conference told me this story: A few months earlier, she and some friends had sprouted a lot of seeds for a taste test of sprouts at an herbal food fest. One of the seeds they sprouted was fenugreek.

After eating several fair-size portions of fenugreek sprouts over the course of several days, one of the women noticed that her breasts seemed somewhat larger. This is called a mastogenic effect. She did not understand what was going on until another woman in the group handed her a copy of my article.

Green Pharmacy for Breast Enlargement

I'm not going to take sides on the issue of breast enlargement. All I know is that quite a few women dream of larger breasts, and many opt for silicone implants. If you read the papers, you know that these implants are very controversial, with many women and some scientists calling them dangerous, while other women and other scientists say that they cause no real problems.

While I can't judge whether silicone breast implants are harmful, I know that if my daughter wanted her breasts enlarged, I'd certainly encourage her to try natural approaches first. Here are several herbs that might prove helpful in providing a modest boost in size.

❧

Bustea

Want a bustier look? Drink Bustea! Here's a tea recipe that will give you a hearty dose of breast-enhancing herbs.

In a saucepan, pour two cups of water over one cup of fenugreek sprouts. Add a dash or two of anise, basil, caraway, dill, fennel, licorice, marjoram and lemongrass. Bring to a boil, then let cool. Add lemon juice and honey to taste. Drink one to two cups a day.

Fennel contains phytoestrogens, plant chemicals similar to the female hormone estrogen. Folklore maintains that the other herbs in this tea can also help enlarge the breasts.

❧

❀❀❀ **Fenugreek** (*Trigonella foenum-graecum*). The seeds and sprouts have a centuries-old folk reputation as breast enlargers. In fact, 100 years ago the herb was a key ingredient in the original formula for Lydia Pinkham's Vegetable Compound, a popular remedy for "female troubles"—everything from menstrual pain to postmenopausal vaginal dryness.

As I learned in Arkansas, there are also modern testimonials for fenugreek's effects on the breasts and good reason to believe this herb really works.

Fenugreek seeds contain a fair amount of diosgenin, a chemical compound that's often used to create semisynthetic forms of the female sex hormone estrogen.

While estrogen has many effects on the body, two relate principally to breast enlargement. The hormone causes growth of breast cells and contributes to water retention. In fact, many women who take the Pill, which contains estrogen, for birth control often experience as a side effect the feeling of breast fullness caused by water retention.

Plant estrogen (phytoestrogen) from sources like fenugreek does not lead to uncomfortable breast fullness. If my daughter wanted to try fenugreek, I might suggest that she drink a formula that I developed for exactly this purpose. I call it Bustea.

Massaging powdered fenugreek into the breasts is also worth a try, since breast tissue can apparently absorb a certain amount of plant chemicals. Not too long ago, two distinguished pharmacognosists (natural product pharmacists) published a paper entitled "Higher Plants as Potential Sources of Galactagogues." (Galactagogues are substances that promote the secretion and flow of breast milk.) These two scientists seemed surprised to find that 68 of the 255 plants used as traditional galactagogues were and are applied topically.

To use powdered fenugreek, grind up seeds or sprouts in a blender, add a dash of vegetable oil and apply the mixture as a paste.

❀❀ **Fennel** (*Foeniculum vulgare*). Fennel is another estrogenic herb that has been used for centuries to promote milk production. You could include it in Bustea to complement the fenugreek. Don't use fennel oil, however. In pregnant women, the oil can cause miscarriage. And in doses greater than about a teaspoon, it can be toxic.

❀❀ **Saw palmetto** (*Serenoa repens*). This plant is best known these days for its ability to shrink an enlarged prostate gland in men. But a century ago, this herb was best known as a folk approach to breast enlargement. Naturopathic physicians continue to recommend it for this purpose. Most people use standardized store-bought capsules (one to two grams) or alcohol extracts. To use this herb, follow the package directions.

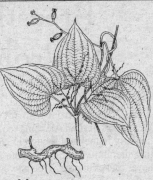

Wild Yam

Also called colic root or rheumatism root, wild yam is a twining perennial that was once used by American Indians to ease the pain of childbirth.

🍂🍂 **Wild yam (*Dioscorea villosa*).** Here's another herb that is reputed to have estrogenic effects. Personally, I've never been that impressed with wild yam because, according to my database, it contains a lot less diosgenin than fenugreek. But I bow to practicing herbalists such as Susun Weed, author of *Breast Cancer? Breast Health!*, who say that they have made salves out of the wild yam. These herbalists maintain that the women who use this salve gain the desired effects. To make a salve, it's best to shave off the outer bark of the root and reduce the inner root bark to paste in a blender.

🍂 **Cumin (*Cuminum cyminum*).** Both common cumin and black cumin (*Nigella sativa*) have been shown to increase the number of mammary cells in laboratory animals. The herb's effects on the human breast are unknown, but mammals tend to have similar reactions to compounds with mammary effects. You could spice up Bustea with more ground cumin. You could also make liberal use of this spice in cooking.

Breastfeeding Problems

I was born in rural Alabama, and I spent my first few months breastfeeding from both my mother and a black wet nurse. Wet nurses in rural Alabama took herbs to promote lactation, particularly fennel and fenugreek. Based on my review of the scientific literature, I'd have to vote for fenugreek over fennel. But it never ceases to amaze me how much wisdom there is in folk wisdom.

Compared with formula, mother's milk is better for mother-child bonding, plus it is easier for babies to digest, does not cause constipation and protects the infant from allergies and several infectious diseases. It also has contraceptive benefits for the mother, although nursing women can get pregnant. For all of these reasons, and after years of touting formula, since the 1980s doctors have switched back to promoting breastfeeding. (Another case of modern medicine reversing itself. Science marches on!) In fact, a new type of specialist, lactation consultant, has sprung up to help new mothers deal with breastfeeding problems: too little milk, too much milk, sore nipples and painful nipple infections (mastitis).

Green Pharmacy for Breastfeeding Problems

I'm no lactation consultant, but permit me to suggest a few herbs that can help make breastfeeding a more rewarding experience.

❧❧❧ **Fenugreek (*Trigonella foenum-graecum*).** Fenugreek seed has been used to increase milk production since biblical times. The herb contains phytoestrogens, which are plant chemicals similar to the female sex hormone estrogen. A key compound, diosgenin, has been shown experimentally to increase milk flow. I would readily wager that dietary levels consumed in some societies—parts of the Middle East, for example—could be shown to increase milk flow.

Because fenugreek is my first-choice herb for promoting milk production, it is also the main ingredient in my Bustea, which I also recommend for breast enlargement. You can find the recipe on page 109.

✿✿✿ **Garlic** (*Allium sativum*). To treat mastitis, doctors often prescribe antibiotics. The problem is that antibiotics get into breast milk, and I'm not so sure it's a good idea to expose infants to these drugs.

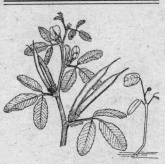

Fenugreek

Also known as Greek hay, fenugreek has long been used to heal sick animals as well as humans.

Missouri naturopath Chris Deatheridge, N.D., has what I think is a better approach. He suggests mixing a dropperful of echinacea tincture, three cloves of raw garlic and four to six ounces of carrot juice in a blender and drinking the mixture every two hours. He reports many quick, permanent cures. I'm not surprised. Garlic is a potent antibiotic.

In addition, garlic helps babies nurse better. If breastfeeding mothers eat a few cloves of garlic within an hour before nursing begins, babies attach to the breast more readily, stay there longer, suck more and drink more milk, according to studies done at the Monell Chemical Senses Center in Philadelphia.

✿✿ **Anise** (*Pimpinella anisum*). Anise is very helpful in promoting lactation, according to Jean Valnet, M.D., a pioneer of aromatherapy and author of *The Practice of Aromatherapy*. Dr. Valnet also recommends caraway, fennel and lemongrass. He's a bit surer than I am, but I'm inclined to accept his recommendations, which is why all of these herbs are incorporated into my Bustea. They also improve the flavor of the active fenugreek.

✿✿ **Chasteberry** (*Vitex agnus-castus*). Talented fourth-generation California herbalist Christopher Hobbs, a botanist whom I respect, suggests using *Vitex* shortly after delivery to promote milk flow. This recommendation goes a bit beyond the usual uses of chasteberry for breast tenderness, PMS and menstrual complaints, but I have no problem suggesting this revered women's herb to enhance lactation. It's probably worth a try. (And it's a handsome ornamental flowering tree, as lovely as lilac.)

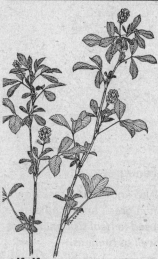

Alfalfa

Alfalfa, a favorite food for cattle, may help stimulate milk production.

Echinacea (*Echinacea*, various species). Echinacea, also known as coneflower, is useful in treating mastitis and nipple fissures, according to Maine herbalist Deb Soule, founder of Avena Botanicals and author of *The Roots of Healing*. I'm not surprised at this recommendation, because echinacea is both an antibiotic and an immune system booster.

I suggest blending a dropperful of echinacea tincture in juice along with a few cloves of garlic; drink it three or four times a day. (Although echinacea can cause the tongue to tingle or go numb temporarily, this effect is harmless.)

Fennel (*Foeniculum vulgare*). Fennel, which research shows has weak properties similar to those of the stronger female hormone estrogen, has been used for centuries to promote lactation. You can try two teaspoons of crushed seeds per cup of boiling water and drink up to three cups a day.

Don't use fennel oil. In pregnant women, the oil can cause miscarriage. And in doses greater than about a teaspoon, it can be toxic.

Peanut (*Arachis hypogaea*). In China, when women produce little milk, herbalists give them peanuts. There just might be something to it. Like so many other legumes, peanuts contain several estrogenic compounds that might spur milk production.

Alfalfa (*Medicago sativa*). Like fenugreek, alfalfa is estrogenic. If you'd like to produce more milk, it probably can't hurt to add heaping handfuls of sprouts to your salads. If you have lupus or a family history of lupus, however, it's a good idea to steer clear of alfalfa sprouts. There's some evidence that they may trigger lupus in sensitive individuals.

❧ **Dandelion** (*Taraxacum officinale*). The Chinese boil about an ounce of minced dandelion root in two to three cups of water until only half the liquid remains, then use compresses of the resulting brew to treat mastitis. This sounds like a good treatment to me. If my daughter had mastitis, I'd suggest that she try it.

❧ **Jasmine** (*Jasminum sambac*). To suppress milk flow, an age-old Indian folk treatment is to apply fresh jasmine flowers to the breasts. In one study, Indian researchers matched this treatment against doses of bromocriptine (Parlodel), a drug that terminates lactation by inhibiting secretion of a hormone involved in milk production. In the study, half of a group of women took bromocriptine, and half applied crushed jasmine to their breasts. Both treatments were equally effective lactation inhibitors, although bromocriptine lowered hormone levels more than the flowers did. I don't see how this could work, but that's what the study showed.

❧ **Parsley** (*Petroselinum crispum*). Eating chopped fresh parsley is an old folk treatment for breast tenderness. It makes sense: Some breast tenderness is caused by water retention, and parsley is diuretic, which means that it helps flush excess water from the body.

The herb's diuretic action probably accounts for Dr. Valnet's recommendation to use parsley to help reduce milk production in preparation for weaning. He also recommends mint and sage for this purpose.

❧ **Sesame** (*Sesamum indicum*). The Chinese roast sesame seeds, grind them and then eat them with a small amount of salt to increase milk flow. I love sesame seeds and can think of no more wholesome food. While I don't know of any research showing that it works, I can't think of a good reason not to give it a try.

❧ **Squaw vine** (*Mitchella repens*). This herb is useful in treating nipple soreness that results from nursing, according to herbalist Paul Bergner, editor of *Medical Herbalism*. His recipe: Boil two ounces of squaw vine in a pint of water, add a pint of heavy cream, then boil the mixture down until it has the consistency of a salve. Let cool and apply after each feeding.

Bronchitis

I'm not personally acquainted with the TV newsman Walter Cronkite, but he and I have something in common. Over a decade ago, on independent trips to China, our hosts gave both of us honeysuckle tea. I was given the tea for flu. He got the tea for bronchitis, the inflammation of the bronchial tubes that causes persistent cough, chest congestion and often the production of a lot of thick, sticky phlegm.

Both of us recovered quickly, and I'm inclined to believe that this ancient herbal remedy helped. Doctors tend to scoff at such statements. Our two case studies are merely what the scientists often dismiss as anecdotal evidence.

Study Confirms Folk Cures

All right, so our cases don't really prove anything. But there's more to honeysuckle—and other herbs—than just anecdotes. And these days, there are a lot of scientific studies to back that up. In 1993, for example, Chinese researchers divided 96 children with bronchiolitis, a children's form of bronchitis, into three groups.

One-third of the children were given the herbal formula *shuang huang lian*, which consists of honeysuckle, forsythia and skullcap. Another third got only antibiotics, and the remaining third were given both herbs and antibiotics.

The children who were given the herbs alone showed improvement in chest symptoms, cough, fever and wheezing. Compared with those on antibiotics, the herbs-only group fared better in some ways: They had fewer days with fever and less wheezing and coughing. No adverse reactions to the herbs were noted.

That's the good news. The bad news, to my way of thinking, is that the herbal infusion was administered intravenously for seven days. Nowhere do I recommend herbal injections. For treating bronchitis, taking herbs in the form of tea or tinctures is safe and often quite effective.

And tell your doctor to save the antibiotics for emergencies. The downside of antibiotics is that they make any "bugs" that survive more resistant to treatment.

This Chinese study is good enough to give me confidence in suggesting honeysuckle and forsythia as treatments for respiratory problems because it confirms centuries of folkloric use. But apparently it hasn't budged the Food and Drug Administration (FDA), which does not list either honeysuckle or forsythia on the list of herbs generally regarded as safe (GRAS), let alone as treatments for bronchitis. The ways of the FDA are a mystery to me. I regard honeysuckle and forsythia as safe and effective, and I wouldn't hesitate to use them for bronchitis and the chest congestion of colds and flu. But because they are not GRAS, all I can say to other people is, try them at your own risk.

Bronchitis has several possible causes. It may be bacterial or viral, or it may be caused by some chronic irritant such as cigarette smoking or exposure to certain chemicals. Children are more likely to develop bronchitis (and asthma) if their parents smoke or if they are exposed to high levels of formaldehyde, one of the chemicals that give cars and home furnishings that "new" smell. Sometimes the germs and irritants work together: A smoker catches a cold and the cough turns into bronchitis.

Green Pharmacy for Bronchitis

Bronchitis may clear up by itself without any treatment, but it can also linger and sometimes become chronic. That's why I favor treating it. Honeysuckle (*Lonicera japonica*) and forsythia (*Forsythia suspensa*) are two of my favorite natural bronchitis remedies, but there are many others. Here are some to try.

✿✿ **Eucalyptus (*Eucalyptus globulus*).** Eucalyptus oil is a good expectorant (a substance that helps loosen phlegm). Commission E, the body of natural medicine experts that makes herbal recommendations to Germany's health advisers, has endorsed inhaling eucalyptus vapors to treat bronchitis and coughs.

Taken internally, eucalyptus leaf tea might have the same benefits. I say this because, after you ingest eucalyptus and your body absorbs it, part of its essential oil is secreted through your lungs. So you get the antiseptic, cooling and expectorant properties of eucalyptus right where you need them.

❧❧ Garlic (*Allium sativum*). Eating a lot of garlic can help prevent bronchitis because garlic is filled with chemicals that are antiviral and antibacterial.

Garlic may also protect you from colds and flu because "garlic breath" keeps people from getting too close to you. (Just joking!) Actually, there is a serious side to garlic breath that serves to demonstrate just how useful this herb is in treating respiratory complaints. In the body, garlic releases aromatic chemicals, including allicin, one of the most potent broad-spectrum plant antiseptics. These aromatic compounds are excreted through the lungs—hence garlic breath. The presence of these compounds in the lungs is good. It means that, as with eucalyptus, you get garlic's active constituents right where you need them.

To minimize garlic breath, you can chew on a few sprigs of parsley.

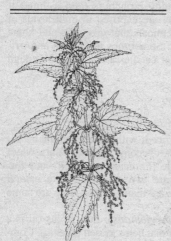

❧❧ Mullein (*Verbascum thapsus*). Mullein has been endorsed by Commission E for respiratory complaints because it has expectorant properties. It can help bring up that sticky phlegm. In fact, mullein has been an herbal favorite for respiratory ailments for thousands of years. In addition to its expectorant action, it soothes the throat, has bactericidal activity and helps stop the muscle spasms that trigger coughs.

❧❧ Stinging nettle (*Urtica dioica*). In recent years, nettle has been increasingly touted for treating bronchitis, asthma and hay fever—and with good reason. The juice of the roots and leaves, mixed with honey or sugar, relieves both bronchitis and asthma. Try

Stinging Nettle

This plant does sting, but the leaves, roots and even nettles (when softened by boiling) have healing powers.

two teaspoons of dried herb per cup of boiling water and steep until cool.

🌿 **Couchgrass (*Agropyron repens* or *Elymus repens*).** This herb is also known by an ironic name, quackgrass, which I love. Despite its name, however, it is not a quack remedy. It works and has long been used for respiratory complaints. Commission E recognizes couchgrass as an effective treatment for respiratory inflammations, including bronchitis.

🌿 **English plantain (*Plantago lanceolata*).** This herb and its plantain relatives have a worldwide reputation as cough suppressants. Commission E recommends it as safe and effective for bronchial conditions. As a bonus, it has antibacterial action. You may use about one teaspoon of dried herb per cup of boiling water and steep until cool.

🌿 **Horehound (*Marrubium vulgare*).** Commission E endorsed horehound for bronchial complaints, so why did the FDA declare it ineffective against coughs? Beats me.

Personally, when it comes to herbal medicine, I'd believe Commission E over the FDA any day. Herbal medicine is far more mainstream in Germany than it is in the United States, and Commission E bases its recommendations on serious scientific research. For bronchitis, I suggest brewing a strong horehound tea with lemon and licorice. Try two teaspoons of horehound per cup of boiling water.

🌿 **Ivy (*Hedera helix*).** Ivy is also useful for treating bronchitis and other respiratory problems, according to Commission E.

🌿 **Knotgrass (*Polygonum aviculare*).** This is another herb with Commission E endorsement. The Commission recommends knotgrass for sore throat and respiratory complaints, including bronchitis.

🌿 **Marsh mallow (*Althaea officinalis*) and other mallows.** The mallows are good respiratory tract soothers (demulcents), according to Commission E. Marsh mallow is particularly good because its demulcent roots also have an anti-inflammatory effect. This probably explains why this herb has been used for centuries as a treatment for bronchitis, colds, coughs and sore throat.

🌿 **Primrose (*Primula veris*).** Here's yet another herbal endorsement from Commission E. I know that I mention their recommendations a lot for certain conditions, but a nod from this body of scientists should be viewed with respect. Their research suggests using about one teaspoon of dried primrose flowers or a half-teaspoon of root in tea as an expectorant for treating bronchitis, colds and cough. I should point out also that this particular recommendation is for primrose, not evening primrose (*Oenothera biennis*), which shows up so often elsewhere in this book.

Soapwort (*Saponaria officinalis*). The root of this herb is a good expectorant for treating respiratory conditions, including bronchitis, according to Commission E. Chemicals in the plant—saponins—reportedly have pain-relieving and anti-inflammatory action, besides helping other compounds get the job done. To make a tea, use one teaspoon of dried herb per cup of boiling water and steep until cool.

Herbal formulas. You can use any of the herbs mentioned in this chapter singly if you'd like, but most herbalists recommend using them in combination. A noted British herbalist whom I respect, David Hoffmann, author of *The Herbal Handbook*, suggests using equal parts of horehound, mullein and elecampane. (Elecampane has a long history of use as an antiseptic and expectorant.)

Another formula that I'd try for bronchitis contains horehound, mullein, plantain, cayenne, chickweed, kelp, licorice, pleurisy root, saw palmetto berries, slippery elm bark and wild cherry bark. American Indians used these herbs for respiratory complaints.

In addition to using herbs that treat bronchitis, I'd also suggest using echinacea, which enhances immunity.

As a snack to munch along with your herbal formula of choice, you can mix up some of my Burning Broncho-Buster Spread. To make it, mix garlic, ginger, mustard, turmeric, chili peppers and horseradish or wasabi. Start with just a little of each and experiment until you find a combination you can live with. I must warn you, however, that this herbal formula is *very* hot. It will open your sinuses as well as your bronchial tubes.

I'm serious about it, though. If you can handle the heat, a little of this mixture spread on crackers or bread will really help. You can also make a piping hot tea containing any or all of these ingredients.

Plants containing vitamin C. In studies, hospital patients with bronchitis recovered faster when they took vitamin C supplements. Daily supplements of 500 milligrams of vitamin C have also been shown to help with allergies and asthma, so there's clearly a link between using this vitamin and a reduction in respiratory infections, nasal congestion and watery eyes.

I feel fine about recommending vitamin C supplements, but I feel even better about endorsing plant foods that are high in this important vitamin, such as red and green peppers, citrus fruits and chili peppers.

✦ **Whole grains, nuts and other foods containing magnesium.** Speaking of vitamins and minerals, the risk for respiratory diseases such as bronchitis increases as magnesium levels decline. The more magnesium in the body, the less wheezing and other respiratory complaints. Naturopaths commonly recommend taking 300 to 600 milligrams daily as a preventive, which sounds like a good idea to me. You might also eat more foods that are rich in magnesium, such as whole grains, soybeans, nuts, fish, dairy products and lean meats.

Bruises

You've probably heard of using raw beefsteak to treat black eyes and other bad bruises. But what about pineapple? If the tropical fruit worked on boxers' bruises, would you be interested?

Two physicians I respect—Melvyn Werbach, M.D., assistant clinical professor of psychiatry at the University of California, Los Angeles, School of Medicine, and naturopath Michael Murray, N.D., co-authors of *Botanical Influences on Illness*—both seem impressed by an old study on bromelain, a protein-digesting (proteolytic) enzyme in pineapple, for treating bruises.

In this study, researchers gave bromelain to 74 boxers with numerous bruises, while 72 other bruised boxers received an inactive substitute (placebo). Among those receiving the placebo, 14 percent healed in four days. But among the boxers taking bromelain, 78 percent healed in four days.

How does it work? Bromelain appears to inhibit the formation of prostaglandin E_2, a chemical in the body that is involved in inflammation. At the same time, it stimulates the production of prostaglandin E_1, an anti-inflammatory chemical.

Pineapple's No Panacea

Those black-and-blue marks known as bruises are actually caused by blood that leaks out of capillaries just under the skin, usually after an injury. Black eyes are more common in men than women, while blue spots occur most frequently on the legs of older women.

If I were a charlatan, I could push pineapple juice or pineapple concentrate as a treatment for this condition. The press releases would be fun to write: "Recent Study Confirms the Folklore: Pineapple Takes the Purple Out of Pugilists' Punched Pupils."

I'm not that strongly in favor of bromelain, however. In fact, I don't think pineapple and bromelain represent the best natural approach to either the prevention or treatment of bruises. Bromelain occurs in very low levels in pineapple, and only about 40 percent of it gets from the digestive tract to other parts of the body.

Then, how about pure bromelain? After all, you can buy it at many natural food stores. Naturopaths, who are big on bromelain, suggest taking 150 to 450 milligrams three times a day on an empty stomach to treat bruises, many sports injuries, swelling and inflammation.

Perhaps it is as effective as the naturopaths say, but personally I'd suggest fruits that are rich in vitamin C and bioflavonoids, such as oranges and other citrus fruits. Bioflavonoids are beneficial nutrients that often show up in foods that are rich in vitamin C, and together these nutrients help strengthen capillary walls, making them more resistant to the blood leakage that causes bruises. When bruises occur, vitamin C and bioflavonoids help capillary walls—and black-and-blue marks—heal more rapidly.

Green Pharmacy for Bruises

While you're feasting on pineapple and citrus fruit, however, you might also try some other traditional herbal treatments that have scientific merit.

🍂 **Arnica (*Arnica montana*).** This herb, also known as mountain daisy, is helpful in treating bruises, according to Commission E, the body of experts that advises the German government about herbs.

Arnica, which has pain-relieving, antiseptic and anti-inflammatory properties, is best reserved for use on the skin. While you should not take it internally to treat bruises, you can make a healing solution using one teaspoon of dried herb per cup of boiling water. Steep until cool and then apply with a clean cloth. Or make the solution using tincture of arnica; a few drops per cup of water will do it. Commercial, mostly homeopathic arnica ointments are also available. Look for a product containing up to 15 percent arnica oil and follow the package directions.

✿ **Comfrey (*Symphytum officinale*).** Comfrey is among the oldest herbal remedies for skin problems, dating back to ancient Greece. Modern researchers have discovered that it contains allantoin, a chemical that promotes skin repair. Allantoin is an ingredient in a number of commercial skin creams.

A review of the scientific literature by Commission E uncovered evidence that comfrey is also anti-inflammatory. That's why the Commission endorsed applying it to the skin to treat bruises, dislocations and sprains.

To treat bruises, medical anthropologist and herb expert John Heinerman recommends first-aid application of ice packs, then a bandage soaked in comfrey tea. Quick action can prevent some discoloration.

It's probably a good idea not to ingest comfrey, however. It contains pyrrolizidine alkaloids, compounds that are toxic to the liver, and there is some controversy about its safety.

✿ **Grape (*Vitis vinifera*).** In recent years, a chemical found in grape seeds and pine bark has become a popular, though expensive, supplement. It is sold under the brand name Pycnogenol. According to some naturopaths, Pycnogenol increases levels of vitamin C in the body's cells and strengthens the capillaries against the kind of traumatic injury that causes bruises. I'm not entirely sold on Pycnogenol, but by blending grape seeds into grape juice, you can get some for free.

✿ **Parsley (*Petroselinum crispum*).** Repeated applications of crushed parsley leaves will usually clear up any black-and-blue marks within a day or so. I plan to try parsley the next time I get a bruise.

✿ **Potato (*Solanum tuberosum*).** Old-timers claim that raw potato is better than beefsteak for a black eye. Me, too. Cheapskate semi-vegetarian that I am, I would surely apply a potato, along with some other herbs mentioned in this chapter, before using beefsteak.

❧ **St.-John's-wort (*Hypericum perforatum*).** This herb has a reddish oil that may ooze out when the plant is handled, making it seem to bleed. According to tradition, it came to be used for skin conditions simply because skin also bleeds. Although such reasons seem silly now, there has been some scientific verification that the herb is useful for treating bruises, burns, cuts and other wounds. Commission E has endorsed it for these uses. Try steeping one to two teaspoons of dried herb in vegetable oil for a few days. Then use the oil to treat bruises.

❧ **Witch hazel (*Hamamelis virginiana*).** The astringency of the leaves and bark of witch hazel made it a popular early American remedy for all sorts of skin conditions, from bruises to varicose veins. Witch hazel water is available at pharmacies.

Bunions

B ecause I'm partial to being barefoot whenever possible, I've managed to completely sidestep painful conditions like corns and bunions that shoe-wearers often get. In fact, I've never had any foot problems except those related to gout and minor bouts with athlete's foot in the distant past.

A bunion is a deformity of the big toe. The base of the toe protrudes outward, forcing the rest of the toe to point inward, sometimes even overlapping the other toes. The bunion is the bump at the base of the big toe.

Bunions are sometimes caused by a hereditary weakness called hallux valgus. (*Hallux* means "big toe," and *valgus* means "bowed.") But more often, especially in women, they result from trying to force the foot into a pointy-toed, high-heeled shoe. The bunion rubs on shoes, causing a thick callus to form.

Green Pharmacy for Bunions

The best advice for bunions is to wear shoes with roomy toe boxes so that the bunion doesn't rub. Cushioned shoe pads also help. While your podiatrist may recommend these remedies as a matter of course, there are other, herbal sources of bunion relief.

Here are some of the herbs that can help some people.

✺✺ Calendula (*Calendula officinalis*). More often used for bruises, cuts and inflammation, this herb is sometimes recommended for bunions. I'd try it by applying a commercial calendula salve or tincture directly to the bunion, maybe two or three times a day for up to a week. You'll know by then if it's going to help.

✺✺ Pineapple (*Ananas comosus*). Naturopaths suggest taking bromelain, a protein-dissolving (proteolytic) enzyme found in pineapple, for inflammatory joint problems such as bunions. I generally prefer a whole-foods approach, but it is possible to buy just the bromelain. Naturopath Michael Murray, N.D., co-author of *Encyclopedia of Natural Medicine* and several other scholarly books on nutritional and naturopathic healing, recommends taking 250 to 750 milligrams three times a day. All indications are that bromelain is extremely safe. In human studies, doses up to 2,000 milligrams have caused no side effects.

You can take commercial bromelain products if you like. I love pineapple and would rather get my bromelain from the natural source. If I had a bunion, I'd eat lots of pineapple in fruit salads with papaya, which also contains a potent proteolytic enzyme (papain), and season it all liberally with ginger, which contains both proteolytic and anti-inflammatory compounds.

✺✺ Red pepper (*Capsicum*, various species). Capsaicin, the hot ingredient in red pepper, is also medically "hot" as a pain reliever for inflammatory conditions. When applied to the skin at the site of pain, capsaicin blocks certain pain nerves by depleting them of substance P, one of the compounds responsible for producing pain. Many studies show that creams containing 0.025 percent capsaicin relieve all sorts of pain after a few weeks of treatment.

If I had a painful bunion, I'd try this herb. At home, I'd bite off one end of a hot pepper and chew it, and I'd rub the other end directly on the bunion. On the road, I'd go with commercial over-the-counter capsaicin preparations, such as Zostrix and Capzasin-P.

If you use a capsaicin cream, be sure to wash your hands thoroughly afterward so that you don't get it in your eyes. Also, since some people are quite sensitive to this compound, you should test it on a small area of skin before using it on a larger area. If it seems to irritate your skin, discontinue use.

✺✺ Turmeric (*Curcuma longa*). Research suggests that like

red pepper, turmeric depletes nerve endings of substance P. Applying about a teaspoon of grated fresh turmeric directly to the bunion twice a day could conceivably be helpful. Other studies show that when ingested, the compound curcumin in turmeric has potent anti-inflammatory effects, another reason that it might help relieve bunion pain.

The standard dose of curcumin is 400 milligrams three times a day, which is the equivalent of about six to eight teaspoons of turmeric. That's way more turmeric than you'd want to use in a curry. To get this herb's anti-inflammatory benefits, you'll have to use capsules.

✸✸ Willow (*Salix*, **various species**). Willow is herbal aspirin, thanks to the compound salicin that it contains. A closely related compound, salicylic acid, is approved by the Food and Drug Administration as a callus remover and for wart treatment. Salicylic acid also shows up in many over-the-counter preparations for treating bunions and corns. Salicylates are absorbed through the skin. If I had a callused bunion, I'd try applying fresh willow by wrapping the inner bark around the bunion. I'd also add some dried bark to my daily herbal teas. If you're allergic to aspirin, however, you probably shouldn't take aspirin-like herbs, either.

✸ Arnica (*Arnica montana*). The flowers of this plant, also known as mountain daisy, are useful for treating muscle and joint complaints, according to Commission E, the body of experts that makes herbal recommendations to the German government. It doesn't take much extrapolation to speculate that this herb might also help deal with bunions.

For a tea, use one to two teaspoons of dried herb per cup of boiling water and steep for ten minutes. Don't drink more than two cups a day for more than three days. For longer-term use, I'd go with an arnica ointment, which is what homeopaths recommend for all sorts of muscle, joint and sports injuries. Many health food stores and pharmacies now carry arnica ointments. Follow the package directions.

✸ Camomile (*Matricaria recutita*). Essential oils of camomile, cypress and juniper have been suggested by aromatherapists for treating bursitis and could conceivably be useful for bunions. Of the three, camomile would be my top choice. It has well-established anti-inflammatory activity that could help keep bunions under control. After you've drunk your camomile tea, apply the spent tea bag directly to the bunion.

If you have hay fever, however, you should use camomile

products cautiously. Camomile is a member of the ragweed family, and in some people, it might trigger allergic reactions. The first time you try it, watch your reaction. If it seems to help, go ahead and use it. But if it seems to cause or aggravate itching or irritation, discontinue use.

✿ **Clove** (*Syzygium aromaticum*). Clove oil is almost pure eugenol, a potent anesthetic widely used by dentists for treating toothache. If I had a bunion and capsaicin were unavailable or ineffective, I might try clove oil by placing a few drops on a cotton bandage and applying it directly to the bunion once or twice a day. If it irritates your skin, discontinue use.

✿ **Ginger** (*Zingiber officinale*). In addition to having some proteolytic activity, spicy ginger is also a pain-relieving anti-inflammatory that might help control the discomfort of bunions, according to Indian researchers. They gave three to seven grams (1½ to 3½ teaspoons) of powdered ginger a day to 28 people with painful and inflamed joints. More than 75 percent experienced noticeable relief from pain and swelling. After up to 30 months, none reported adverse effects from this dosage of ginger.

For bunions, I'd suggest drinking ginger tea made with one teaspoon of grated fresh ginger per cup of boiling water. I would drink this every day and apply grated ginger directly to the bunion once or twice a day as well.

✿ **Sundew** (*Drosera*, **various species**). This herb has a long folk reputation as a treatment for bunions, corns and warts. About 15 years ago, scientists learned why: It has proteolytic activity. To use this herb, crush the fresh plant and apply it directly to the bunion once or twice a day for up to a week. The fresh herb is readily available in many parts of the country: I know places in peat bogs where it grows so abundantly that it's almost a weed. Elsewhere, however, it's often listed as a locally endangered species, so you shouldn't pick it unless you've grown it on your own property.

Burns

M y wife is no real fan of herbal medicine. She'd rather go to doctors and take pills than have anything to do with the herbal concoctions and healing vegetable soups that I mix up, messing up her kitchen. But like so many homemakers, my herbally skeptical Peggy still has a small potted aloe plant on her kitchen windowsill, and she's used its gel to treat burns several times over the years.

My secretary is also a fan of aloe for burns. Once she fell asleep outdoors and wound up with a nasty sunburn on her feet and ankles. She reached for her aloe and got effective relief.

Burns by the Numbers

Burns come in three degrees of severity. First-degree burns injure only the outermost layer of skin. An ordinary sunburn, for example, is a first-degree burn.

When a burn develops blisters, the injury has penetrated deeper into the skin, and you have a very painful second-degree burn.

The worst type of burn, a third-degree burn, is, oddly, often not painful at all. That's because the injury penetrates so deeply that it destroys the nerves that transmit pain signals to the brain.

Third-degree burns are medical emergencies that always require professional care and typically necessitate hospitalization. And any second-degree burn that covers an area of skin larger than a quarter should receive medical attention.

Green Pharmacy for Burns

For first-degree and smaller second-degree burns, there are a number of herbal treatments that can soothe the burn and help bring relief.

Aloe (*Aloe vera*). Aloe has been used to treat burns and other wounds since ancient times. But it's not just a folk remedy. Many studies have shown that the gel obtained by slitting open the succulent's fat, leathery leaves relieves burns, including burns caused by radiation treatments for cancer.

My friend Varro Tyler, Ph.D., dean and professor emeritus of pharmacognosy (natural product pharmacy) at Purdue University in West Lafayette, Indiana, cites many studies showing that aloe gel is useful in treating burns, wounds and frostbite.

Scientists are still not certain how aloe speeds the healing of burns, but the herb appears to have several beneficial effects.

One study showed that aloe increases the amount of blood flowing to areas of burned tissue, which brings more of the body's healing resources to the area where they're needed.

Aloe also contains enzymes, carboxypeptidase and bradykininase, that relieve pain, reduce inflammation and decrease redness and swelling. In addition, aloe gel has antibacterial and antifungal properties, which might help prevent burns from getting infected.

Aloe belongs in every kitchen, the place where most household burns occur. It's my first-choice herb for burns. Unfortunately, the Food and Drug Administration (FDA) does not share my opinion. Two FDA advisory panels found "insufficient evidence" that aloe is useful for burns.

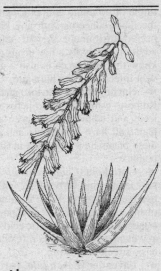

Aloe

Aloe, which is easily grown indoors on a windowsill, has been used medicinally since biblical times.

When the FDA says "insufficient evidence," it doesn't mean that the evidence isn't out there—it clearly is, and lots of it. It means only that years ago, when the panels were considering over-the-counter drugs (and when U.S. herbalism was at a low ebb), no one sent the panels enough studies to convince them. And why should they? The herbal believers are already convinced, and there's no economic incentive for drug companies to get aloe approved when anyone can grow it and the companies can't make any money on it.

❧ **Echinacea (*Echinacea*, various species).** Most people familiar with herbs know that echinacea (also known as coneflower) stimulates immune responses. Because it does, if I had a burn, I'd take out my tincture of echinacea and drink a teaspoon or two. (Although echinacea can cause your tongue to tingle or go numb temporarily, this effect is harmless.) One of the main concerns with any kind of burn is infection, and a beefed-up immune system helps guard against infection. In addition, I'd apply a few drops directly to the burn. Few people know that echinacea is also a gentle antiseptic that helps prevent infection at the burn site.

✱ Garlic (*Allium sativum*) and onion (*A. cepa*). From Africa to Rome to America, these herbs or their close relatives (chives, leeks and scallions) have been applied directly to burns. These plants all have undeniable antiseptic properties. To use any of these plants on a burn, just mash them and apply the paste as a poultice.

✱ Gotu kola (*Centella asiatica*). Naturopathic physicians suggest taking this herb (along with foods high in vitamin C) for treatment of burns. There is some evidence that the combination of the vitamin and three compounds in gotu kola—asiatic acid, asiaticoside and madecassic acid—stimulate collagen synthesis, a key element in skin repair. (Collagen is a protein that forms the basic structure of skin.)

✱ Lavender (*Lavandula*, various species). During the 1920s, French perfume chemist René-Maurice Gattefossé burned his hand in his laboratory. He plunged it into the nearest liquid—a container of lavender oil. The pain subsided quickly and the burn healed with no scarring. This incident may have led to the development of aromatherapy, the use in healing of various essential oils taken from plants.

Other essential oils, such as camomile, camphor, eucalyptus, geranium, onion, peppermint, rosemary and sage, have also been touted as burn treatments. But aromatherapists I know reserve their highest praise for lavender oil. Consider placing a vial on your kitchen windowsill right next to the aloe plant. (Remember, though, that you should never ingest essential oils, as even a small amount can be toxic.)

✱ Plantain (*Plantago*, various species). Plantain is one of the most popular folk herbal remedies for burns in the United States. Juice from the fresh leaves of this plant is applied directly to mild burns. I've used it many times and found it soothing.

✱ St.-John's-wort (*Hypericum perforatum*). Germany's Commission E, the scientists who advise the German government about herbal treatments, praised St.-John's-wort as an anti-inflammatory external treatment for first-degree burns. One German study showed that St.-John's-wort salves speeded up burn healing time and helped reduce scarring. You may need to beat the bushes to find a salve containing this herb in America, but tinctures are readily available. You can also make a suitable preparation by steeping one to two teaspoons of dried herb (preferably the flowering tops) in a few ounces of vegetable oil.

Bursitis and Tendinitis

A few years back, the *New York Times* published a story about my lifelong love affair with medicinal plants. Some time after it ran, I got a call from a *Times* employee who said that something like 20 percent of the newspaper's employees who banged away daily on computer keyboards were experiencing problems with inflamed joints, including tendinitis in their wrists or shoulders or bursitis of the shoulder.

He said that he was looking into alternative medical treatments, came across my name in the *Times* archives and called me. I sent him what I had, and my sympathy as well. I've had bursitis myself and can vouch for the pain and disability it causes. Like the man at the *Times*, I, too, spend hours on end working at a computer. I also enjoy playing the guitar and bass fiddle and do a fair amount of driving and lawn mowing, all of which can aggravate bursitis and tendinitis.

These two disorders are often lumped together, but they're actually two distinct conditions. Bursitis is an inflammation of the bursae, the fluid-filled sacs that help lubricate the joints in places where muscles and tendons meet bone. Tendinitis is an inflammation of the tendons, the tough, elastic, fibrous tissues that connect muscles to bones.

The two terms are often used interchangeably because the bursae are located near tendon-bone connections, and both conditions cause pain in and around the joints. Bursitis and tendinitis also have the same cause—overuse of a particular joint. These kinds of problems show up as a result of sports, as in tennis elbow, and in jobs that require repetitive movement, such as carpentry and butchering. Whatever you call them, though, bursitis and tendinitis really hurt. And interestingly enough, they both respond to the same kinds of treatments.

Physicians generally treat bursitis, tendinitis and related problems with rest and medications that relieve pain and reduce inflammation—aspirin and other nonsteroidal anti-inflammatory drugs and corticosteroids.

Green Pharmacy for Bursitis and Tendinitis

I think resting a joint that has been affected by tendinitis or bursitis is a great idea. Ice packs might also help control the pain and inflammation. But don't count on an ice pack to provide complete relief. And while taking aspirin and related drugs is fine, you should be aware that there are also a number of natural alternatives.

Willow (*Salix*, various species) and other natural pain relievers. Willow bark is herbal aspirin. So are meadowsweet and wintergreen. They all contain salicylates, natural precursors of aspirin. To make a tea, I suggest using one to two teaspoons of dried herb per cup of water and boiling it for about 20 minutes. Have a cup two or three times a day. Or try a teaspoon of tincture of any of these herbs three times a day. Remember, though, that if you're allergic to aspirin, you probably shouldn't take aspirin-like herbs, either.

Ginger (*Zingiber officinale*). Ginger has a long folk history in Asia as a bursitis treatment. Since I like ginger, I suggest trying it in combination with pineapple and a little licorice (both discussed below) for recurring bursitis.

Echinacea (*Echinacea*, various species). This herb, also called coneflower, is good for connective tissue injuries such as tennis elbow, skier's knee and jogger's ankle, according to Michael Moore, author of *Medicinal Plants of the Desert and Canyon West* and one of the nation's leading herbalists. All of these injuries are, in fact, types of tendinitis. He recommends taking up to a half-ounce of echinacea tincture daily until the swelling and pain are reduced. That's a lot of tincture, but echinacea is not hazardous (although it may cause your tongue to tingle or become numb), so it's probably worth a try.

Horsetail (*Equisetum arvense*). This herb is one of Nature's richest sources of the element silicon, and some say that it is in a form that is especially easy for your body to use. A number of studies show that silicon plays an important role in the health and resilience of both cartilage and connective tissues such as tendons. (Cartilage forms a significant portion of joints.)

I can't say that I'm entirely sold on high-silicon herbs and foods for treating bursitis and tendinitis, but two scientists I respect, herbal pharmacologist Daniel Mowrey, Ph.D., author of *The Scientific Validation of Herbal Medicine* and *Herbal Tonic Therapies*, and Forrest Nielsen, M.D., director of the Grand Forks USDA Human Nutrition Research Center in North Dakota, tout silicon. So I think it's worth trying, although you should not use this herb without the guidance of a holistic practitioner.

If you're advised to take this herb, you can make a tea by putting five teaspoons of dried horsetail, one teaspoon of sugar and one quart of water in a pot. (The sugar will pull more silicon out of the plant.) Bring it to a boil, then reduce the heat and let it simmer for about three hours. Strain the tea and let it cool before drinking it.

Other plants high in silicon include barley, chickweed, cucumbers, parsley, stinging nettle, walnuts, Brazil nuts, cashews, pistachios, string beans and turnips.

❧ **Licorice (*Glycyrrhiza glabra*).** Licorice can be every bit as effective a treatment for bursitis and tendinitis as the commonly prescribed drug hydrocortisone, according to Dr. Mowrey. Plus, the herb has none of the usual side effects, such as weight gain, indigestion, insomnia and lowered resistance to infection, that are associated with cortisone and hydrocortisone. From what I know of licorice's anti-inflammatory effects, I believe this herb is worth trying. (While licorice and its extracts are safe for normal use in moderate amounts—up to about three cups of tea a day—long-term use or ingestion of larger amounts can produce headache, lethargy, sodium and water retention, excessive loss of potassium and high blood pressure.)

❧ **Pineapple (*Ananas comosus*).** This tasty fruit contains enzymes that break down protein. One of these enzymes, bromelain, is particularly important because it has anti-inflammatory properties. Pineapple reduces swelling, bruising and pain and speeds the healing of joint and tendon injuries.

Many athletes believe that pineapple helps heal sprains and tendinitis. Some eat lots of pineapple before and after strenuous workouts to help protect their tendons, as tendinitis is a major problem for them. Does it work? I don't have a definite answer for that, but my colleague James Gordon, M.D., president and director of the Center for Mind-Body Medicine in Washington, D.C., told me that he was amazed at how pineapple alleviated his chronic back condition that involved pain and inflammation.

The bromelain content of pineapple is not all that high, but if I had bursitis or tendinitis, I'd try this approach. It probably can't hurt to add fresh pineapple and pineapple juice to your menu while you're getting over an episode of tendinitis or bursitis. Papaya contains enzymes similar to those in pineapple, so you might want to add some of this fresh fruit to your menu as well.

❧ **Purslane (*Portulaca oleracea*) and other foods containing magnesium.** Magnesium is an important mineral for muscles, bones and connective tissues. And since leafy green vegetables are a good source of magnesium, I've created a Magnesium Medley Salad. To make it, include any of the following ingredients to which you have access, in whatever amounts are pleasing to you: fresh purslane, green beans, spinach and lettuce. And throw some poppy seeds into the dressing; they also contain magnesium.

❧ **Stinging nettle (*Urtica dioica*).** This silicon-rich herb has strong folkloric support as a treatment for gout and rheumatism, which means it's long been used to treat inflammatory conditions that affect the joints. So it seems promising as a treatment for bursitis and tendinitis as well.

❧ **Turmeric (*Curcuma longa*).** Joseph Pizzorno, N.D., president of Bastyr University in Seattle, and naturopath Michael Murray, N.D., co-authors of *A Textbook of Natural Medicine*, are just two of the herbal scholars who note that curcumin, a compound abundant in turmeric, has proved as effective as cortisone in the treatment of some kinds of inflammation. They suggest taking both 250 to 500 milligrams of curcumin and 250 milligrams of bromelain three times a day, between meals.

You can purchase these isolated compounds in natural food stores, but I have a suggestion that you might enjoy more. Try preparing ripe pineapple, for bromelain, with turmeric, for a generous amount of curcumin. Come to think of it, a fruit cocktail made of pineapple and papaya spiced with ginger and turmeric would taste pretty darn good.

I always take a whole-foods approach whenever possible. I think that generally, whole foods have more healing power going for them than any individual ingredients that have been isolated from them.

Cancer Prevention

It gives me great pleasure to be alive and well in my late sixties. I must admit that I had a hard time during my 65th year. You see, I was haunted by one disturbing health statistic in my family. My father and two of his brothers all died at age 65 of colon cancer or cancer of the gastrointestinal tract. Now it so happens that they also retired at that age, so I decided that I was going to try another tactic. Maybe if I didn't retire, I wouldn't die, either. So I worked another year at the U.S. Department of Agriculture (USDA) and made it to 66 without developing colon cancer.

In truth, I think I do know why my dad and uncles developed their cancers and I did not. They all grew up as good old boys in rural Alabama, eating what rednecks used to eat—a high-fiber, low-fat country diet. But then they became successful insurance salesmen and began eating more meat and potatoes (more meat than potatoes).

I think that changing their diet like that killed them. It's as simple as that. It was especially bad that they abandoned the cornbread, peas, cabbage, green beans, lima beans and collard and turnip greens of their youth. Rebellious son that I am, I cut way down on the meats and returned to all the high-fiber, low-fat foods that my dad had stopped eating. It turns out that this is a diet rich in cancer-preventing chemicals from plants (phytochemicals).

Food as Preventive Medicine

You're probably expecting me to discuss a number of individual herbs in this chapter, as I do in all the other chapters, but I simply can't do that here. One definition of *herb*—the one I favor—is any plant that can be used as a healing agent. As our understanding of the healing power of plants continues to grow, so does the number of plants that can be called herbs. If these days the definition embraces many of our foods, so be it.

When it comes to preventing cancer, the key seems to be eating as wide a variety of fruits and vegetables as possible. In a sense, then, if you want to lower your risk of cancer, you can create a whole diet—excluding or minimizing meats and dairy products—that consists of healing herbs. So singling out individual plants would be giving you a false picture of how to use herbs to prevent cancer.

I was one of the first of the high-fiber "flakes," back before nutritionists discovered the importance of what they used to call roughage. As a matter of fact, my everyday diet turned out to be higher in fiber than the high-fiber diets that were fed to the volunteers in five formal USDA studies. I know, because I was one of the subjects in those studies.

Of course, I can't *prove* that my dad's high-fat diet killed him, nor that my plant-based diet has spared me from becoming a cancer statistic. But the research is very clear. As fat and meat consumption increases, cancer rates rise. But as fruit and vegetable consumption increases, thereby lowering fat in the diet and increasing the amount of fiber and helpful phytochemicals, cancer rates fall.

Fighting the Wrong Battles

The National Cancer Institute (NCI) has been waging its war on cancer for 30 years now. But in every year reported up until 1996, cancer deaths were increasing, according to NCI statistics. Some of the increases have to do with the fact that fewer people are dying of heart disease and stroke, so they live long enough to get cancer. But considering all the money and all the effort this country has invested in beating cancer, we don't have a whole lot to show for it.

❧❧
Lifestyle Keys to Locking Out Cancer

Cancer prevention involves many of the same wise moves involved in preventing many other diseases. You should make the effort to get:

• More vegetables and fruits, less fat and red meat.
• Greater variety in your diet, less monotony.

- More cereals and whole grains, less processed sugar.
- More natural food colors, fewer artificial colors.
- More herbal spices, fewer artificial flavorings.
- More natural, whole foods, fewer processed foods.
- More estrogen-like chemicals from plants (phyto-estrogens), fewer synthetic hormones.
- More fruit and vegetable juices, fewer alcoholic beverages.
- More fresh air, less smoke- and pollution-filled air.
- More tranquillity, less stress.
- More exercise, less television.
- More public greenery, less pavement.
- More organic gardens and farms, fewer pesticides.
- More herbal alternatives, fewer pharmaceutical "magic bullets."

❦

Over the years, many new chemotherapy drugs have been developed, and some work pretty well to extend life, although they don't cure cancer. And some of the best of those new chemotherapeutics come from plants: Taxol, a treatment for ovarian and breast cancer, originally from the Pacific yew tree; etoposide, a treatment for testicular cancer and small-cell lung cancer, from the mayapple; and vinblastine and vincristine, which treat Hodgkin's disease, leukemias and lymphomas, both from the Madagascar periwinkle.

But as far as I'm concerned, something is very wrong with the way the NCI has approached cancer. The vast majority of NCI research money—our tax dollars—has gone for the development of chemotherapeutics, with comparatively little devoted to prevention.

Chemotherapeutics have their place in the grand scheme of things, but they're not cures. They are usually life-extenders that add a few months or years to average survival. But those months or years are often lower-quality time because of the many side effects that chemotherapy drugs cause.

From 1977 to 1982, I was involved with the NCI's cancer

screening program, a multiyear effort that investigated the cancer treatment potential of thousands of plant compounds and gave us the ones mentioned above. I've also been involved with the embryonic Designer Food Program of the National Institutes of Health (NIH), which is attempting to design foods high in healthful phytochemicals that prevent cancer.

I have a greater respect for the potential of the food program than I do for the results of the drug-finding program. Clearly, cancer prevention programs can save more lives than treatment programs can, and at a fraction of the cost. Still the 30-year-old cure-oriented war on cancer gets the most tax dollars, while prevention programs get very little.

ᡒᡈ·ᡈᢣ

Strive-for-Fiveade

I recently concocted a most attractive Fiveade. First I diced one apple, two carrots and sections of one lime and one pink grapefruit. Then I tossed them in the blender and just covered them with water. The resulting beverage was the color of orange sherbet, just like the artificial orange sherbet my dad used to buy me in Durham.

By drinking the Fiveade for breakfast, I did all of my striving for five before lunch. Then I made another batch and divided it: I froze some like sherbert and some as ice pops with sticks. I can't wait to try it on my grandkids. They would want it sweeter, I'm sure, but I could fool them with stevia, an herb that's a good substitute for sugar and artificial sweetener. It's available in herb shops; you can open a tea bag and add a pinch to beverages.

ᡒᡈ·ᡈᢣ

Almost all of my documents on cancer have to do with prevention. Yes, by all means, let us develop effective, gentle treatments, but I think it's more important, and more cost-effective, to work to prevent this disease.

Green Pharmacy for Cancer Prevention

Twenty years ago, long before scientists reached a consensus on the fact that a diet high in fruits and vegetables helps prevent cancer, and long before the NIH began urging everyone to "strive for five"—five servings of fruits and vegetables a day—*Prevention* magazine asked me for ideas on cancer prevention. I came up with several: a big green salad or coleslaw (coleslaw being a redneck favorite in my family), a big bowl of mine-strone soup and a Cancer Prevention Herbal Salad.

I'm sure you know how to make a fine green salad, and plenty of good slaw and minestrone recipes are available, so I won't dwell on them here except to say that it's impossible to use too many different vegetables. Try to include as great a variety of fruits and vegetables in these dishes—and in your diet—as you possibly can.

My herbal salad recipe is a little more obscure, so I'll discuss it more fully.

🍀🍀🍀 **Cancer Prevention Herbal Salad.** At the core of the recipe are several plants I lifted (with thanks) from Jonathan Hartwell's ethnobotanical classic *Plants Used against Cancer*, a compendium of about 3,000 plants cited in the medical-folk-loric literature for treating cancer. More than half of Hartwell's plants turned out to contain a compound useful in the treatment of some types of cancers, at least in the test tube.

My Cancer Prevention Herbal Salad now includes garlic, onions, red peppers, tomatoes, red clover flowers, chopped cooked beets, fresh calendula flowers, celery, fresh chicory flowers, chives, cucumbers, cumin, peanuts, pokesalad, purslane and sage.

In addition, I came up with a cancer prevention dressing to use with this salad. It includes flaxseed oil, evening primrose oil, garlic, rosemary, a dash of lemon juice and that Latin American favorite, hot peppers.

Fifteen years after I developed my salad, late in 1989, Herbert Pierson, Ph.D., of the NIH called to invite my participation in the Designer Food Program for cancer prevention. This was a major national effort to manipulate foods to increase their content of nutraceuticals (nutrients with medicinal value). The idea was to enhance the amount of cancer-fighting chemicals in foods, either by manipulating the plants' genes or by coming up with necessary techniques that would preserve or enhance the desired medicinal effects.

Dr. Pierson was most interested in my database of medicinal phytochemicals in food plants and herbs, which includes anti-cancer compounds—the same ever-evolving database on which this book is based. He invited me to attend a meeting where experts would explain the cancer-prevention benefits of various plants.

Imagine my delight when my colleagues and fellow researchers spoke about the anti-cancer phytochemicals that they were finding in plants. My fellow scientists gave presentations on the sulfides in garlic, the capsaicin in red peppers, the limonene in citrus fruits and the lycopene in tomatoes. They touted the cancer-fighting potential of such herbs as flax, licorice and rosemary. (Ever since that conference, I've been adding rosemary to my salad dressing.)

The Designer Food Program clearly had a lot going for it. I got excited about the program and eagerly anticipated five years of helping the NIH in this area. But alas, Dr. Pierson left the NIH, and the program now seems much less visible and exciting.

Fortunately, research on the medicinal potential of foods is going forward in other programs and institutions throughout the nation. Over the next several years, you'll be hearing a lot more about nutraceuticals, phytochemicals and meals that heal. Foods and traditional medicinal herbs clearly have healing properties, including the ability to prevent cancer.

Canker Sores

Early American settlers introduced myrrh to the New World. Although most of us associate myrrh with the Christmas tale of the Three Wise Men's gifts to the baby Jesus, these early settlers weren't carrying myrrh for religious purposes. They used it as a treatment for canker sores and other kinds of mouth sores, according to Walter Lewis, Ph.D., and Memory Elvin-Lewis, Ph.D., both professors at Washington University in St. Louis and co-authors of the classic book, *Medical Botany*.

Canker sores are painful, craterlike ulcers that form in the mouth or on the inner lips. Also known as aphthous ulcers, canker sores usually clear up by themselves within a week or so, but they often recur, sometimes in the form of multiple sores. Estimates vary, but somewhere between 20 and 50 percent of Americans know the pain of canker sores.

Folk Treatments: The Way to Go

Doctors don't have much to offer people with canker sores. They often prescribe antibiotics or corticosteroids, medications that help relieve pain and inflammation. But neither of these treatments helps much. So even doctors tend to recommend traditional relief—ice to alleviate the pain and rinsing the mouth with warm saltwater several times a day.

Doctors also suggest eliminating things that sometimes trigger or aggravate canker sores, such as alcohol, chewing gum, citrus fruits, coffee, dairy products, meat, pineapple, spicy foods, tomatoes, toothpaste and vinegar and other acidic foods. (If you're not sure which foods are acidic, just put anything that tastes sour on the list.)

Doctors also suggest avoiding anything that you happen to be allergic to. People often indulge in "just a taste" of something to which they know they have a mild allergy, but nibbling these "forbidden" foods is a notorious cause of canker sores.

Green Pharmacy for Canker Sores

I'm all for using ice and rinsing your mouth with saltwater. And I think it's a great idea—as well as obvious—to avoid possible canker sore triggers whenever possible. I myself would also try these herbal alternatives.

Myrrh (*Commiphora*, various species). Myrrh is more than just a folk remedy for canker sores. Germany's Commission E, the body of scientists that provides advice on herbal matters, has endorsed powdered myrrh for the treatment of mild inflammations of the mouth and throat because it contains high amounts of tannins.

Tannin, the common name for tannic acid, is a constituent of many plants and gives foods an astringent taste. An antiseptic with broad-spectrum antibacterial and antiviral action, it's especially helpful for treating mouth sores, which could be caused by a bacterium, a fungus, a virus or an allergy.

To use powdered myrrh, just open a capsule (available at health food stores) and dab a little directly on the sore.

❧❧ **Tea (*Camellia sinensis*).** Myrrh isn't the only herb that's high in tannin: Regular beverage tea also has a rich supply. Try placing a spent tea bag on your canker sores. Or make tea from some of the other herbs that are high in tannin, such as bearberry, eucalyptus, St.-John's-wort, sage, raspberry, peppermint and licorice.

❧ **Cankerroot (*Coptis groenlandica*).** This plant got its name because of its traditional use as a treatment for canker sores. American Indians and early settlers alike used cankerroot as a tea to treat both sore throat and canker sores. Penobscot Indians chewed raw root for canker sores and fever blisters.

The plant, which is also known as goldthread, shares many of the active ingredients and healing properties of the more familiar goldenseal, barberry and Oregon grape.

❧ **Goldenseal (*Hydrastis canadensis*).** This herb was an American Indian favorite for treating all sorts of wounds. When scientists looked at this herb, they found that the Indians were on to something. It turns out that goldenseal contains astringent, antiseptic chemicals that help treat wounds and infections.

To make a canker sore mouthwash, use two teaspoons of dried goldenseal per cup of boiling water and steep until cool. Use it as a mouth rinse three or four times a day. Barberry and Oregon grape have similar constituents and healing effects.

❧ **Licorice (*Glycyrrhiza glabra*).** In one study that looked at the power of licorice to heal canker sores, a mouthwash containing this herb provided relief for 75 percent of the people who used it. Those who got relief noted substantial improvement within one day and complete healing by the third day. This study was cited by Melvyn Werbach, M.D., assistant clinical professor of psychiatry at the University of California, Los Angeles, School of Medicine, in his insightful book *Nutritional Influences on Illness*.

In addition to tannin, licorice has two other things going for it: the compounds glycyrrhetinic-acid and glycyrrhizin, both of which help speed the healing of sores. You might sweeten the teas recommended here with licorice.

❧ **Sage (*Salvia officinalis*).** Although it is not among the richest sources of tannin, many herbalists suggest making a strong sage tea to treat inflammations of the mouth and throat. To make this tea, use two teaspoons of dried herb per cup of boiling water. Let it steep until cool and then gargle with it.

You should not drink too much of this tea. Sage contains a fair amount of thujone, a compound that in very high doses may cause convulsions. Although sage is an excellent healing herb, and weak sage tea preparations are recommended elsewhere in this book, sage is just one of those things—like aspirin—that is good in small amounts and not so good in large amounts.

❧ **Wild geranium (*Geranium maculatum*).** The root of this common plant was well-used medicinally by American Indians and early settlers. The Cherokee, for example, used it as an astringent to stop the bleeding of open wounds and as a wash to treat canker sores. Given its wide folk use to treat mouth sores, I think this high-tannin herb is worth trying.

Cardiac Arrhythmia

A very frightened father called me asking for help. His six-year-old daughter had been diagnosed with a seriously irregular heartbeat (cardiac arrhythmia).

Arrhythmias are much worse than the more common heart palpitations, a condition in which the heart occasionally seems to skip a beat or two. Heart palpitations are often minor and self-correcting. Cardiac arrhythmias are not. They often don't normalize by themselves, and they can lead to a potentially fatal heart attack. Arrhythmias are usually diagnosed in people over 50, but here was a father telling me that his little girl had this problem.

He told me that his daughter had been taking a calcium channel blocker, a standard type of heart medication, but that it hadn't helped. "Oh, no," I thought. "Now you want to switch to an herbal medicine, and you want me to tell you which one and how much to take."

So I took a breath and was about to deliver my usual spiel: "I don't prescribe, especially for something as potentially serious as cardiac arrhythmia. See your doctor."

But it turned out that when the calcium channel blocker

didn't do the trick, the daughter's doctor, of all people, had suggested adding a few natural alternatives to her treatment regimen: hawthorn, coenzyme Q_{10} and magnesium.

The Natural Route

The herb hawthorn is a traditional heart tonic. And coenzyme Q_{10} and magnesium have been shown in several studies to help the heart. The father followed the doctor's advice, and he said that the natural approach was working better than the calcium channel blocker had. But now that the daughter was taking hawthorn regularly, the father was naturally concerned about its potential long-term toxicity.

❧

Improving the Beat

In addition to herbs, a healthy lifestyle helps prevent and treat arrhythmia. Here are the basics.
• Eat a low-fat diet.
• Exercise regularly.
• Don't smoke.
• Manage your stress.
• Manage your blood pressure and cholesterol levels.

Unless you have some medical reason to avoid alcohol, by all means have one or two drinks a day. Some 30 studies suggest that this level of alcohol consumption reduces heart attack risk by 25 to 40 percent. But don't exceed that two-drink limit: Heavier drinking may increase the risk of heart disease.

❧

I went to my database and reference books and faxed him what I could find. Hawthorn appeared to be safe for long-term use, but I learned that most people who use it for heart problems (primarily Europeans) are older adults, not children. Curiously, none of my sources at hand said that hawthorn helped treat arrhythmias. In fact, one source said it might cause them. But I found no case reports of heart attacks resulting from using this herb, so I told the worried father that I'd rather give my daughter hawthorn than a calcium channel blocker.

A few months later, the girl's father called again, elated, to share his good news. Just in time for Christmas, his daughter was off the calcium channel blocker completely, thanks to the hawthorn, coenzyme Q_{10} and magnesium. At her last checkup, her doctor detected no arrhythmia at all. I suggested that he plant a hawthorn tree in his yard to show to people when he recounts his story.

Problems with Rhythm

Cardiac arrhythmia simply means that the heart rhythm is irregular, either too fast or too slow. When your heart beats too fast—more than 100 beats per minute—the condition is known as tachycardia. When it beats too slowly—fewer than 60 beats per minute—you have bradycardia.

Arrhythmias are also named according to the part of the heart that is affected. Atrial arrhythmias disturb the heart's ability to pump the blood from its upper chambers, which results in the "pooling" of blood. This stagnant blood can form clots and trigger heart attack or stroke. Ventricular arrhythmias, which affect the heart's larger, lower chambers, can lead to a condition called ventricular fibrillation, a condition in which the chambers quiver weakly instead of contracting vigorously. Ventricular fibrillation is the underlying cause of a substantial proportion of heart attack deaths.

Green Pharmacy for Cardiac Arrhythmia

Cardiac arrhythmia is a serious condition that should be treated by a physician. If I had it, I would certainly take the medications my doctor prescribed. But in consultation with my

physician—and many are increasingly open to herbal remedies—I might also try some medicinal herbs.

🌿🌿🌿 **Angelica (*Angelica archangelica*).** This herb contains
at least 14 anti-arrhythmic compounds, one of which is said to be
as active as verapamil (Calan, Isoptin), a popular calcium channel
blocker. I suggest taking angelica in the form of my Anti-arrhythmic Angelade. To make this tasty cocktail, put angelica, carrots,
celery, fennel, garlic and parsnips through your juicer. You may
have to add some water and spices to make it drinkable. Heavy
with carrots and garlic, it can be quite tasty. I suggest drinking one
or two eight-ounce glasses.

Celery contains calcium blockers and other plant chemicals
(phytochemicals) such as apigenin, apiin, magnesium and
potassium that help prevent and treat arrhythmias, plus other
compounds that help lower blood pressure and cholesterol.
Garlic also appears to be a potent anti-arrhythmic agent. In
studies, laboratory animals that ate garlic powder showed less
ventricular tachycardia and fibrillation.

🌿🌿🌿 **Cinchona (*Cinchona*, various species).** This is the
source of quinine, which is famous as a treatment for malaria.
Quinine started to gain attention as a remedy for heart problems
about a century ago. Legend has it that a Dutch merchant with
atrial fibrillation consulted several doctors, who told him there
was no remedy. He sought his own remedy and took a gram of
quinine. When he returned to his doctors the next day, so the
story goes, his pulse was regular.

The key compound is quinidine, now a standard anti-arrhythmic medication. Quinidine is not the only helpful compound in
the herb, however; there are more than a dozen. Since you get
a few of these compounds when you drink tonic water, I'd drink
plenty of tonic if I had arrhythmia.

🌿🌿🌿 **Hawthorn (*Crataegus*, various species).** Hawthorn is
a centuries-old heart tonic, and modern research has confirmed
its traditional use. Many studies show that it helps prevent heart
problems, gently strengthening the heart muscle, improving
blood circulation through the heart and reducing the heart's
need for oxygen. It also helps the heart circulate blood with less
effort.

Naturopathic physicians recommend taking standardized
extracts. The kind of extracts is important, and I'm going to
include these details so that you can discuss them with your
physician and make sure you are getting the right herbal med-

ication if your doctor gives you the go-ahead to try this. (Notice that naturopaths do not recommend using raw hawthorn. Also note that many states do not require naturopaths to be licensed. If you have any hint of a heart condition, you *must* look into your naturopath's credentials and training. If you're not sure whether to proceed, discuss it with your regular physician.)

The recommended extracts contain 1.8 percent vitexin-4-rhamnoside or 10 percent oligomeric procyanidins (OPCs) in dosages of 120 to 240 milligrams three times a day. If the extracts are standardized to 18 percent OPCs, the recommended dosage is 240 to 480 milligrams once a day. To obtain these extracts, you must consult a naturopath.

There have been scattered reports that hawthorn may increase arrhythmias in some cases. I don't put much stock in these reports, but it's better to be safe than sorry. You really need to be monitored by a doctor if you try this herb.

✴✴ Canola (*Brassica*, various species). Australian cardiologists have shown that dietary canola oil helps prevent cardiac arrhythmias in laboratory animals. I bet that it would also help in people.

✴✴ Khella (*Ammi majus*). Khella is the source of amiodarone (Cordarone), one of the key anti-arrhythmia medications. London cardiologist Arthur Hollman, M.D., tells the story of the development of this drug in his book *Cardiology from Nature*, which is a tribute to the powers of natural medicine.

Back in 1946, a technician in the medical research laboratory of G. V. Anrepin, M.D., developed a kidney problem and treated himself with a Middle Eastern herbal remedy, khella.

As fate would have it, the technician also had angina, which improved dramatically while he was taking the herb. Intrigued by this unexpected benefit, Dr. Anrepin studied the plant and isolated its active ingredient, khellin. Further work elsewhere led to the development of khellin-derived amiodarone, which was originally used to treat angina. Eventually, in 1974, its unique anti-arrhythmic activity was discovered.

It is possible to get some benefit from taking the herb itself to treat arrhythmia. The usual recommendation calls for pouring boiling water over about a quarter-teaspoon of powdered khella fruits. Steep for five minutes and drink the tea after straining.

✴ Astragalus (*Astragalus*, various species). Also known as *huang qi*, astragalus is best known as an immune stimulant. According to California herbalist Kathi Keville, author of *The

Illustrated Herb Encyclopedia and *Herbs for Health and Healing*, it is also a heart tonic that helps prevent and treat arrhythmia. You can try a tea made with one to two teaspoons of dried herb steeped in boiling water.

❦ **Barberry (*Berberis vulgaris*).** Barberry is best known as an herbal antibiotic because it contains berberine, a compound also found in goldenseal. Berberine also helps prevent and treat ventricular arrhythmias, according to Melvyn Werbach, M.D., assistant clinical professor of psychiatry at the University of California, Los Angeles, School of Medicine and author of *Nutritional Influences on Illness*.

In one Chinese study, berberine reduced ventricular arrhythmias by more than 50 percent in more than half of the people who used it. In addition to goldenseal, other herbs with berberine include Oregon grape and goldthread.

The best way to take this herb is to buy a standardized herbal extract at a health food store or herb shop and follow the package directions. It is possible to make a tea using a teaspoon or two of the dried herb to a cup of boiling water.

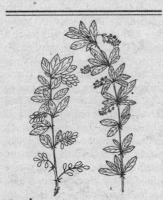

Barberry

Along with its close relative Oregon grape, barberry may stimulate the immune system and help fight damage from free radicals.

❦ **Ginkgo (*Ginkgo biloba*).** Ginkgo is a favorite Chinese heart tonic. I know of no studies showing that ginkgo has anti-arrhythmic effects, but like hawthorn, it improves blood flow to the heart and lessens coronary demand for oxygen, thus reducing shortness of breath and chest pain. If I had an arrhythmia, I would include ginkgo among my herbal treatments.

You can buy ginkgo extracts at many health food stores; follow the package directions. You can try 60 to 240 milligrams a day, but don't go any higher. In large amounts, ginkgo may cause diarrhea, irritability and restlessness.

❦ **Horehound (*Marrubium vulgare*).** Horehound is best known as a treatment for coughs and colds because the two key compounds it contains, marrubiin and marrubic acid, are good expectorants. But these compounds also have a normalizing effect on heart rhythm. You can make a tea using two to three teaspoons of the herb and drink a cup after lunch and dinner.

❦ **Motherwort (*Leonurus cardiaca*).** With a name like *cardiaca*, this herb might be expected to help heart problems, and science confirms that it does. Chinese studies show that it slows a rapid heartbeat, generally improving cardiac activity. It also helps tranquilize the nervous system, reducing the anxiety, nervous tension and stress that may accompany or trigger heart problems.

The Chinese reportedly consume as much as nine ounces (250 grams) a day. That sounds like a bit much to me. I'd suggest trying about a half-ounce in three cups of boiling water for two or three days to see if it helps.

❦ **Purslane (*Portulaca oleracea*) and other plants containing magnesium.** According to estimates I've seen, more than 70 percent of Americans may get insufficient magnesium. Maybe that's why we have so much arrhythmia. Scientists note that magnesium, at doses of 250 milligrams a day, helps prevent cardiac arrhythmia.

Purslane is very rich in magnesium (nearly 2 percent on a dry-weight basis). Green beans, poppy seeds, oats, cowpeas and spinach are also good sources. In season, I cook purslane like spinach and eat several ounces at a time.

❦ **Reishi (*Ganoderma lucidum*).** Sixteenth-century Ming Dynasty texts say that this marvelous Chinese medicinal mushroom "mends the heart." And my good friend, pharmacognosist (natural product pharmacist) Albert Leung, Ph.D., says in his *Better Health with (Mostly) Chinese Herbs and Food* that reishi has considerable value in preventing and treating arrhythmia.

Reishi is a heart tonic, like hawthorn and ginkgo. It improves blood flow to the heart, reduces coronary demand for oxygen and helps ease the chest pain of angina. I make reishi tea using three to six teaspoons of dried herb per cup of boiling water.

❦ **Scotch broom (*Cytisus scoparius*).** This herb is useful as a heart tonic, according to Commission E, the German expert committee that judges the safety and effectiveness of herbal medicines. The principal active constituent is an anti-arrhythmic compound, sparteine.

You can make a tea using one teaspoon of dried herb per cup

of boiling water. Drink up to two cups a day. One note of caution: Scotch broom also contains the compound tyramine, which means that it should not be used with the class of antidepressant medications known as MAO inhibitors. If you take an antidepressant, find out if it's an MAO inhibitor, and if it is, don't use this herb.

❧ **Valerian** (*Valeriana officinalis*). Valerian is best known as an herbal sleep aid, and with good reason. But herbal pharmacologist Daniel Mowrey, Ph.D., author of *The Scientific Validation of Herbal Medicine* and *Herbal Tonic Therapies*, says that valerian also contains proven anti-arrhythmic compounds. In fact, this herb was used for arrhythmias and palpitations in Roman times.

Valerian also has other heart benefits: It lowers blood pressure, increases blood flow to the heart and improves the heart's pumping ability.

This herb smells pretty foul, but in spite of this, I'd try a tea made with one to two teaspoons of dried herb per cup of boiling water. Drink two to three cups a day. If you can't handle the taste, try capsules or a tincture instead. Both the dried herb and tincture are available at health food stores or herb shops. Follow the package directions.

Carpal Tunnel Syndrome

K athi Keville is a California herbalist whom I like and respect. Like me, she often spends days chained to her computer. Unlike me, she developed carpal tunnel syndrome (CTS), caused by compression of the nerve that passes through the "tunnel" formed by the wrist bones. The symptoms of CTS are pain, weakness, finger stiffness and a pins-and-needles sensation.

As Keville's CTS went from bad to worse, she had to give up her massage practice and stop playing the recorder because she lost so much sensation in her fingers. She could barely finish typing the manuscript for her book, *The Illustrated Herb Ency-*

clopedia. Finally, her CTS got so bad that she lost the ability to turn the doorknob to her house.

That's when Keville got a gentle reminder from an herbalist friend about practicing what she preached. She adopted an aggressive natural healing program. She consulted an excellent osteopath, who manipulated her wrists and encouraged her to exercise, use more herbs and manage her stress more effectively. She received regular massages with relaxing aromatherapy oils. She took her own herbal nerve pain formula and also slathered liberal amounts of herbal oils on her wrists throughout the day.

Her recovery was slow, but she did recover, and without the wrist surgery that is frequently performed for CTS.

Repetitive Movements Hit Home

I may use a computer as much as Keville, or even more—sometimes as much as 14 hours a day. Why haven't I developed CTS?

Being a man is certainly a factor. Women develop carpal tunnel problems more than men do because the cyclical hormone fluctuations of the menstrual cycle, pregnancy and menopause can contribute to swelling of the tissues surrounding the carpal tunnel. But I also think my hand exercises have something to do with it. Adopting a Chinese technique that improves flexibility, I hold two steel balls in one hand and roll them around when I'm not typing. The Chinese balls provide a gentle form of exercise, and the rolling motion massages the tiny

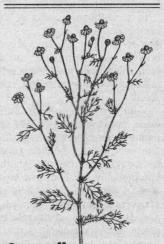

Camomile
Camomile flowers are used to make a sleep-inducing tincture and a tea with anti-inflammatory properties.

muscles and ligaments of the hands and wrists. When I'm at the computer, I take frequent breaks to twirl the Chinese balls in each hand.

Carpal tunnel syndrome is considered a repetitive motion injury—cumulative trauma associated with constant rapid use of the fingers (low-intensity, high-frequency finger work). CTS has been around for decades, the occupational hazard of bookkeepers and supermarket checkout clerks who punched buttons all day long. But it did not become a household word until the 1980s, when personal computers came to dominate so many workplaces. Suddenly millions of people's jobs required the kind of steady, rapid finger movements that can cause repetitive motion injuries like CTS. It is also a problem for some musicians, factory workers and other people who must constantly use their hands.

Green Pharmacy for Carpal Tunnel Syndrome

Fortunately, there are quite a few herbs that can help alleviate this problem.

🌿🌿🌿 **Willow (Salix, various species).** Willow bark, the original source of aspirin, contains chemicals (salicylates) that both relieve pain and reduce inflammation. You might also try other herbs rich in salicylates, notably meadowsweet and wintergreen.

With any of these herbs, I'd steep one to two teaspoons of dried, powdered bark or five teaspoons of fresh bark for ten minutes or so, then strain out the plant material. You can add lemonade to mask the bitter taste and drink two to three cups of tea a day. Remember, though, that if you're allergic to aspirin, you probably shouldn't take aspirin-like herbs, either.

🌿🌿 **Camomile (Matricaria recutita).** Camomile tea is best known as a tasty way to calm jangled nerves. But its active compounds (bisabolol, chamazulene and cyclic ethers) also have potent anti-inflammatory action. Camomile is widely used in Europe for many inflammatory diseases. If I had CTS, I'd drink several cups of camomile tea a day.

🌿🌿 **Pineapple (Ananas comosus).** Pineapple contains a protein-dissolving (proteolytic) enzyme, bromelain, that is often recommended for CTS.

"Bromelain has well-documented effects on virtually all inflammatory conditions, regardless of cause," according to naturopaths Joseph Pizzorno, N.D., president of Bastyr University in Seattle, and Michael Murray, N.D., co-authors of *A Textbook of Natural Medicine*. "Bromelain can reduce swelling, inflammation and pain. Bromelain is extremely safe to use. In human studies, very large doses (nearly two grams) have been given without side effects."

Naturopaths suggest taking 250 to 1,500 milligrams of pure bromelain a day, between meals, to treat inflammatory conditions such as CTS. Bromelain is available at many health food stores. Since I favor food sources, however, I prefer to get my bromelain from pineapple itself. Ginger and papaya also contain helpful proteolytic enzymes. You might enjoy a Proteolytic CTS Fruit Salad composed of pineapple and papaya and spiced with grated ginger.

❧❧ **Red pepper (*Capsicum*, various species).** Also known as cayenne, red pepper contains six pain-relieving compounds and seven that are anti-inflammatory. Especially noteworthy is capsaicin. Commercial salves containing capsaicin, such as Zostrix and Capzasin-P, are widely used to treat pain.

I would try this herb if I had CTS. You might add several teaspoons of powdered cayenne to a quarter-cup of skin lotion and rub it on your wrists. Or you could make a capsaicin lotion by steeping five to ten red peppers in two pints of rubbing alcohol for a few days. Just wash your hands thoroughly after using any topical capsaicin treatment, as you don't want to get it in your eyes. Also, since some people are quite sensitive to this compound, you should test it on a small area of skin before using it on a larger area. If it seems to irritate your skin, discontinue use.

I'd also suggest adding a few drops of lavender oil to your red-pepper salve. Lavender oil is a mainstay of aromatherapy, useful for treating inflammation and burns. Its aroma is also quite relaxing, which helps when you're feeling the pain of CTS.

❧❧ **Turmeric (*Curcuma longa*).** This herb contains curcumin, a potent anti-inflammatory chemical. Some studies suggest that curcumin is only about half as effective as the pharmaceutical anti-inflammatory medication cortisone, but consider that cortisone is expensive and can have nasty side effects. Turmeric is much easier on the system and the pocketbook, not to mention a lot tastier.

Naturopaths suggest taking 250 to 500 milligrams of pure curcumin a day, between meals. Dried turmeric contains about

1 to 4 percent curcumin, so to get the dose that naturopaths recommend, you would have to consume 10 to 50 grams (5 to 25 teaspoons) of dried turmeric. That's a lot more than even I would add to a curried rice dish. Instead, try using turmeric liberally on food and then taking some more in capsules.

❦ Comfrey (*Symphytum officinale*). My good friends, pharmacognosist (natural product pharmacist) Albert·Leung, Ph.D., and noted Arkansas herbalist and photographer Steven Foster, in their excellent *Encyclopedia of Common Natural Ingredients*, explain that applying comfrey to the skin can help relieve pain, swelling and inflammation. This has been confirmed through studies using laboratory animals. The active compounds are allantoin and rosmarinic acid.

Comfrey has gotten a lot of bad press in recent years because it also contains pyrrolizidine alkaloids, compounds that may cause liver damage when the herb is ingested. But there's no evidence that comfrey is risky when applied to the skin, which is what I would suggest for CTS (and arthritis). Add a few teaspoons of dried, powdered comfrey to the recipe mentioned above for red pepper or to any favorite skin cream.

❦ Cumin (*Cuminum cyminum*). Cumin is used liberally in Mexican foods. My former U.S. Department of Agriculture colleague, molecular biologist Stephen Beckstrom-Sternberg, Ph.D., and I once studied the properties of this spice and discovered seven pain-relieving compounds, three that are anti-inflammatory and four that combat swelling. If I had CTS, I'd use lots of cumin on food and add it to my curried rice.

❦ Sage (*Salvia officinalis*). Dr. Beckstrom-Sternberg and I identified six anti-inflammatory compounds in sage. If I had CTS, I'd use this spice liberally in all sorts of foods, not just turkey stuffing.

❦ Foods high in vitamin B_6. Naturopaths suggest getting 40 to 80 milligrams of vitamin B_6 twice a day to treat CTS. In one study of people with this condition, two-thirds of those using this amount of B_6 reported improvement.

Foods high in B_6 include cauliflower, watercress, spinach, bananas and okra. It would be difficult to get enough B_6 to treat CTS solely from food. If you have this condition, you might consider a supplement. The Daily Value is only 2 milligrams, however, and getting too much of this vitamin has been linked to nerve disorders. If you'd like to try this therapy, please discuss it with your doctor.

Cataracts

Some time back, I published a magazine article entitled "Catnip and Cataracts," which explored the possibility that the herb most cats find intoxicating might also help prevent the common—and potentially blinding—eye disease. It was a speculative piece, and I played it that way, not making any big promises.

This notion is still speculative, but as time has passed, I've become increasingly persuaded that catnip is a three-star herb for cataract prevention. And I think several other herbs can help as well.

I should say right away that herbs can't cure cataracts. This condition is serious, and anyone with even the first hint of cataracts should definitely be under a doctor's care. But I do believe that herbs can help prevent them.

Clouded Vision

Cataracts are cloudy areas that develop in the normally clear lens of the eye. An estimated 20 percent of the world's population, mostly the elderly, has cataracts. Some four million Americans have sight-impairing cataracts, and at least 40,000 have become legally blind before receiving surgical treatment.

In the United States, cataracts afflict around 5 percent of those ages 52 to 64, 18 percent of those ages 65 to 74 and half of those 75 and older. But the faint beginnings of the condition can be detected in about three-quarters of Americans.

The mainstream medical treatment for cataracts is surgery. The clouded lens is removed from the eye, and an artificial one is inserted. More than 500,000 cataract operations are performed each year. They usually restore reasonably good vision, but they cost the nation a fortune—more than $3.5 billion a year.

Cloud Factors

Scientists used to think that cataracts were caused by old age, along with the bad luck of being susceptible to the condition. Then researchers noticed that certain groups are unusually likely to get cataracts. Smokers face a much greater than normal risk of developing the condition. Those with diabetes or heavy metal poisoning and people who have been using steroids for a long time are also at increased risk.

Now we know why. What clouds the eye lens is the damage from oxidation, a biochemical process set in motion when a highly reactive form of oxygen changes within our cells. Smoking and other risk factors all increase oxidative damage. According to one study, for instance, a group of women who smoked 30 cigarettes a day showed a 60 percent greater risk of developing cataracts.

Can anything prevent cataracts? You bet—antioxidants.

Antioxidants are chemical substances that prevent oxidative damage by neutralizing free radicals, the renegade oxygen molecules that are so damaging to the body. Among the best antioxidants is vitamin A, which we get from food in the form of carotenoids like beta-carotene. Other antioxidants include vitamins C and E, the vitamin-like flavonoids, and the mineral selenium.

Several studies have shown that diets rich in vitamins C and E help prevent cataracts. For example, one study showed that taking 1,000 milligrams of vitamin C a day can slow the development of cataracts. Which brings me back to my magazine article about catnip. Its leaves, and the leaves of many mint relatives like rosemary, contain generous amounts of vitamins C and E, some of which can be extracted in catnip tea or a mixed mint tea like my Cataractea.

In addition to antioxidants, the trace minerals magnesium and manganese appear to play a role in cataract prevention. Enzymes containing these minerals help dispose of proteins damaged by oxidation that contribute to eye clouding. Catnip and the other mints contain both of these essential trace minerals.

Finally, catnip and other mints are also rich in flavonoids, and several studies have now shown how important flavonoids are.

Although flavonoids have only recently been praised for

their properties, they were identified decades ago. Albert Szent-Gyorgyi, the researcher who first discovered vitamin C in 1928, was also a champion of flavonoids. He called them vitamin P.

Green Pharmacy for Cataracts

There are a number of herbs that can help prevent cataracts.

❧❧❧ **Bilberry (*Vaccinium myrtillus*).** As far back as World War I, British fliers munched bilberries before missions to sharpen their vision. Bilberry has many botanical relatives, including blueberry, cranberry and huckleberry, and similar chemicals occur in other fruits such as blackberry, raspberry, grape, plum and wild cherry. All have reputations for aiding vision.

Modern research shows that these fruits contain compounds known as anthocyanosides, which do indeed contribute to visual acuity. A group of Italian researchers showed that a mixture of anthocyanosides from bilberry plus vitamin E halted the progression of lens clouding in a remarkable 97 percent of people with early-stage cataracts.

Naturopaths recommend taking a standardized bilberry extract (containing 25 percent anthocyanidin) at a dose of 80 to 160 milligrams three times a day. This extract should be available wherever high-quality herbal formulations are sold.

I prefer a cup of blueberries, which are more readily available than bilberries. German herbalists suggest a tea made with two to four tablespoons of crushed blueberries.

❧❧❧ **Catnip (*Nepeta cataria*).** I'm not yet ready to say that catnip tea is guaranteed to prevent cataracts. But I think that two cups of catnip (or mint) tea a day should significantly reduce your likelihood of developing this problem.

Hot catnip tea in winter and iced catnip tea in summer are quite tasty. In addition to helping prevent cataracts, this herb is a mild tranquilizer, so not only will you stop worrying about cataracts quite as much, you'll also reduce your worries in general.

❧❧❧ **Rosemary (*Rosmarinus officinalis*).** A mint relative of catnip, rosemary contains more than a dozen antioxidants. It also contains at least four other known cataract fighters. That's why I include it in my Cararactea. I'd also suggest using rosemary liberally in cooking. It's especially good on roasted potatoes and is often used in chicken dishes.

❧❧ **Brazil nut (*Bertholettia excelsa*).** These nuts contain gen-

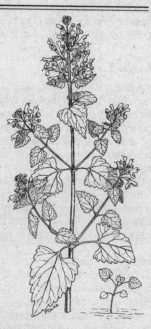

Catnip

Catnip, a member of the mint family, releases a distinctive aroma when it's made into an herbal tea.

erous amounts of vitamin E, plus the essential trace mineral selenium, which boosts vitamin E's antioxidant benefits. Selenium levels in the eye lenses of people with cataracts are a mere 15 percent of normal, suggesting that selenium supplementation or the selenium from Brazil nuts might help prevent cataracts. At least, it might slow their progression. The average Brazil nut contains the Daily Value for selenium.

✿✿ **Carrot (*Daucus carota*).** There's a fair amount of folklore that carrots are good for vision. As it turns out, it's more than folklore. One researcher at the pharmaceutical firm Hoffmann-La Roche cites more than 30 studies providing evidence that carotenoids help prevent what he calls the three Cs: cancer, cardiovascular disease and cataracts. Carotenoids (including beta-carotene) are the compounds that give carrots their orange color.

This conclusion is supported by a decade-long Harvard study indicating that by getting 50 milligrams of carotenoids every other day, you can significantly reduce the risk of cancer, cardiovascular disease and cataracts.

It would take seven good-size carrots to provide 50 milligrams of carotenoids. But if you don't like munching on carrots, whip up some of my Candied Carotenoids. Or simply eat more orange, yellow and dark green fruits and vegetables, all of which are high in carotenoids.

❧

Candied Carotenoids

If you're looking for a spectacular way to enjoy many of the eye-protecting yellow vegetables, this recipe can't be beat. In fact, take it to a Thanksgiving family potluck. Any elderly relatives with the beginnings of cataracts will be particularly interested in the recipe.

- 2 cups canned pumpkin
- 2 cups finely chopped orange sections
- 1½ cups pink grapefruit juice
- 1 cup chopped carrots
- 1 cup chopped sweet potatoes
- 2 teaspoons grated orange rind
  Dash of salt
  Dash of paprika
  Dash of turmeric
  Sugar (optional)
- 1 teaspoon grated coconut

In a large saucepan, combine the pumpkin, oranges, grapefruit juice, carrots, sweet potatoes, orange rind, salt, paprika and turmeric. Bring to a simmer over medium heat. Cover and cook for 20 minutes, or until the vegetables are tender.

Working in batches, transfer the mixture to a blender and puree. Return the mixture to the saucepan. Taste and add a small amount of sugar if needed. If the soup is too thin, simmer until it reaches the desired consistency. Serve sprinkled with the coconut.

Makes 6 servings

❧

❧❧ **Onion (*Allium cepa*).** Onion is one of our best sources of quercetin, a compound that has been shown in studies to help prevent cataracts in people with diabetes. While I suspect that it works for all kinds of cataracts, no research yet confirms this.

In any case, it's a good idea to use more onions. When you make stews and soups, leave the onion skin on while cooking to allow as much quercetin as possible to make its way into the food. Discard the skin before serving the dish.

Cataractea

Are you interested in protecting your vision as you age? Learn to enjoy this tea daily, and there's a good chance it will help you do just that.

To make the tea, boil two quarts of water. Remove from the heat and add one handful each of catnip, rosemary and lemon balm (also known as melissa). Add a few teaspoons of grated ginger and a dash or two of turmeric. Steep for 20 minutes and drink warm or cold with lemon juice and honey.

❧❧ **Purslane (*Portulaca oleracea*).** Purslane is high in all of the nutrients that help prevent cataracts—vitamin C, vitamin E, carotenoids and other potent antioxidants, notably one known as glutathione. Just a half-cup of fresh purslane contains healthy amounts of beta-carotene and vitamins C and E.

Fresh purslane can be awfully hard to come by if you don't grow it yourself. If you have a garden, however, you might consider including it in your next planting. I recently transplanted a thick bed of purslane seedlings to the main part of my garden. I'll eat it in soups and salads or like spinach for the rest of the year.

🌺🌺 **Turmeric (*Curcuma longa*).** In addition to good amounts of vitamins C and E and carotenoids, turmeric contains many other antioxidants. Turmeric is a key ingredient in many curry spice blends. Experiment with it in cooking.

🌺 **Capers (*Capparis spinosa*).** My own research at the U.S. Department of Agriculture with molecular biologist Stephen Beckstrom-Sternberg, Ph.D., shows that capers are a very rich source of cataract-preventing compounds known as aldose-reductose inhibitors. Use capers whenever you want extra zing in cooking.

🌺 **Ginger (*Zingiber officinale*).** Ginger is another good source of antioxidants. It also makes my Cataractea tastier.

Chronic Fatigue Syndrome

Fatigue used to be considered only a symptom, but in the last decade or so, chronic fatigue syndrome (CFS) has become one of the nation's most controversial illnesses. Depending on whom you talk to, this disease either doesn't exist at all or it's an epidemic.

All sorts of things have been fingered as causes: allergies, food intolerances, drug reactions, yeast infection, psychological problems and chronic infection with the Epstein-Barr virus (the culprit that causes mononucleosis), just to name a few.

According to some estimates, 3 million Americans—90 million people worldwide—suffer from the well-defined group of symptoms that seem to be associated with CFS. These symptoms, doctors say, include profound lethargy not alleviated by sleep, plus depression, headache, fevers, malaise, memory loss, mental confusion, poor concentration, pain and weakness of the joints and muscles, recurring infections, severe exhaustion from minor activities, sore throat, stomach distress and swollen lymph glands. Oddly enough, even the people who have all of these symptoms do not appear to be sick—doctors find little, if anything, wrong during a physical exam, and laboratory tests frequently fail to find any abnormalities.

The National Institutes of Health estimates that the people who are most at risk for CFS are white, middle-class women.

I believe CFS is a very real condition. I also agree with many experts in the field that it's very confusing. Any number of infections, allergies, foods, drugs, nutritional deficiencies and other illnesses might contribute to it. Because CFS is so multi-faceted, I shy away from anyone who claims to understand completely *the* cause or *the* cure.

I'd advise anyone with chronic fatigue to find a good physician who understands the condition and follow the doctor's advice to help explore all possible causes. To see what helps and what hurts you, by all means have your doctor test you for allergies, including food allergies.

One more note before we get to the herbs: Almost every CFS expert recommends trying a whole-food, vegetarian or near-vegetarian diet to see if it helps. Even if it doesn't cure your fatigue, it should reduce your risk of heart disease, cancer, obesity, high blood pressure and many other serious conditions. And any of these conditions will certainly contribute to chronic fatigue, even if they don't cause it.

Green Pharmacy for Chronic Fatigue Syndrome

There are a number of herbs that may prove helpful.

✺✺ Assorted antiviral herbs. Several herbalists I respect claim to relieve chronic fatigue successfully in a high percentage of people with combinations of antiviral herbs: echinacea, goldenseal, licorice, lemon balm (also known as melissa) and ginger. I think this approach is worth a try. You can make a blend of equal amounts of these herbs or use varying amounts, adjusting the blend to your personal taste. Make a tea using a teaspoon or two of your favorite blend and have a cup two or three times a day. Such herb teas can be energizing.

✺ Asian ginseng (*Panax ginseng*) and Siberian ginseng (*Eleutherococcus senticosus*). Commission E, the group of scientists that advises the German government about herbs, endorses ginseng "as a tonic to combat feelings of lassitude and debility, lack of energy and ability to concentrate, and during convalescence." The suggested daily dose is about one teaspoon steeped in a cup of boiling water to make a tea.

Clinical studies indicate that ginseng improves athletic performance, although it takes up to a month of regular use to notice this herb's benefits. Ginseng also stimulates the immune system, an effect that's been repeatedly confirmed in experiments with animals.

Revered in Asia for thousands of years as an energy-boosting tonic, ginseng is used today by Russian cosmonauts and Asian Olympic athletes as an "adaptogen," an herb that increases general resistance to all types of stress. It does this in addition to reducing fatigue and improving alertness, coordination, memory and stress-coping abilities.

AR. PHARM.

Asian Ginseng

A root primarily imported from China and Kenya, this type of ginseng won mythic renown for increasing longevity.

Some years ago, a co-worker asked if there were any caffeine in an "energy preparation" that he was taking to combat fatigue. The formula included damiana, ginseng, royal jelly and saw palmetto. He said it was really helping him, but he was afraid it was getting him up earlier in the morning. And when he woke up, he said, he had a tremendous urge to go to work.

Nope, I told him, no caffeine in there. But I added that ginseng can be quite a stimulant. I told him to keep taking it and to get up and work whenever the urge struck him. (Don't let that energy go to waste.)

❧ **Mate (*Ilex paraguayensis*).** Commission E approves using one to two teaspoons a day in tea for banishing mental and physical fatigue. Most of mate's energy-boosting activity comes from its caffeine content. While it may be good as an occasional picker-upper, however, I wouldn't recommend taking it daily to treat CFS.

❧ **Purslane (*Portulaca oleracea*) and other foods containing magnesium.** People who advocate juicing for health often stress the importance of getting magnesium from greens to boost stamina and energy. If you want to get more magnesium, try purslane, string beans, spinach, cowpeas, lettuce, stinging nettle, poppy seeds, licorice root and coriander.

You could just take a magnesium supplement (the Daily Value is 400 milligrams), but personally, I'd much rather eat a purslane/string bean/spinach salad with poppyseed dressing. With supplements, you get one mineral or a few plant chemicals (phytochemicals), but with whole herbs, you get every therapeutic phytochemical in the plant—possibly hundreds.

❧ **Spinach (*Spinacia oleracea*) and other foods containing folate.** Although I prefer to recommend that you get your vitamins and minerals from foods rather than supplements, deficiencies of folate (the naturally occurring form of folic acid) are quite common, and you might need a folic acid supplement. The average American consumes only 61 percent of the Daily Value of 400 micrograms of folate. Whether or not you take a supplement, however, don't neglect good food sources such as spinach, pinto beans, asparagus, broccoli, okra and brussels sprouts.

❧ **Wheatgrass (*Agropyron*, various species) and other grasses.** Juice advocates often recommend wheatgrass juice for fatigue. Personally, I think any juiced wholesome grass, including barley, oats, couchgrass or wheat, would be helpful.

Colds and Flu

Cathy Wilkinson Barash, a friend of mine who lives in Cold Spring Harbor, New York, is the author of *Edible Flowers: From Garden to Palate*. In a letter asking me to review her list of edible flowers before her book went to press, she mentioned: "I have followed the advice you gave me about echinacea when we met at the New York Botanical Garden dinner at Auntie Yuan's restaurant in Manhattan." My advice was to take echinacea at the first sign of sniffles, and Barash says she hasn't had a single cold since she started following that advice.

For centuries, American Indians of the Great Plains chewed

echinacea root or used it in tea to treat colds, flu and many other ailments. Over the last few years, publicity in many magazines has turned echinacea into the hottest health food store cold remedy.

Not too long ago, a leading health magazine heaped praise on echinacea as a cold remedy, quoting anecdotal evidence from several of my herbal buddies. Mark Blumenthal, executive director of the American Botanical Council in Austin, Texas, said, "I haven't had a cold in four years thanks to garlic, echinacea, astragalus and goldenseal." Steven Foster, noted Arkansas herbalist, photographer and co-author of *Encyclopedia of Common Natural Ingredients*, said, "I've gone two or three years without a cold or flu by taking echinacea." And herb advocate Andrew Weil, M.D., professor at the University of Arizona College of Medicine in Tucson and author of *Natural Health, Natural Medicine*, agreed: "Some years I don't get any . . . I eat raw garlic. I take echinacea."

Universal Sniffling and Sneezing

The common cold, an infection of the upper respiratory tract, is caused by any of 200 different viruses. The viral infection and the immune system's battle against it produce the all-too-familiar symptoms: sore throat, nasal congestion, runny nose, watery eyes, hacking cough and sometimes fever.

Colds are spread directly from person to person by coughing or sneezing or by hand-to-hand contact. The virus gets on one person's hands and can spread to the hands of others. If your virus-contaminated hands touch your nose or eyes, you catch the cold. The virus can also live for several hours on everyday surfaces like counters and doorknobs. Your hands can literally pick it up that way as well. (That's a good reason to wash your hands often during cold and flu season.)

The average American adult suffers two to three colds a year; the average young child has as many as nine. That adds up to something like one billion colds a year.

If you are getting more than your fair share of colds, your immune system may need help. Maybe the right herbs can help you as they have me. I definitely take these herbs, and I catch fewer colds than my wife and kids and grandkids.

Green Pharmacy for Colds and Flu

There are quite a few herbs that can help boost your immune system's cold-fighting power.

✺·✺·✺ Echinacea (*Echinacea*, various species). I use echinacea, also known as coneflower, myself. There's good research, most of it German, to show that it strengthens the immune system against cold viruses and many other germs as well. Echinacea increases levels of a chemical in the body called properdin, which activates the part of the immune system responsible for increasing defense mechanisms against viruses and bacteria.

Echinacea root extracts also possess antiviral activity against influenza, herpes and other viruses. In a study of 180 people with flu, one scientist found that 900 milligrams of an echinacea extract significantly reduced symptoms.

There's one odd thing about good echinacea: Shortly after ingesting a tea or tincture, it makes the tongue numb or tingly. Don't worry, though: This reaction is harmless.

But as effective as echinacea can be, it's no miracle cold cure. Even if you take this herb on a regular basis, you still might catch some colds. In fact, some herbalists caution that you should not use echinacea every day as an immune-enhancing tonic but should take it only when you feel a cold coming on or when those close to you have one. I'm still debating with myself on this.

✺·✺·✺ Garlic (*Allium sativum*). Eat enough garlic, and most people (along with their cold germs) will stay away from you. I'm just joking, and there really are some excellent reasons to use this herb to prevent colds and flu. Garlic contains several helpful compounds, including allicin, one of the plant kingdom's most potent, broad-spectrum antibiotics.

As anyone who has ever had garlic breath knows, this herb's aromatic compounds are readily released from the lungs and respiratory tract, putting garlic's active ingredients right where they can be most effective against cold viruses.

✺·✺·✺ Ginger (*Zingiber officinale*). Pouring a cup of boiling water onto a couple of tablespoons of fresh, shredded ginger root to make a good hot tea really makes a lot of sense as a cold treatment. That's because this herb contains nearly a dozen antiviral compounds.

Scientists have isolated several chemicals (sesquiterpenes) in ginger that have specific effects against the most common family of cold viruses, the rhinoviruses. Some of these chemicals are remarkably potent in their anti-rhinovirus effects.

Still other constituents in ginger, gingerols and shogaols, help relieve cold symptoms because they reduce pain and fever, suppress coughing and have a mild sedative effect that encourages rest.

Ginger has one more thing going for it—it's tasty. I'd say there are a lot of good reasons to make ginger a regular part of your cold-treatment arsenal.

Black cherry (*Prunus serotina*). During their summer season, I add crushed cherries to my lemonade. Basic teas have been used for colds, but I prefer the fruits. They contain vitamin C and benzaldehyde, and they taste good, too, really improving my pink lemonade.

Citrus fruits and other foods containing vitamin C. Like the late Linus Pauling, Ph.D., many herbalists and physicians suggest taking 500 milligrams of vitamin C four times a day for the relief of symptoms. Several studies done by Elliot Dick, Ph.D., epidemiologist at the Respiratory Virus Research Laboratory at the University of Wisconsin in Madison have shown that it works. (Some people develop diarrhea after taking as little as 1,200 milligrams of vitamin C a day, but this is rare. If you'd like to try this therapy, cut back on the amount of vitamin C if you develop diarrhea.)

I take vitamin C for colds, but I do it without using many pills. I prefer to get mine from camu-camu (*Myrciaria dubia*), the Amazonian fruit that has the world's highest vitamin C content. You undoubtedly won't have

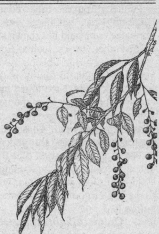

Black Cherry

Black cherry, a member of the rose family, is a vitamin C–rich addition that will make your lemonade less tart.

access yet to this amazing fruit, but other good sources of this vitamin include acerola, bell peppers, cantaloupe, citrus and pineapple.

🌿🌿 **Elderberry (*Sambucus nigra*).** This herb contains two compounds that are active against flu viruses. It also prevents the virus from invading respiratory tract cells.

A patented Israeli drug (Sambucol) that contains elderberry is active against various strains of viruses. At Kibbutz Aza in Israel, a flu outbreak provided a good opportunity to test Sambucol. Twenty percent of flu sufferers who used it showed significant relief of fever, muscle aches and other symptoms within 24 hours, and another 73 percent felt better after the second day. In three days, 90 percent were reported completely cured. In a similar group that received an inactive treatment (a placebo), only 26 percent were improved in two days, and it took most of them six days to feel well again.

Publicity from this trial sold more than 30,000 bottles of Sambucol in Israel within a year. Sambucol also stimulates the immune system and has shown some activity in preliminary trials against other viruses, such as Epstein-Barr, herpes and even HIV.

Sambucol has just become available in the United States, and you may be able to find it on the shelves at your pharmacy or health food store. Next time I have the flu, I intend to try it. You can also make a tea from the herb itself.

🌿🌿 **Forsythia (*Forsythia suspensa*) and honeysuckle (*Lonicera japonica*).** These herbs are the traditional Chinese approach to colds, flu and other viruses. Reviewing the research, I'm persuaded that they have real antiviral benefits. When I feel a cold or flu coming on, I mix honeysuckle and forsythia with lemon balm tea, which also has antiviral action. I find a hot tea combination of the three herbs especially nice just before bed.

🌿🌿 **Onion (*Allium cepa*).** Onion is a close relative of garlic and contains many similar antiviral chemicals. One old folk remedy for colds recommends steeping raw onion slices overnight in honey, then taking the resulting mixture at intervals like a cough syrup. Of course, you could also simply use more onions in cooking whenever you have a cold.

🌿 **Anise (*Pimpinella anisum*).** Commission E, the body of experts that makes recommendations about herbs to the German government, endorses aniseed as an expectorant for getting rid of phlegm. In large doses, it also has some antiviral benefits.

You can make a tea by steeping one to two teaspoons of crushed aniseed in a cup or two of boiling water for 10 to 15 minutes. Then strain it. Suggested dose: one cup of tea, morning and/or night. This should help you cough up whatever's loose and also help you fight the cold. (It also tastes good.)

❦ **Ephedra (*Ephedra sinica*).** Also known as *ma huang* or Chinese ephedra, ephedra is a powerful decongestant. It contains chemicals, ephedrine and pseudoephedrine, that open up the bronchial passages. Pseudoephedrine works so well that it is used in many over-the-counter decongestants and inspired the commonly known brand name Sudafed.

Along with its decongestant action, however, ephedra is also a powerful stimulant that can raise blood pressure and cause insomnia and jitters. In fact, within the last few years, a number of people died from abusing this herb when they overdosed in a misguided attempt to get high, and the Food and Drug Administration has taken measures to remove ephedrine supplements from the market. Because of ephedra's stimulant action and those unfortunate fatalities, this herb is controversial, and some herbalists discourage using it at all.

To me, ephedra is still the herbal decongestant of choice. It is safe when used responsibly, but because of its many potential side effects, I hesitate to recommend it without this proviso: Before taking ephedra, please discuss it with your doctor. To be on the safe side, start with a weak tea.

❦ **Goldenseal (*Hydrastis canadensis*).** Both antiseptic and immune stimulating, goldenseal reportedly increases the blood supply to the spleen, an organ that's the staging area for the fighting cells of your immune system.

The major healing component in goldenseal, berberine, activates special white blood cells (macrophages) that are responsible for destroying bacteria, fungi, viruses and tumor cells. Several related chemicals in the herb appear to help the berberine do its job.

❦ **Licorice (*Glycyrrhiza glabra*)** Licorice contains antiviral compounds that induce the release of interferons, the body's own antiviral constituents. Licorice also has a pleasantly sweet taste that offsets the bitterness of several of the other cold herbs (goldenseal and willow), so it's good in combination with them.

❦ **Marsh mallow (*Althaea officinalis*) and other mallows.** Marsh mallow has been used for thousands of years as a soothing herb for cold-related cough and sore throat and other respiratory conditions. Marsh mallow roots contain a spongy material called mucilage that soothes inflamed mucous membranes, perhaps because of anti-inflammatory and antiseptic compounds that the plant is known to contain.

Commission E endorses marsh mallow, hollyhock and other mallows for cough and sore throat.

Most members of the mallow family, including okra and roselle (the red in Red Zinger tea), contain soothing mucilage. This son of Alabama suggests that you try—at least once—adding a lot of okra to your chicken soup. It adds something extra to the soup's cold-relieving benefits.

❧ **Mullein (*Verbascum thapsus*).** A tea made with mullein flowers provides throat-soothing mucilage and also has an expectorant effect. The plant reportedly contains compounds that inhibit flu viruses. I have had good success with mullein leaf teas as well.

❧ **Seneca snakeroot (*Polygala senega*).** Commission E recommends seneca snakeroot as an expectorant for reducing upper respiratory phlegm. To make a tea, use about one teaspoon per cup of boiling water. (This herb is also recommended for treatment of bronchitis and emphysema.)

❧ **Slippery elm (*Ulmus rubra*).** Finally, the Food and Drug Administration got something right. It has declared slippery elm a safe and effective throat and respiratory soother. Slippery elm was a medical mainstay in this country for more than 150 years and was long listed in the nation's official guides to therapeutics. The bark contains large quantities of a mucilage that acts as an effective throat soother and cough suppressant.

❧ **Watercress (*Nasturtium officinale*).** Commission E suggests using two to three teaspoons of dry watercress to make a tea for treating cold-related runny nose and cough. Or try an ounce of fresh watercress—it makes a great addition to a salad.

Ginger and watercress make a piquant combination. For colds in summer, when fresh watercress is abundant, I'd suggest combining them.

❧ **Willow (*Salix*, various species).** Willow bark is an herbal source of aspirin; the compound salicin, which is found in willow, is a chemical precursor of modern aspirin that has a virtually identical effect. Commission E recognizes willow bark as a pain reliever and anti-inflammatory fever reducer that helps relieve many cold and flu symptoms, including sore throat, fever, headache and other aches.

Many herbalists recommend the bark of the white willow (*S. alba*), but it doesn't contain much salicin—only 0.5 to 1 percent on a dry-weight basis. Other species contain much more herbal aspirin. These include violet willow (*S. daphnoides*), crack willow (*S. fragilis*) and purple osier (*S. purpurea*). If possible, use these more salicin-rich willows. But in a pinch, you can use white willow. It takes only about a half-teaspoon to a teaspoon of dried herb made into a tea to provide 100 milligrams of salicin, which should be enough to relieve the aches related to colds. Remember, though, that if you're allergic to aspirin, you probably shouldn't take aspirin-like herbs, either.

Also remember that you should not give either aspirin or its natural herbal alternatives to children with colds. When children take aspirin-like drugs for viral infections (especially colds, flu and chicken pox), there's a chance that they might develop Reye's syndrome, a potentially fatal condition that damages the liver and brain.

❧ **Garlic-and-onion chicken soup.** I heartily agree with the folkloric tradition that hot, spicy chicken soup is good for colds and flu. Just make sure you use lots of garlic and onions. And along with your vegetables, throw in some ginger and hot red pepper. Good food—and good medicine.

Constipation

A few years ago, I was interviewed for Dan Rather's *Eye on America* program on CBS. In another segment of the same program, Rather interviewed the commissioner of the Food and Drug Administration (FDA), David Kessler, M.D. The program showed me in my habitual fieldwork environment, on location in Ecuador, wearing my exotic jungle garb. Dr. Kessler was shown in his office wearing his usual coat and tie. Although we never actually met or debated on that program, the difference in our garb spoke volumes.

Dr. Kessler and I disagreed about herbs and nutritional supplements. He has come down rather hard on them, while I am convinced that they can be useful. They're a cheap way to prevent some conditions, ameliorate others and even cure a few. But the FDA does not allow any medicinal claims for herbs and supplements unless they have been proven to FDA satisfaction with extensive clinical trials.

As of 1995, it cost $500 million to jump through the FDA hoops to prove any new drug, herb or supplement to be safe and effective. Few marketers of herbs or supplements have that kind of spending money. Drug companies, which do have the money, can justify the expense because once they get a new drug approved, they usually have a patent entitling them to exclusive marketing rights for many years. During that time they can recoup many times over the investment made in the approval process. But who in their right mind would spend hundreds of millions to prove that prune juice is a good laxative? (It is.) You can't patent prunes, so you could never make your money back.

In Praise of Prunes

When Dan Rather's producer called, he asked me what questions Rather should ask Dr. Kessler. I told him to have Rather offer Dr. Kessler a bottle of prune juice and ask if he considered it a safe, effective laxative. If he answered no, I suggested that Rather request that Dr. Kessler drink some and experience the results for himself. If he answered yes, I suggested that Rather ask why FDA labeling regulations prohibit prune juice marketers from stating that prune juice is a safe, effective, gentle laxative.

At my supermarket, prune juice costs only $1.30 a quart, making it probably the cheapest, least unpleasant laxative now available. At my nearby herb store, effective botanical laxatives—rhubarb root, cascara sagrada bark, senna pods and leaves and psyllium seeds and husks—are almost as cheap, but they don't taste half as good.

Meanwhile, FDA-approved commercial laxatives, many of which have senna, cascara sagrada or psyllium in them, are comparatively costly. And many Americans *do* use prune juice as a laxative. So why won't the FDA allow it to be labeled as such?

Facts on Fiber

The sad fact is that most Americans probably wouldn't need a laxative, herbal or otherwise, if they ate right. Doctors know that a high-fiber diet controls constipation by keeping things moving through the intestine.

Thanks to a family history of colon cancer, I was already a high-fiber freak when I first heard a talk by Denis Burkitt, M.D., a respected British surgeon who has spent a lifetime working in East Africa. Dr. Burkitt noted that in nonindustrial societies, among them the African communities where he worked, people eat a very high-fiber diet and rarely suffer from constipation. In fact, the only people Dr. Burkitt ever saw with constipation while in Africa were wealthy people who ate the same low-fiber diet that so many Americans eat.

Here's a sure-fire formula to create a problem with constipation: Take all the fiber-rich fruits, vegetables and whole grains out of your diet. In their place eat lots of meats, fats and dairy foods. No wonder an estimated 10 percent of Americans suffer from constipation, with at least 20 percent of the elderly complaining of it.

When I say that diet can control constipation, I'm not just talking about prune juice. Every whole-grain item and every fiber-rich fruit and vegetable helps prevent and relieve constipation. In folk medicine the foods that get special recognition as laxatives include almonds, apples, avocados, chicory, dandelion, dates, endive, figs, flaxseed, grapes, mangos, papayas, parsley, persimmons, pineapple, prunes, rhubarb, rutabagas, soybeans, turnips, walnuts and watercress. You might easily contrive any number of soups and salads from this list.

If you are constipated, the first thing you should do is change your diet to the "double high five" by eating five fruits and five vegetables a day. If you are still constipated after two days, increase your fruit and veggie intake while diminishing your intake of low-fiber foods like meats and refined breads. Also, I'd recommend that you avoid tea if constipation is a problem for you. Tea is rich in tannins, which is one reason that it is recommended as a treatment for diarrhea. Tannins help bind stools and hold back bowel movements.

Fruit and vegetable juices also work, especially those that retain much of their fiber. Prune juice tops the list, of course, but some juice advocates say that apple-pear juice is a particularly good laxative. Among vegetable juices, asparagus, jícama and potato have been suggested.

Some people who favor juicing use machines that eject most of the fiber. When it comes to treating constipation, that's a big mistake, because fiber is precisely what you want.

Green Pharmacy for Constipation

Several herbs can also help prevent and treat constipation.

✷✷ Flax (*Linum usitatissimum*). Also known as linseed, flaxseed as an herbal treatment for constipation gets an endorsement from Commission E, the body of scientists that provides advice on herbal treatments to Germany's equivalent of the FDA. Commission E suggests taking one to three tablespoons of whole or crushed flaxseed two or three times a day for chronic constipation.

A special word of warning: If you try this remedy, make sure that you also get plenty of water—at least eight full glasses a day—to keep all that bulk moving through your digestive system.

✷✷ Psyllium (*Plantago ovata*). Tiny psyllium seeds contain a fiber called mucilage, which absorbs a great deal of fluid in the gut. This makes the seeds swell. They add bulk to stool, and as stool becomes bulkier, it presses on the colon wall, triggering the muscle contractions we experience as "the urge." Psyllium is quite popular in Germany, and Commission E approves taking three to ten tablespoons a day for chronic constipation.

As with flaxseed, psyllium needs water to work, and if you take it without water, it might obstruct your digestive tract.

And if you have asthma, don't take this herb. There have been several reports of allergic reactions to psyllium, including a few serious asthma attacks from inhaled seed dust.

You should also watch how you react to this herb if you have allergies. If allergic symptoms develop after you take it once, don't use it again.

✷ Aloe (*Aloe*, various species), buckthorn (*Rhamnus catharticus*), cascara sagrada (*Rhamnus purshianus*), frangula (*Frangula alnus*) and senna (*Cassia senna*). These herbs all contain powerful natural laxative chemicals called anthraquinones. With certain reservations, Commission E endorses all of these herbs for treating chronic constipation.

I suggest trying any of these anthraquinone herbs only as a last resort. You should try a high-fiber diet and other, gentler herbs before reaching for any of these. Any herb that contains anthraquinones can be unpleasantly powerful.

If you use buckthorn, cascara sagrada or frangula, which are all barks, insist on aged bark. The anthraquinones in fresh bark irritate the digestive tract and may cause bloody diarrhea and vomiting.

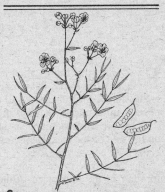

Senna

Leaflets and seed pods of senna are used to make a powerful laxative.

Anthraquinone laxatives should not be taken over long periods of time or during pregnancy or nursing. If you take these laxatives for long periods, you may become dependent on them. That's why I call them a last resort.

❧ **Fenugreek (*Trigonella foenum-graecum*).** Like psyllium, fenugreek seeds contain fluid-absorbing mucilage. If you use fenugreek seeds, make sure you drink plenty of water to keep things moving along. And don't use more than two teaspoons at a time, as any more may cause abdominal distress.

❧ **Rhubarb (*Rheum officinale*).** I like this constipation-relief recipe from physician Ronald Hoffman, M.D., that was published in *Parade* magazine: Puree three stalks of rhubarb without the leaves. Add one cup of apple juice, a quarter of a peeled lemon and one tablespoon of honey. It will make a thick, tart drink that should do the trick.

Dr. Hoffman is right about rhubarb. It contains a natural laxative chemical that's roughly equivalent to that in cascara sagrada and senna. It's also high in fiber. Remember, though, that its laxative action can be pretty powerful; you should probably try some other methods first.

Corns

It's strange, this thing called heredity. My father was always bothered by corns, but I've never had any trouble. Then again, maybe lifestyle makes all the difference in this case. Dad never went barefoot; I always did.

Corns are hardened, mound-shaped areas of increased growth on the skin of the toes. Hard corns occur on the toes, while soft corns arise between the toes.

The best way to deal with corns is to prevent them from forming in the first place. Almost always, they're caused by shoes that fit too tightly, bunching up the toes and irritating the skin. Many people, especially women, wear shoes that are too small for them in the belief that small feet make them appear daintier. But in my opinion, the pain just isn't worth it. (Personally, I'd rather be with a happy, healthy woman in shoes that fit her than with a woman who cripples herself in the name of daintiness.)

Green Pharmacy for Corns

If you can't prevent corns, then I'd suggest some herbal treatments that should help.

❦

Celandine Corn Remover

Here's a gentle herbal remedy that you can make yourself for softening and removing corns. The herb celandine has a worldwide reputation as a corn remover.

    6 cups water
    1 teaspoon potassium chloride
    4 ounces fresh celandine, chopped
    1 cup glycerin

Put the water in a medium saucepan and add the potassium chloride. Heat and stir until the potassium chloride dissolves. Remove from the heat, add the celandine and let stand for 2 hours.

Return the pan to the heat and bring the mixture to a boil. Reduce the heat and simmer for 20 minutes.

Using a sieve or wire strainer, strain the liquid into a medium bowl. Discard the plant material.

Return the liquid to the pan and let it simmer until it is reduced to 1½ cups. Add the glycerin and continue simmering until the liquid is reduced to 2 cups. Strain the liquid, place it in a bottle and store it in cool place. Apply it to corns twice a day—for example, before you leave for work and before you go to bed.

Note: Potassium chloride is available at supermarkets as a commercial salt substitute.

❧

━━━━━━━━━━━━━━━━━━━━━━━━━━━━━━━━

❧ **Celandine (*Chelidonium majus*).** Everywhere I go, from Connecticut to China, herbalists I respect tell me about using celandine to treat corns. I confess that I have not yet tried it, but if I ever get a corn, I plan to. In fact, I've got the formula all ready for a Celandine Corn Remover.

❧ **Fig (*Ficus carica*), papaya (*Carica papaya*) and pineapple (*Ananas comosus*).** When King Solomon developed boils, his physicians applied figs; this is one of the very few descriptions of the medicinal use of herbs in the Bible. Figs contain protein-dissolving enzymes that help dissolve unwanted skin growths, including corns. Papaya and pineapple contain similar enzymes, and all three fruits have age-old reputations for reducing corns and warts.

Here's a recipe culled from my database that I might try if I ever abandoned my barefoot ways and got a corn. Open a fresh fig and tape the pulp to the corn overnight. Or cut a square of pineapple peel and tape the inner side to the corn overnight. The following morning, remove the herb and soak the foot in hot water. After an hour or so, try to remove the corn. It should come off fairly easily, but you can rub it gently with a pumice stone if necessary.

"Some stubborn cases, however, may require four to five overnight treatments," warns medical anthropologist John Heinerman, Ph.D., author of *Heinerman's Encyclopedia of Fruits, Vegetables and Herbs*. Folklore attests to some fairly similar procedures using papaya.

❦ **Willow (*Salix*, various species).** Willow contains aspirin-like compounds known as salicylates that relieve pain. But salicylates are also powerful acids that can help dissolve corns and warts. Just use this herb carefully, placing willow bark poultices directly on the corn itself; don't let the herb come in contact with the surrounding skin. Because they're acidic, salicylates may cause skin inflammation.

❦ **Wintergreen (*Gaultheria procumbens*).** This is another good source of salicylates. Some herbalists recommend that you apply wintergreen oil to remove calluses, corns, cysts and warts. I'd probably try it for corns, both to dissolve hardened skin and to relieve pain. Again, to make sure you avoid irritation, apply the oil only to the corn itself and not to the surrounding skin.

Remember, though, to keep wintergreen oil (or any product containing it) out of the reach of children. The minty smell can be very tempting, but ingesting even small amounts can prove fatal to young children.

Coughing

The common cough is perhaps more common than the common cold. Roughly half of the people seeking medical care in winter suffer from inflammation of the respiratory tract, with cough and other related symptoms. No matter what the cause, coughing is pretty much the same—productive coughs bring up mucus, while nonproductive or dry, hacking coughs do not.

Remember, if you have a cough that just won't go away, it means that your body is sending you some kind of message. It could be something as simple as "stop smoking" or "get that sinus infection cleared up." While you're treating your cough, you also need to pay attention to what your body is trying to tell you. If home remedies don't seem to help and your cough persists for several days, see your doctor.

Green Pharmacy for Coughing

Regardless of the cause, however, herbs can provide some relief. Herbal cough treatments have been recommended since ancient times. Here are some that I'd recommend.

Coltsfoot (*Tussilago farfara*). Christopher Hobbs, a fourth-generation California herbalist and author of several fine books on herbal medicines, suggests a tea made with four parts coltsfoot, four parts plantain, one part licorice, one part marsh mallow and two parts thyme, plus a little of the immune-boosting herb echinacea. Sounds like a winner to me.

Coltsfoot has been used as a cough remedy since ancient times. In fact, its generic name, *Tussilago*, comes from the Latin for "cough." But coltsfoot, like several other herbs, contains chemicals called pyrrolizidine alkaloids (PAs). At high doses, these chemicals can damage the liver, and long-term use can conceivably lead to liver cancer. As a result, some herbalists have gone on record as saying that herbs like coltsfoot that contain PAs should never be ingested.

But Commission E, the body of experts that advises the German government about herb safety and effectiveness, endorses using up to three teaspoons of coltsfoot a day to make a tea to treat a cough. At that dose, you won't consume more than ten milligrams of PAs, a level that the group sees as safe for occasional use as a cough treatment.

Personally, I see nothing wrong with a little coltsfoot now and then. I use it myself from time to time. It soothes the throat, reducing the urge to cough. But don't use this herb if you take a lot of medications, because you'll stress your liver as you're clearing medications from the body. And don't use it if you have a history of liver disease or alcohol abuse.

Elderberry (*Sambucus nigra*). Israeli scientists praise elderberry for treating colds, cough and fever. An Israeli study showed that a drug (Sambucol, which is now available in the United States) made from elderberry is effective against flu, including the cough that goes with it. You can also purchase an elderberry tincture or use the dried herb to make a tea. I would not hesitate to use American elderberry instead.

❧❧ **Ginger (*Zingiber officinale*).** Several chemicals in ginger (gingerols and shogaols) have been shown in studies using laboratory animals to have cough-suppressing, pain-relieving and fever-reducing action. Similar effects in humans have not been demonstrated, but I believe that ginger can help relieve a cough. You can try adding it to whatever you take for coughs.

❧❧ **Lemon (*Citrus limon*).** Here's another Chris Hobbs cough formula: Steep 2 teaspoons of organic lemon rinds, 1 teaspoon of sage and ½ teaspoon of thyme in boiling water for 15 minutes. Then add the juice of ½ lemon and 1 tablespoon of honey. I'm quite partial to lemonade, and I think this remedy is definitely worth trying. In fact, drink it two or three times a day. (Hobbs calls for organic rinds because it is just about impossible to wash away the pesticides that are commonly used on citrus fruits.)

❧❧ **Licorice (*Glycyrrhiza glabra*).** Among its many beneficial properties, licorice soothes mucous membranes and has a long history of use for coughs and asthma. You might try licorice tea (made with one teaspoon of dried root per cup of boiling water) or add some licorice root to other herbal cough formulas.

Licorice and its extracts are safe for normal use in moderate amounts—up to about three cups of tea a day. However, long-term use or ingestion of larger amounts can produce headache, lethargy, sodium and water retention, excessive loss of potassium and high blood pressure.

❧❧ **Slippery elm (*Ulmus rubra*).** The Food and Drug Administration has declared slippery elm a safe, effective cough soother. The bark contains large quantities of a mucilage that acts as an effective throat soother and cough suppressant. You can buy commercially prepared throat lozenges containing slippery elm, or you can use the dried herb to make a tea.

❧ **Anise (*Pimpinella anisum*).** Commission E endorses aniseed as an expectorant for removing phlegm in the respiratory tract and as a cough suppressant.

You could try a tea made with one to two teaspoons of crushed aniseed per cup of boiling water. Steep for 10 to 15 minutes, then strain. Suggested dose: one cup, morning and evening.

❦ Burnet-saxifrage (*Pimpinella·major*). Commission E approves burnet-saxifrage root (three to six teaspoons) for ailments of the upper respiratory tract. Studies show that it has the properties of an expectorant and cough suppressant. It is widely used to treat bronchitis, hoarseness and sore throat.

❦ Marsh mallow (*Althaea officinalis*). I find marsh mallow's soothing roots and extracts, which also contain mucilage, quite useful for relieving cough and sore throat. Commission E recommends marsh mallow root for treating irritation of the mucous membranes of the throat and any associated dry cough. You can make a tea with two teaspoons of dried herb per cup of boiling water.

❦ Mullein (*Verbascum thapsus*). Like marsh mallow, mullein contains throat-soothing mucilage. It also has chemicals called saponins that have an expectorant effect. Commission E approves mullein flowers for treating coughs.

Members of my family have used mullein leaves to treat cough, and I think of it as safe and effective. I'd suggest straining the tea to remove the hairs, which can be irritating, and adding lemon, honey and other herbs to mask the bitter taste.

❦ Primrose (*Primula veris*). Commission E endorses using one to two teaspoons of dried primrose flowers to make a cup of tea for relieving coughs. Note, however, that this particular recommendation is for primrose, not evening primrose (*Oenothera biennis*).

❦ Stinging nettle (*Urtica dioica*). Tea made from this herb is an old standby for coughs. Nettle also has a long history of use as a treatment for colds, whooping cough (pertussis) and tuberculosis. It's certainly worth trying. I'd suggest a tea made from the leaves for coughs and hay fever.

❦ Sundew (*Drosera*, various species). Here's another herb with the Commission E seal of approval. You can try making a tea with one to two teaspoons of dried herb per cup of boiling water. Drink once a day.

Sundew has been used for hundreds of years to treat bronchitis, cough, whooping cough and especially dry, irritating coughs in children. Modern research has validated these uses, showing that this herb has expectorant, cough-suppressing and bronchial-soothing properties.

Cuts, Scrapes and Abscesses

I hope you never have an abscess like the one I had on my left leg 30 years ago in the rain forest of Panama. In the jungle, minor cuts seem to turn into major infections almost overnight. This one started out as a little nick above my left ankle. Almost before you could say "suppurating"—the medical term for the oozing pus produced by infected wounds—my abscess turned into a perfect example of what Hollywood movies about the tropics used to call jungle rot.

My lower leg was a painful mess, with an angry, spreading wound dripping disgusting green pus, the viscous debris of my immune system's fight against the bacteria that had taken up residence in my calf.

In the sleepy little province of Darien near the Colombian border, where my cut turned into an abscess, my Panamanian friends shook their heads knowingly. They said my infection had been caused by too close an encounter with tropical dumbcane (*Dieffenbachia seguine*), which is the same as the familiar palmlike *Dieffenbachia* houseplant. My friends assumed that some of the caustic resin from cut stems of dumbcane had entered a minor cut. That sounded possible, especially since I tended to go barefoot on the slippery slopes of the rivers, trying not to embarrass myself by falling down. But I'll never know for sure. All I knew was that as the ulcer grew larger, I became feverish—and scared.

I put on a brave face, but skin infections in the tropics can quickly become serious. Three decades ago, I was not quite as confident of the Green Pharmacy as I am today. I figured I should see an American physician at a hospital in the Canal Zone.

The doctor confirmed my worst fears. After one look at my abscess, he said that if I didn't get intravenous antibiotics immediately, I might lose my leg. He gave me some antibiotics, but even that was not enough, in his view. If I wanted to save the leg, he said, I should return to the United States for continued treatment.

To further complicate my decision, that was just the time when the American military offered me a king's ransom to return to the rain forest as a botanical consultant. What to do? I wanted that job more than anything. But I also wanted to keep my leg.

Trusting Bush Medicine

I called my friend Narciso "Chicho" Bristan, an African-Panamanian who had accompanied me on several jungle trips. He, too, would enjoy a financial windfall by joining the new expedition into the bush.

Chicho took me hobbling to see his sister, Carmen, a Darien nurse with an extensive knowledge of bush medicine. She had seen ulcers like mine before. Yes, I needed immediate treatment, but no, I didn't need to be hospitalized or receive intravenous antibiotics.

Carmen said I could treat my abscess with "flowers," but not the botanical kind. She meant flowers (purified powder) of sulfur. She recommended flushing out my interconnected sores with hydrogen peroxide, a good disinfectant, drying them in the sun and finally sprinkling on flowers of sulfur.

I decided to take a chance on bush medicine. Soon after that visit, I limped back into the jungle, still leaning on Chicho. But I didn't have to lean on him for long. Carmen's program and her flowers of sulfur quickly healed that angry abscess. Within a month, all I had left was a scar that I bear to this day, testimony to my first leg-threatening encounter with jungle rot.

Today, Chicho is the watchman in Darien's Cerro Pirre National Forest, my favorite Central American rain forest preserve. And thanks in part to my experience in treating that abscess with bush medicine, I was able to perform a 30-year stint as the U.S. Department of Agriculture's expert on herbal medicine.

I've spent 5 of the last 30 years tromping around the tropics looking for medicinal plants. And while I've found quite a few, I've also learned that you don't have to venture off into the Panamanian rain forest to find effective medicinal herbs. Some are much closer to home. Many of our best medicines are right here in our own backyards.

Green Pharmacy for Cuts, Scrapes and Abscesses

Everyone develops skin infections of one kind or another at some point in life. Chances are that yours won't become as serious as mine did, but if a cut becomes more red, tender or painful after a day or two or starts oozing fluid, it means that you have an infection that should be treated by a doctor.

Here are several herbs that can be very effective in treating minor cuts. If you'd like to try them on more serious cuts and abscesses (they do work), please discuss it with your physician before doing so.

✿✿✿ **Teatree (*Melaleuca*, various species).** Teatree oil was used by Australian aborigines and early settlers to treat abrasions, athlete's foot, bug bites, burns and cuts. Its use as a wound treatment has spread around the world. There's good reason for this, as it contains the powerful antiseptic compound terpinen-4-ol.

Varro Tyler, Ph.D., dean and professor emeritus of pharmacognosy (natural product pharmacy) at Purdue University in West Lafayette, Indiana, recommends teatree oil as a wound treatment.

✿✿

Blisterine All-Purpose Herbal Antiseptic

I call this recipe Blisterine because I've used it to prevent and treat infections in popped blisters. But you can also think of it as Better than Listerine, because I believe it is.

I begin with a handful of fresh thyme or horsebalm because they contain the compound thymol, the very same active ingredient found in the commercial mouthwash Listerine. Then I add handfuls of other plants that contain potent herbal antiseptics: eucalyptus or rosemary, which contain cineole; one of the many mints that contain menthol; and cherry birch or wintergreen, which contain the aspirin-like compound methyl-salicylate. (These are only the main antiseptic chemicals. Each plant actually contains more than 20.)

Crush the herbs, put them all in a glass jar and cover them with vodka. After a few days, strain out the plant material and keep the liquid in your medicine chest or first-aid kit to use on cuts and scrapes. If you accidentally mistake this liquid for your after-dinner brandy, never fear. Not only will it not hurt you, it actually tastes pretty good. (Take all things, however, including herbal liqueurs, in moderation.)

❧·❧

I have personally used teatree oil as an externally applied antiseptic for abscesses, and I can attest to its value. It is well-proven as an antiseptic against bacteria and fungi. In fact, teatree oil is just as good as any of those nonherbal antiseptics Mother used to use—iodine and mercurochrome.

People who are sensitive to it may find that the pure oil irritates their skin. I suggest diluting it by putting several drops in a couple of tablespoons of any vegetable oil. If you find that the oil irritates your skin, dilute it further or discontinue use. And don't take teatree oil, or any essential oils, internally. They are extremely concentrated, and even small quantities of many of them are poisonous.

❧·❧ **Calendula (*Calendula officinalis*).** Commission E, the expert committee of German medicinal herb experts that advises the German government, endorses calendula for reducing inflammation and promoting wound healing. It does both.

To make a wash to treat cuts, pour a cup of boiling water over a teaspoon of dry petals and steep for ten minutes. Then soak a clean cloth in the liquid and apply it as a compress on the wound.

Calendula may be even more effective in creams. You can buy commercial skin treatment products containing calendula in many health food stores.

❧·❧ **Comfrey (*Symphytum officinale*).** This herb contains a compound, allantoin, that helps heal wounds. Its astringent tannic acids may also contribute to wound healing.

Comfrey has gotten some bad press recently because it contains chemicals called pyrrolizidine alkaloids, which can damage the liver. Many authorities warn against ingesting it. But there's little if any risk in applying comfrey externally. It's still my first line of defense against sores that are slow to heal. To use it, you can take some fresh leaves and rub them directly on the affected area. You can also find commercial skin-care products containing comfrey in many health food stores.

✒✒ Echinacea (*Echinacea*, various species). Echinacea has potent immune-stimulating properties that help the body heal wounds. Commission E approves applying echinacea preparations externally to treat superficial wounds.

I think of this herb as only a mild antiseptic when it's applied externally. If I had an infected cut, I'd take some tincture or drink echinacea tea to strengthen my immune system so my body could heal the infection. (Although echinacea can cause your tongue to tingle or go numb temporarily, this effect is harmless.)

✒✒ Goldenseal (*Hydrastis canadensis*). Like several other yellow-rooted species—barberry, goldthread, Oregon grape and yellowroot—goldenseal contains several antiseptic compounds, notably berberine and hydrastine. I would not hesitate to apply a poultice of crushed goldenseal root if I got cut in the forest and didn't have any other antiseptics handy.

✒✒ Gotu kola (*Centella asiatica*). Gotu kola contains asiatic acid, a compound that spurs the development of the connective tissue that must form in order for wounds to heal. In clinical trials, external applications of gotu kola extract have proven useful in treating wounds, skin grafts, surgical incisions and even gangrene.

✒✒ Horsebalm (*Monarda punctata*). Since I have horsebalm growing in my backyard in Maryland, I simply make a wound-healing tincture by filling a glass with the crushed leaves and covering them with cheap vodka. Cold alcohol seems to capture more of the antiseptic compounds found in this plant than does warm alcohol. I let it steep for a few days. Then the liquid can be applied to cuts as an antiseptic wash.

If you decide to try this herb, feel free to soak bandages in the tincture and lay the wet dressing directly on top of infected wounds. Then cover the wet dressing with a clean, dry bandage. Change the dressing every few hours as it dries. You can also apply tincture-soaked wet dressings to cuts that are not infected to keep them infection-free and help speed their healing.

You can use this same general recipe to make tinctures of the other herbs listed in this chapter.

✇ **Aloe (*Aloe vera*).** While I am quick to use aloe for burns, I'm not so sure I want to use it for wounds that are much more than a scrape or scratch. Studies show that it has little benefit in treating deep, incision-type wounds. It has proved useful for treating superficial cuts, however.

✇ **Arnica (*Arnica montana*).** This herb, also known as mountain daisy, is useful for treating and disinfecting cuts and other types of wounds, according to Norman G. Bisset, Ph.D., professor of pharmacy at King's College at the University of London and author of the excellent book, *Herbal Drugs and Phytopharmaceuticals*.

Commission E agrees, approving external application of arnica flowers as a quick fix for wounds, bruises, dislocations and sprains. Suggested dosage: For a compress, use one to two teaspoons per cup of boiling water. Steep until cool. Soak a clean cloth in it and apply.

✇ **Clove (*Syzygium aromaticum*).** The dried flower buds of this tropical tree can be found on your spice rack, and oil of clove is a staple in aromatherapy and in dentists' offices. That's because clove oil is rich in eugenol, a chemical that serves double duty as both an antiseptic and a painkiller. You can sprinkle powdered cloves on a cut to keep it from becoming infected.

✇ **Garlic (*Allium sativum*).** Once when I had an infected earlobe and no access to a doctor, I applied garlic, taping a cut clove directly over the affected area. It looked a little silly, but the treatment worked. Garlic reduced the infection and accompanying swelling.

Applying garlic to the skin can cause skin irritation in some people, but garlic is one fine antibiotic. If you opt for this treatment and it irritates your skin, however, discontinue use immediately.

Garlic is not the only herbal antibiotic. Its close relatives, onion and chives, are also loaded with antiseptic compounds.

✇ **Marsh mallow (*Althaea officinalis*).** Poultices of marsh mallow have been used for thousands of years to treat wounds. The herb's root contains a soluble fiber (mucilage) that expands into a spongy, soothing gel in water. It's probably worth a try.

✇ **Melilot (*Melilotus officinalis*).** Experiments using laboratory animals have shown that this herb accelerates wound healing. The active constituent appears to be the compound coumarin. In Germany, powdered melilot is mixed with an equal amount of water to make a poultice for treating hemorrhoids. It seems reasonable to me to try this poultice to treat minor cuts and wounds. ,

❧ **Honey.** While not exactly an herb, honey is made from flowers, and I think this treatment deserves a mention. In many folk medicine traditions around the world, honey is dabbed on wounds because it dries to form a natural bandage.

Actually, medical science has demonstrated that honey does even more. Several studies of surgical wounds show that honey accelerates healing. I've never used it myself, but I've seen Indians in Panama and Peru use it quite successfully.

Dandruff

I've rarely been bothered by dandruff. And although I can't be sure, I think I know why—it's all the biotin I eat.

Biotin, an important vitamin-like nutrient that the body uses in many ways, shows up in my database as a major anti-dandruff compound. Naturopaths recommend getting six milligrams a day for prevention and treatment of both dandruff and the related condition seborrhea.

My database tells me that soybeans are very high in biotin (750 parts per million). That means I'd need only a handful to provide the six milligrams I'd need to save my scalp from dandruff and seborrhea. I have often eaten that many soybeans as I wandered through the soybean fields at the U.S. Department of Agriculture Agricultural Research Station in Beltsville, Maryland, where I've spent the last 30 years trying to spread the word about the healing powers of plants.

Then again, maybe I'm dandruff-free not just because of biotin but also due to the breakfasts I eat. I tend to begin my mornings with things like a sandwich made with Brazil nut butter and coleslaw with tomatoes, washed down with vegetable juice. My breakfasts contain a lot of other anti-dandruff ingredients: selenium, sulfur, lecithin and zinc in the Brazil nut butter, citric acid in the vegetable juice and red pepper in the slaw.

Green Pharmacy for Dandruff

Dandruff is a common scalp condition that causes unsightly white flakes to appear in the scalp and hair. The white flakes are dead scalp skin. Dandruff is often the result of seborrhea, an inflammation (dermatitis) of the scalp. Here are some herbs you might try for preventing and treating dandruff.

✿✿✿ **Soybean (*Glycine max*) and other foods containing biotin.** While there seems to be some biotin in just about all plants, my database reveals some standouts. Soybeans have the most, followed by garlic, American ginseng, oats, barley, Asian ginseng, avocado, cottonseed, alfalfa, sesame, corn, fava beans and elderberry.

Lamentably, my database can't provide the whole story, because science just doesn't know all that much about the biotin content of plants. That's due to the amazing fact that no one has ever been funded to do detailed analyses of the minor constituents of all those fruits, nuts and veggies that the government is urging us to consume. (You might want to contact your Congressional representative to request funding for more detailed nutritional studies.)

✿ **Burdock (*Arctium lappa*).** Seborrhea often responds to massaging burdock root oil into the scalp, according to Rudolf Fritz Weiss, M.D., the dean of German medical herbalists and author of *Herbal Medicine*.

✿ **Celandine (*Chelidonium majus*).** I learned about this one from Edward E. Shook's *Advanced Treatise in Herbology*. Shook maintains that celandine works not only for dandruff but also for dry skin, hives, corns and warts.

Using celandine to treat dandruff involves brewing up an herbal scalp rinse. Into six cups of water, place one teaspoon of potassium chloride (available at supermarkets as a salt substitute). Heat and stir until the potassium chloride dissolves. Then chop four ounces of fresh celandine and add it to the solution. (If fresh celandine isn't available, you can use a half-cup of the dried herb instead.) Let stand for two hours, then boil slowly for 20 minutes. Strain the plant material out and simmer, reducing the liquid to 1½ cups. Add eight ounces of glycerin and continue simmering, reducing the liquid slowly to two cups. Strain the result, bottle it and store it in cool place. Use it once or twice a day as a hair rinse.

✿ **Comfrey (*Symphytum officinale*).** Allantoin, a chemical in this herb, has anti-dandruff properties, according to *Hunting's Encyclopedia of Shampoo Ingredients*. You might be able to find a commercial shampoo that contains comfrey at a health food store. If not, you can add a couple of drops of comfrey tincture to your favorite herbal shampoo.

❧ **Ginger (*Zingiber officinale*) and sesame (*Sesamum indicum*).** Medical anthropologist John Heinerman, Ph.D., author of *Heinerman's Encyclopedia of Fruits, Vegetables and Herbs*, shares the following Egyptian dandruff/seborrhea treatment: Take one to two tablespoons of ginger juice (squeezed from about two grated roots) and mix it with three tablespoons of sesame oil and a half-teaspoon of lemon juice. Rub the mixture into the scalp three times a week. I think it sounds interesting, although sesame oil can be expensive. If I had dandruff, I might give this one a try.

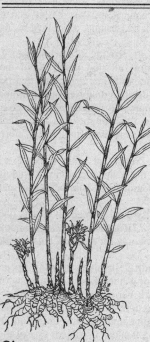

Ginger

This spice, used by the ancient Greeks and Romans as a digestive aid, has many other uses as well.

❧ **Licorice (*Glycyrrhiza glabra*).** Licorice contains glycyrrhizin, a compound that can minimize the scalp's secretion of oils, according to the *Lawrence Review of Natural Products*, a respected newsletter. Keeping oil production down should help control dandruff. You can steep a couple of handfuls of dried herb in a bottle of vinegar and use it as a hair rinse.

❧ **Plantain (*Plantago*, various species).** Like comfrey, plantain contains allantoin. You could make a strong tea and use it as a hair rinse.

❧ **Teatree (*Melaleuca*, various species).** Teatree oil, an antiseptic favored among aromatherapists, contains substances known as terpenes that penetrate the top layers of the scalp and carry their disinfectant activities deeper than most emollients. You might mix a few drops into a couple of tablespoons of herbal shampoo. Just don't take teatree oil, or any essential oil, internally. They are extremely concentrated, and even small quantities of many of them can be poisonous.

❧ **Scarborough Shampoo.** Many herbalists recommend the old standard—one ounce each of dried sage and rosemary infused in two cups of water for 24 hours and used daily as a hair rinse. I think I'd also add thyme as an even more powerful antiseptic. Add parsley and you have the herbal combination made famous by the folk song "Scarborough Fair"—parsley, sage, rosemary and thyme. You can create what I call Scarborough Shampoo by adding a few drops of tincture of each of these herbs to a good commercial herbal shampoo.

❧ **Vinegar and apple cider.** These are both old folk remedies for dandruff. Warm one or both and apply the liquid directly to the scalp, then shampoo.

Depression

On my first trip to Macchu Picchu, Peru, one of my colleagues confided that he'd suffered debilitating episodes of depression. He'd had all the classic symptoms: profound sadness, feelings of helplessness and hopelessness, poor concentration, disturbed eating, sleeping and bowel habits, and an inability to derive pleasure from normally pleasurable activities.

All modern drugs had failed him. I braced myself for the usual question: "Know any herbs that might help?" When he asked, I answered with my usual cautious reply: "If I had depression, I'd try St.-John's-wort." But I might just as easily have said "licorice." Both are three-star champs in the Green Pharmacy.

Green Pharmacy for Depression

It goes without saying that everyone gets the blues from time to time. Depression that won't let up, however, is a serious disorder. If you suffer from ongoing depression, you should see your doctor for treatment. In the meantime, there are also a number of herbs that can prove helpful.

❧

Be Careful
with MAO Inhibitors

People who are taking MAO inhibitors, or using herbs that contain MAO inhibitors, on a regular basis need to avoid certain foods and medications. The foods to avoid are alcoholic beverages and anything that is smoked or pickled. The medications to stay away from are cold and hay fever remedies, amphetamines, narcotics, tryptophan and tyrosine.

❧

❧❧❧ **Licorice** (*Glycyrrhiza glabra*). No plant in my database has more antidepressant compounds than licorice, but it does not have St.-John's-wort's folk history of use as an antidepressant. Strange. At least eight licorice compounds are monoamine oxidase (MAO) inhibitors, which are compounds capable of potent antidepressant action.

If you'd like to try licorice to beat depression, simply add some to any of the other herbal teas suggested in this chapter. (While licorice and its extracts are safe for normal use in moderate amounts—up to about three cups of tea a day—long-term use or ingestion of larger amounts can produce headache, lethargy, sodium and water retention, excessive loss of potassium and high blood pressure.)

❧❧❧ **St.-John's-wort** (*Hypericum perforatum*). This herb

got its name because the plant flowers on St. John's day, June 24. (*Wort* is Old English for "plant.") Its star-shaped yellow flowers, which turn red when bruised, are beautiful enough to make anyone with the blues feel happier. But this herb also has a long history of folk use for treating anxiety and depression. Modern science has shown that generations of folk herbalists were right.

Clinical studies show that treatment with just one of the active compounds in this herb, hypericin, results in significant improvement in anxiety, depression and feelings of worthlessness. Some studies show that it's a more powerful antidepressant than some pharmaceutical drugs such as amitriptyline (Elavil) and imiprimine (Tofranil). What's more, it has fewer side effects. Some researchers say that it has no side effects at all.

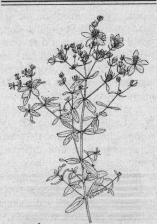

St.-John's-wort

This herb, once used to ward off evil spirits and treat snakebite, has been extensively researched as an antidepressant in Germany and the former Soviet Union.

Studies also show that St.-John's-wort improves sleep quality, often a major problem for people who are seriously depressed. In one study, German researchers gave St.-John's-wort to 105 people with moderate depression. Compared with a similar group not receiving the herb, they slept better and exhibited less sadness, helplessness, hopelessness, exhaustion and headache. They also reported no side effects.

While some researchers attribute the benefits of the herb to its MAO inhibitors, other studies downplay this activity. Jerry Cott, Ph.D., director of the Polytherapeutic Medication Development Program of the National Institute of Mental Health in Bethesda, Maryland, tells me that even though *Hypericum* is a leading antidepressant, it has much less MAO inhibitor activity than we had previously believed.

Commission E, the body of scientific experts that advises the German government on the safety and effectiveness of herbs, heaps praise on St.-John's-wort as a treatment for depression. If you'd like to try it, I'd suggest a tea made by steeping one to two teaspoons of dried herb in a cup of boiling water for ten minutes. St.-John's-wort appears to be most effective if you take one to two cups of tea a day for four to six weeks, according to Varro Tyler, Ph.D., dean and professor emeritus of pharmacognosy (natural product pharmacy) at Purdue University in West Lafayette, Indiana. Dr. Tyler says that different chemical compounds in St.-John's-wort work together to relieve mild depression in several different ways. The advantage of this combined action is fewer side effects, because the total response is not due to a single strong action.

Do not take St.-John's-wort if you're pregnant. And avoid intense sun exposure while using it, since this herb can make the skin more sensitive to sunlight.

❧

Activating the Tryptophan Trigger

Is it possible to use nutrition to banish depression?

Bear with me a moment while I trip through some biochemistry: The body converts carbohydrates—sugars and starches in your diet—to glucose, a type of sugar commonly called blood sugar. Glucose triggers the pancreas to release insulin. Insulin in turn raises brain levels of the amino acid tryptophan, a raw material in the production of the neurotransmitter chemical called serotonin.

Neurotransmitter chemicals are used by nerves to communicate with each other and to function properly. High levels of serotonin produce a very particular effect: The neurotransmitter elevates mood and enhances feelings of well-being and satiety.

If you follow this logic just one step further, it sounds as if a high-carbohydrate diet should help relieve depression. And one study suggests that it can do just that. After eating high-carbohydrate biscuits, people with mild depression—including people trying to quit smoking and premenstrual women—reported feeling more mellow.

So go ahead: Eat more biscuits, bagels and pasta and see if it doesn't make you feel better.

You could also boost your intake of tryptophan. Sunflower seeds, pumpkin seeds and evening primrose seeds (*Oenothera biennis*) are all high in this feel-good amino acid.

Enhancing the amount of serotonin in the body is, by the way, one of the accepted medical approaches to treating depression. Fluoxetine (Prozac), the popular antidepressant drug, works by helping the body hold onto its serotonin.

❦

Ginger (*Zingiber officinale*). In addition to its uplifting flavor, there are other good reasons to take ginger along with any other antidepressant herbs that you are taking. Ginger has a long folk history of use for treating anxiety and depression, and I've heard enough about its good effects to make me a believer.

Purslane (*Portulaca oleracea*). Many people get the urge to eat when they are depressed. And eating just might help—if you eat the right foods. Foods containing the minerals magnesium and potassium have been shown to have antidepressant effects. Purslane, which is very rich in these minerals, is also high in other constituents with antidepressant value, including calcium, folate (the naturally occurring form of folic acid) and lithium. In fact, purslane contains up to a whopping 16 percent antidepressant compounds, figured on a dry-weight basis.

Working with my database, it's clear that purslane is just one of several salad ingredients that might help relieve depression. Hence, my Un-Sad Salad: lettuce, pigweed, purslane, lamb's-quarters and watercress. I'd also be sure to use a little thyme in the dressing, as it's very high in the antidepressant mineral lithium.

Rosemary (*Rosmarinus officinalis*). Rosemary essential oil is a favorite among aromatherapists for treating depression. A massage with a few drops of rosemary oil in vegetable oil or massage lotion probably can't hurt. It contains the compound cineole, which has been shown to stimulate the central nervous system.

Other herb oils that aromatherapists recommend for treating depression include bergamot, basil, camomile, clary sage, jasmine, lavender, neroli, nutmeg and ylang-ylang. Remember, though, that these oils are for external use only.

✤ **Ginkgo (*Ginkgo biloba*).** Studies have shown that ginkgo may help relieve depression, especially in the elderly who suffer reduced blood flow to the brain.

In one study, European scientists recruited a group of 40 depressed elderly people with cerebral blood flow problems who did not respond to pharmaceutical antidepressants. The researchers gave them 80 milligrams of ginkgo extract three times a day. Their depression and mental faculties both improved significantly.

In fact, European studies have confirmed the use of standardized ginkgo leaf extract for a wide variety of conditions associated with aging, including memory loss and poor circulation.

One standard ginkgo preparation, a 50:1 extract, uses 50 parts leaves to come up with 1 part extract. Such 50:1 extracts are available in health food stores. If you want to try ginkgo, this is the way to go. You can try 60 to 240 milligrams a day, but don't go any higher than that. In large amounts, ginkgo may cause diarrhea, irritability and restlessness.

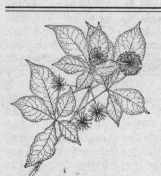

Siberian Ginseng

This is not true ginseng, but it has similar healing properties and is frequently used in the United States.

✤ **Siberian ginseng (*Eleutherococcus senticosus*).** In studies using laboratory animals, Siberian ginseng has been shown to act as an MAO inhibitor. In people with depression, the herb helps improve their sense of well-being. You might try either capsules or standardized extracts.

Other herbs with MAO inhibitor activity include caraway, celery, coriander, dill, fennel and nutmeg.

✤ **Foods rich in B vitamins.** Neurotransmitters, the chemicals that allow nerve cells to communicate and function properly, play a role in depression. Nutritionists suggest getting enough of certain B vitamins—folate and vitamins B_6 and B_{12}—to keep neurotransmitter levels high.

Good sources of folate include pinto beans, navy beans, asparagus, spinach, broccoli, okra and brussels sprouts. As far as vitamin B_6 is concerned, high levels occur in cauliflower, watercress, spinach, bananas, okra, onions, broccoli, squash, kale, kohlrabi, brussels sprouts, peas and radishes.

You might also try adding the amino acid phenylalanine to your diet. In one study, more than 75 percent of people with severe depression showed rapid improvement while taking supplements of phenylalanine and vitamin B_6. Since I generally prefer getting nutrients from foods, I'd recommend the four richest food sources—sunflower seeds, black beans, watercress and soybeans. How about a black bean-soybean soup with watercress, garnished with a sprinkling of sunflower seeds?

Diabetes

In 1989, a physician from Florida wrote to Walter Mertz, M.D., then director of the U.S. Department of Agriculture (USDA) Human Nutrition Research Center in Beltsville, Maryland: "Enclosed is a sample of a 'weed.' A diabetic patient of mine brought it back from the island of Trinidad. She has adultonset diabetes and was taking insulin until she began using this plant. Now she reports that she adds the weed to vermouth and takes small sips of the mixture twice a day. This has resulted in normalization of her blood sugars over the past six months. I am hoping you will be able to identify the plant and to determine its effective ingredient."

Knowing of my interest in herbal medicine, Dr. Mertz sent me the letter and the specimen, which I identified as jackass bitters (*Neurolaena lobata*), a tall perennial weed vaguely resembling American ragweed. Its tincture is a time-honored Creole-Caribbean treatment for diabetes and several other ailments, among them colds, fever, malaria and menstrual cramps.

I'm not sure whether this herb really helps with all those other complaints, but there is good research to show that jackass bitters helps regulate blood sugar (glucose) levels. So it really does help manage diabetes. In several studies using experimental animals, a tincture of the plant has been shown to be anti-hyperglycemic, which is the medical term for anything, including insulin, that lowers blood sugar. It is high blood sugar that is responsible for the serious complications in people who have diabetes.

If the animal dose can be applied to humans, a 150-pound person would have to consume about an ounce of the herb to gain significant anti-hyperglycemic benefits. But based on the letter to Dr. Mertz, apparently some people gain real benefits from taking considerably less. While the herb is difficult to find in the United States, some health food stores and mail-order companies do carry it.

Problems with Fuel Supply

More than 2,000 years ago, the ancients noticed that some people produced copious amounts of strangely sweet-tasting urine that attracted ants. (Tasting urine was a diagnostic tool in many cultures.) They named the condition *diabetes mellitus*, from the Greek for "fountain" and the Latin for "honey."

Diabetes occurs either when the pancreas stops producing the hormone insulin or the body becomes unable to use the insulin it produces. Glucose, the body's major fuel, cannot enter our cells unless insulin is present and working. Without insulin, glucose builds up in the bloodstream and eventually turns up in the urine, causing the sweet taste that the ancients noticed. The sugar imbalance also leads to increased urination and thirst.

Diabetes also causes narrowing of the small blood vessels throughout the body. It seems that the higher the blood sugar level, the more the small blood vessels narrow. As this happens, the blood vessels carry less blood, and circulation is impaired. Poor circulation in turn leads to the complications of poorly controlled diabetes: kidney disease, poor wound healing and foot and eye problems.

Diabetic limb problems are the cause of about half of all U.S.

amputations not caused by injury. Diabetes also alters fat metabolism, increasing the risk that cholesterol-laden plaque will build up in the large blood vessels. This means that people who have diabetes are at considerable risk for heart disease.

Two Conditions, Two Approaches

There are actually two kinds of diabetes—Type I (insulin-dependent) and Type II (non-insulin-dependent).

People who have Type I diabetes must inject themselves with insulin daily to control their blood sugar. People with Type II produce their own insulin, but their cells don't respond to it properly.

Type II is by far the more prevalent form of diabetes, accounting for 85 to 90 percent of cases. It is typically associated with obesity. People with Type II diabetes can usually control their blood sugar through weight loss and diet, sometimes in combination with oral medication that boosts the effect of their own insulin.

It is often possible for people with Type II diabetes to avoid taking drugs, and I favor this approach whenever possible. My review of the literature tells me that dietary approaches are cheaper, more effective and more pleasant than most of the pharmaceutical alternatives.

Some six million Americans are under treatment for diabetes. Almost as many have it and don't know it. Like heart disease and many cancers, diabetes is strongly associated with Western culture and diet. As members of non-Western cultures, notably American Indians and Australian aborigines, have switched from their traditional diets to a more Westernized diet, their rates of diabetes have soared.

Natural Tactics to Beat Diabetes

Diabetes is a serious condition. If you have this disease, you should definitely be under a physician's care. But there's a great deal that you can do to help manage the condition.

Because obesity is so strongly associated with Type II diabetes, weight control is an important element of diabetes self-care. A low-fat diet and regular moderate exercise is the way to go. I'd suggest gradually working up to the point where you can walk briskly for an hour every day. You already know how to walk, and you don't have to buy any special equipment or join a health club. If you've never been physically active, don't despair. Walking and other moderate exercise programs produce the greatest benefits in those who have been the least active.

There's also good evidence that supplementation can help prevent some diabetic complications. I suggest that you ask your doctor for a referral to a clinical nutritionist who can help you design the supplementation program that's right for you. Supplements that may help include vitamins B_6, C and E, chromium picolinate, magnesium, manganese, phosphorus and zinc, plus omega-3 and omega-6 fatty acids.

Green Pharmacy for Diabetes

In addition to exercising and taking supplements, you can try many herbs to help normalize blood sugar levels. The first, jackass bitters, I've already described. Here are the others in the lineup.

✿✿✿ **Fenugreek (*Trigonella foenum-graecum*)**. About half of fenugreek seed (by weight) is a soluble fiber called mucilage. It contains six compounds that help regulate blood sugar levels.

Fenugreek also increases blood levels of HDL ("good") cholesterol while lowering total cholesterol, so it can help prevent cardiovascular disease, a particular hazard for people with diabetes.

✿✿✿ **Onion (*Allium cepa*)**. Onions have a long folk history of use as a dietary supplement to treat diabetes in Asia, Europe and the Middle East. I'm not surprised. Onions—especially the skins—are one of our best sources of the compound quercetin, which has been shown to help with eye problems that are often associated with diabetes, such as diabetic retinopathy.

✿✿ **Beans (*Phaseolus*, various species)**. Many studies demonstrate that eating foods that are high in soluble fiber, notably beans, reduces the rise in blood sugar after meals and delays the drop in blood sugar later on, thus helping to maintain blood sugar at close to desired levels.

If I had diabetes, I would eat lots of beans and bean soups. (For the benefits of both beans and onions, try my recipe for Dia-Beanie Soup.)

❦

Dia-beanie Soup

Beans contain a type of fiber that is particularly useful for controlling blood sugar levels, and onion skin is particularly rich in the beneficial compound quercetin, which serves the same purpose. Leaving the onion skin on while the soup cooks means that more of the compound will end up in the soup bowl, where you want it.

 2 cups water
 1 unpeeled onion, quartered
 1 can (16 ounces) kidney beans, rinsed
   and drained
 1 small carrot, diced
 ½ cup peanuts
 ¼ cup fenugreek sprouts or ½ teaspoon
   fenugreek seeds
 2 bay leaves
 4 cloves garlic, chopped
   Dash of ground cinnamon
   Dash of ground cloves
   Dash of turmeric

In a large saucepan over medium heat, bring the water and onions to a boil. Add the beans, carrots, peanuts, fenugreek sprouts or seeds, bay leaves, garlic, cinnamon, cloves and turmeric.

Bring to a simmer. Cover and cook for 30 minutes, or until the onions are very tender. Remove the onion pieces with a slotted spoon; peel off and discard the skins. Lightly mash the onions with a fork and return to the saucepan. Remove and discard the bay leaves.

Makes 4 servings

❦

✹✹ **Bitter gourd** (*Momordica charantia*). Also known as balsam pear, this herb has attracted considerable interest for its ability to regulate blood sugar. The research was first published in India in the 1960s, and since then several studies have shown that bitter gourd can help control diabetes.

In one trial, five grams (about two teaspoons) of powdered bitter gourd a day decreased blood sugar by 54 percent. In another, taking 50 milliliters (about a quarter-cup) of bitter gourd extract reduced high blood sugar by some 20 percent.

If you'd rather not fiddle with extracts, it's okay to just eat bitter gourd as a side dish, according to Melvyn Werbach, M.D., assistant clinical professor of psychiatry at the University of California, Los Angeles, School of Medicine, and Michael Murray, N.D., co-authors of *Botanical Influences on Illness*.

You could also try juicing it. Or make a decoction by gently boiling four ounces of chopped fresh bitter gourd in a pint of water until about half the liquid has boiled off. Take it once a day.

✹✹ **Garlic** (*Allium sativum*). Like onions, garlic has a significant ability to control blood sugar levels. Eat more garlic—raw, if possible, or lightly cooked in food.

✹✹ **Macadamia nut** (*Macadamia*, **various species**). Since 1986, dietary recommendations for people with Type II diabetes have called for a diet with 15 to 20 percent of calories from protein, less than 35 percent from fat and 55 to 60 percent from carbohydrates. More recent studies show that substituting certain healthy oils—monounsaturated fatty acids (MUFAs)—for some of the carbohydrates can improve blood sugar control while not increasing cholesterol levels.

✹✹

Insulinade

There are a number of spices that research shows can help the body use insulin more efficiently. These include bay leaf, cinnamon, cloves and turmeric.

I'd simply add a pinch or two of each of them to a pot of black tea and steep for ten minutes, then ice the tea. I might also add a pinch of coriander and cumin. The research is not as strong on these two spices, but in animal studies, both have been shown to lower blood sugar somewhat. Those who like fenugreek might add a pinch of that as well.

❧❧

Olive oil is the most noted source of MUFAs. But if you don't like olive oil or simply want to expand your MUFA horizons, try macadamia nuts. They are up to 59 percent MUFAs. Other good sources of MUFAs include avocados, pistachio nuts, cashews, peanuts and Brazil nuts.

❧❧ **Marsh mallow (*Althaea officinalis*).** Marsh mallow root is very high in a soluble plant fiber known as pectin (35 percent on a dry-weight basis). Taking pectin is an effective way to keep blood sugar levels down.

I'd steep the rather fibrous roots in water overnight, or better yet, buy a commercial product. Other good sources of pectin include white-flowered gourd, carrots, rosehips, apples and figs.

❧❧ **Peanut (*Arachis hypogaea*).** Like beans, peanuts have the ability to keep blood sugar levels down. They are criticized for being high in fat, but I love them, munch them frequently and like to spread the news of their value.

❧❧ **Tea (*Camellia sinensis*).** Indian researchers have shown anti-diabetic activity for black tea. In studies, extracts of black tea significantly reduced blood sugar levels in laboratory animals. If I had diabetes, I'd drink lots of tea. You might add blood-sugar-lowering spices to the tea for a little extra help. In fact, give my Insulinade a try.

❧ **Bay (*Laurus nobilis*) and other spices.** My former USDA colleague, Richard Anderson, Ph.D., has demonstrated that bay leaves help the body use insulin more efficiently at levels as low as 500 milligrams (about a half-teaspoon). The leaves have been shown to lower blood sugar levels in experimental animals. I include a few bay leaves in my Dia-Beanie Soup as well as cinnamon, clove and turmeric, which are good at controlling blood sugar levels.

❧ **Gurmar (*Gymnema sylvestre*).** There have been at least four Indian studies on this herb, an Indian folk favorite for treating diabetes. The tea seems to boost insulin production. There is also some intriguing evidence that it may actually increase the number of islets of Langerhans, the cells in the pancreas that produce insulin. A few forward-looking herbal dealers are already marketing this herb in the United States.

Diarrhea

B ack in my musical days, I spent a summer playing bass fiddle with a trio at the Ocean Forest Hotel north of Myrtle Beach, South Carolina. Our vocalist was also a drummer, but for some strange reason, the musicians' union would not allow us to have three instruments. So the vocalist just used drummer's brushes on a folded newspaper on the piano. We told the union, "Look, only two instruments, a bass and a piano."

What a summer that was. My bandmates and I had day jobs painting signs, and then we played music at night. We drank too much and didn't eat enough good food. Our systems were so thrown off-kilter that we all developed bad cases of diarrhea. We honored our affliction by calling the band Three Squirts in the Fountain.

The Dire Discomfort

Everyone knows what diarrhea is. Many serious diseases can cause it. And infectious diarrhea, caused by viruses or bacteria, still ranks as a leading killer of Third World children. But this chapter is devoted to common, run-of-the-mill diarrhea that usually clears up within 48 hours.

The most important thing to do for diarrhea is to drink fluids, but a lot of people do just the opposite. They cut down in the mistaken belief that refraining from drinking fluids will help the body stop producing them.

How well I remember one of our ecotourists at Machu Picchu. She was so convinced that her diarrhea was caused by the water that she refused to drink any. The physicians who accompanied us had a tough job convincing her to drink even bottled water.

The fact is, the main medical risk of ordinary diarrhea is dehydration. So keep getting fluids by sipping water or astringent iced tea throughout the day.

Green Pharmacy for Diarrhea

There are a number of herbal approaches to clearing up a bout of diarrhea. All of these herbs contain one or more of three natural ingredients, tannin, pectin and mucilage.

Tannins are the chemicals that give some herbs their astringency—that is, the ability to bind up or contract tissues. Tannins' astringent action reduces intestinal inflammation. The tannins bind to the protein layer of the inflamed mucous membranes and cause them to thicken, hence slowing resorption of toxic materials and restricting secretions.

Pectin is a soluble fiber that adds bulk to stool and soothes the gut. The "pectate" in the over-the-counter antidiarrheal medicine Kaopectate contains pectin.

Mucilage soothes the digestive tract and adds bulk to stool by absorbing water and swelling considerably.

Here are several of the many herbs that can be helpful.

🐛 **Agrimony (*Agrimonia eupatoria*).** Commission E endorses agrimony for common diarrhea, probably due to its high tannin content. Try using two to three teaspoons of leaves to make a tea.

🐛 **Apple (*Malus domestica*).** Apple pulp is rich in pectin. That's why apples and applesauce are a hallowed folk remedy for diarrhea. (Apple pectin also helps treat constipation because it acts as a gentle stool softener. Like psyllium, it's amphoteric, which means that it works in either direction, plugging you up if your bowels are loose or loosening you up if you are constipated.)

🐛 **Bilberry and blueberry (*Vaccinium*, various species).** Dried (not fresh) fruits of bilberry and blueberry help relieve diarrhea because they are rich in both tannins and pectin.

🐛 **Blackberry and raspberry (*Rubus*, various species).** Commission E, the body of scientists that advises the German government about herbs, suggests making an astringent tea with two teaspoons of blackberry leaf. Oddly, it does not mention raspberry leaf, which is a close botanical relative that is also high in tannin. I've used both and found them effective.

☙ **Carob** (*Ceratonia siliqua*). Years ago in Panama, I had an acute attack of salmonella, a type of food poisoning, after I'd handled fresh-water turtles that harbor the bacteria. My Panamanian doctor prescribed powdered carob for the diarrhea, and it seemed to work. That was nearly 30 years ago.

Then just a few months ago, I reviewed a study of 41 infants with bacterial or viral diarrhea. Children given an inactive substance (a placebo) had diarrhea for an average of nearly four days. Children given carob powder had it for only two days.

☙ **Carrot** (*Daucus carota*). I like the idea of using cooked carrots to treat infant diarrhea. When they're cooked, carrots seem to soothe the digestive tract and control the diarrhea while also providing nutrients that are lost during the attack.

☙ **Fenugreek** (*Trigonella foenum-graecum*). The seeds of this herb contain up to 50 percent mucilage, so they swell in the gut, thus relieving diarrhea. (They also help relieve constipation by softening stool.) Just don't use more than two teaspoons at a time, as more may cause abdominal distress.

☙ **Oak** (*Quercus*, **various species**). Commission E recommends using one to two teaspoons of dried oak bark to make an astringent tea.

☙ **Pomegranate** (*Punica granatum*). Pomegranate, an herb mentioned in the Bible, is often used to treat diarrhea. I'm not surprised, because the seeds are astringent.

☙ **Psyllium** (*Plantago ovata*). Psyllium is useful for relieving constipation. Its high mucilage content also makes it useful for treating diarrhea. By absorbing a great deal of water, psyllium adds bulk to stool. (In constipation, it speeds up transit time by increasing the volume of bowel content.) You should watch how you react to this herb if you have allergies, however. If allergic symptoms develop after you take it once, don't use it again.

☙ **Tea** (*Camellia sinensis*). One of the most astringent plants around is conventional tea in conventional tea bags. Under Food and Drug Administration regulations, Lipton can't make medicinal claims. But the next time you have diarrhea, try a nice cup of tea.

Diverticulitis

Back in 1972, during an administrative stint at the U.S. Department of Agriculture, I had a hard-working secretary who was plagued by diverticulitis. It manifested itself as abdominal pain and cramping, usually on the lower left side, plus occasional fever and bloody stool. I felt for her. My younger brother had also had diverticulitis.

At the time, dietary treatment for diverticulitis was quite controversial. Doctors had been recommending a low-fiber diet to treat it for about 50 years, and my secretary's doctors told her to avoid fruits and vegetables. But that didn't make much sense to the then-small group of natural medicine advocates, including yours truly, who were into high-fiber whole foods.

Even a cursory look at how people eat around the world showed that cultures with a high-fiber diet had little or no diverticulitis (and little or no constipation). Meanwhile, in the industrial West, with its processed foods and low-fiber diet, diverticulitis was common. (And incidentally, constipation was rampant.)

My secretary felt torn between the advice of those advocating high fiber and low fiber, and not knowing what to do added a good deal of stress to her already unpleasant situation. As luck would have it, that very year British researcher Neil Painter, M.D., of Manor House Hospital, London, published a study in the *British Medical Journal* that all but proved that diverticular disease was caused by a low-fiber diet. He recruited some 70 people with diverticulitis and placed them on a diet of whole-wheat bread, high-bran cereals and plenty of fruits and vegetables. That high-fiber diet cured or substantially relieved symptoms in 89 percent of the study participants.

I showed my secretary the study, and I hope she took it to heart. But alas, our careers took us in different directions, and I lost track of her, so I don't know how she fared.

Prevention with Fiber

Today, of course, doctors know that a high-fiber diet is the way to go. I've always eaten that way—lots of fruits, vegetables, breads and herbs—which is why, unlike my brother and secretary, I've never been bothered by either diverticulitis or constipation.

Our ancestors ate lots of fiber, and our colons evolved to handle it. Without enough fiber, we know, strange things begin to happen down there. Food moves more slowly through the colon, causing constipation, and little pockets known as diverticula develop in the colon wall. Sometimes diverticula become plugged with little bits of digested food and often little seeds. If diverticula become inflamed and swell, they cause pain and the other symptoms of diverticulitis.

More than half of those over 60 have noninflamed, painless diverticula, while an estimated 10 percent develop the inflammation of diverticulitis.

To reduce your risk of diverticulitis, the two most important factors are a high-fiber diet and exercise, according to Walid H. Aldoori, M.D., professor in the Department of Nutrition at the Harvard School of Public Health. But while you're eating more whole grains and fresh fruits and vegetables, you should watch some other dietary factors as well. Be sure to drink plenty of nonalcoholic fluids to keep things moving efficiently through your digestive tract. And if you've had diverticulitis, you should steer clear of some small, indigestible seeds—poppy, sesame, raspberry and strawberry—which can plug diverticula and aggravate the condition.

Finally, natural medicine expert and herb advocate Andrew Weil, M.D., professor at the University of Arizona College of Medicine in Tucson and author of *Natural Health, Natural Medicine*, suggests eliminating tobacco, which is good advice even if you don't have diverticulitis.

Green Pharmacy for Diverticulitis

There are many herbs that can help. Here are my favorites.
❧❧❧ **Flax (*Linum usitatissimum*).** Commission E, the German expert panel that passes on the safety, effectiveness and dosage of medicinal herbs for the German government,

approves using one to three tablespoons of crushed flaxseed two or three times a day (with lots of water) to treat diverticulitis.

❧❧❧ **Psyllium** (*Plantago ovata*). Powdery, high-fiber psyllium seed is the major ingredient in Metamucil and a few other bulk-forming commercial laxatives. A few tablespoons a day (with plenty of water) provide a healthy amount of diverticulitis-preventing fiber. Watch how you react to this herb if you have allergies, however. If allergic symptoms develop after you take it once, don't use it again.

❧❧❧ **Wheat** (*Triticum aestivum*). Dr. Painter, whose study found a high-fiber diet to be the cure for diverticulitis, estimated that wheat bran contains five times the fiber of whole-wheat bread, making it the fiber-lover's fiber. He's not alone in his endorsement of wheat bran.

"Bran is the safest, cheapest and most physiologically effective method of treating and preventing constipation," says gastroenterologist W. Grant Thompson, M.D., professor at the University of Ottawa. And, I might add, when you're avoiding constipation you're also avoiding diverticulitis.

❧❧ **Slippery elm** (*Ulmus rubra*). Dr. Weil suggests using slippery elm bark powder to treat diverticulitis. The fibrous bark contains large quantities of a gentle laxative that soothes the digestive tract while keeping things moving.

The Food and Drug Administration has declared slippery elm to be a safe and effective digestive soother. Prepare it like oatmeal, adding hot milk or water to the powdered bark to make a cereal.

❧ **Camomile** (*Matricaria recutita*). British herbalist David Hoffmann, author of *The Herbal Handbook*, suggests sipping on camomile tea throughout the day. This herb is particularly valuable in treating diverticulitis because its anti-inflammatory action soothes the entire digestive system, he says. I suggest making a tea with two teaspoons of dried camomile per cup of boiling water. Steep for five to ten minutes.

❧ **Prune** (*Prunus dulcis*). Prunes combine lots of fiber with a sweet, delicious taste. They've been a folk remedy for constipation for ages. If I had diverticulitis, I'd eat plenty of prunes or drink prune juice.

❧ **Wild yam** (*Dioscorea villosa*). According to California herbalist Kathi Keville, author of *The Illustrated Herb Encyclopedia* and *Herbs for Health and Healing*, whom I highly respect, wild yam helps relieve the pain and inflammation of diverticulitis. I like her formula: two parts wild yam, (anti-inflammatory and antispasmodic), one part valerian (relaxing digestive tract soother), one part black haw (antispasmodic) and one part peppermint (anti-inflammatory and antispasmodic).

If I had diverticulitis, I might use a couple of tablespoons of this herb mixture brewed in a quart or so of water.

Dizziness

Once when Mrs. Duke was experiencing dizziness, she went to the doctor. She came home with an $18 packet of Trans-Derm Scōp—stick-on patches produced by Ciba Geigy that administered the drug scopolamine by absorption through the skin. For quite a while, scopolamine was the standard medication for dizziness and motion sickness.

Little did Peggy know that she could have gotten scopolamine much more cheaply by gathering some plants in our front yard. My jimsonweed (*Datura stramonium*) and cultivated ornamental *Datura* species all contain scopolamine, although perhaps less than the pharmaceutical.

Personally, I wouldn't recommend scopolamine, even from natural sources, for dizziness. It may work, but it can also cause side effects such as blurred vision, dry mouth, hallucinations and heart palpitations. I prefer ginger for seasickness, motion sickness, morning sickness and anything else that can cause dizziness or vertigo.

⟨❧⟩

Ginger Needs More Testing

I'm a big believer in ginger for dizziness, seasickness and all sorts of stomach distress. Centuries of folk use and several good studies support this use. But not every study has been favorable.

One study, sponsored by the pharmaceutical industry, I suspect, concluded that ginger was ineffective and the anti-dizziness medication scopolamine was effective. Personally, I don't buy into the results of a single study, but without an unbiased comparative study, I may never know which of these alternatives is more effective.

Unless the U.S. government sponsors studies comparing new drugs (synthetic and natural) not only with placebos but also with the best herbal alternatives, we may not be getting the best medicines. I want the best, whatever it is.

❧❧

The terms *dizziness* and *vertigo* are often used interchangeably, but technically there is a distinction. Dizziness simply means unsteadiness. Vertigo is worse. It is a disorienting illusion of movement, as if the world were whirling around you, or you around it.

Green Pharmacy for Dizziness

If you have chronic dizziness, see a physician. Prolonged or recurring bouts of dizziness can be a sign of inner ear infection, cardiac arryhthmia, high blood pressure or some other serious problems. For occasional bouts of dizziness, there are several herbs that might prove helpful.

❧❧❧ **Ginger** (*Zingiber officinale*). Chinese sailors chewed ginger root for seasickness thousands of years ago, and as they traveled, their remedy did, too—from Asia to India to the Middle East and on to Europe.

Modern science has shown that there is some validity to this ancient remedy. One study of 80 naval cadets, for example, showed that taking one gram (a half-teaspoon) of powdered ginger shortly before shoving off reduced symptoms of seasickness—including dizziness—by 38 percent and frequency of vomiting by 72 percent.

In earlier studies on land with 18 healthy subjects, one gram of ginger relieved vertigo and motion sickness better than the standard drug, dimenhydrinate (Dramamine).

"To prevent motion sickness, swallow two capsules 30 minutes before departure and then one to two more as symptoms begin to occur, probably about every four hours," suggests Varro Tyler, Ph.D., dean and professor emeritus of pharmacognosy (natural product pharmacy) at Purdue University in West Lafayette, Indiana. Ginger capsules are available at health food stores and other supplement outlets.

You can also try fresh ginger tea or slices of candied ginger, according to herb advocate Andrew Weil, M.D., professor at the University of Arizona College of Medicine in Tucson and author of *Natural Health, Natural Medicine*.

🌿🌿 **Ginkgo (*Ginkgo biloba*).** Ginkgo extract is prescribed extensively in Europe for vertigo, among many other conditions. One French study of 70 people with chronic vertigo showed that 47 percent improved while taking ginkgo. You can try 60 to 240 milligrams a day, but don't go any higher than that. In large amounts, ginkgo may cause diarrhea, irritability and restlessness.

🌿 **Celery (*Apium graveolens*).** Celery seed has a long history of use in traditional Chinese medicine as a treatment for dizziness.

🌿 **Pumpkin (*Cucurbita pepo*).** Some herbalists I respect claim that pumpkin seeds help relieve dizziness. If I were going to take this remedy myself, I'd have some pumpkin seed butter.

🌿 **Assorted herbs.** Recipe writer that I am, I can't resist combining all of the anti-dizziness herbs with a few flavor herbs in a Stomach Settler Tea. Combine four teaspoons of ginger with dashes of ground pumpkin seeds, celery seeds, camomile flowers, fennel, orange rind, peppermint and spearmint and steep for 15 minutes.

Dry Mouth

The Tupi Guarani Indians of Brazil have a plant called jaborandi that causes salivation. In fact, in the Tupi language, *jaborandi* means "that which causes slobbering."

When researchers at the National Institute on Dental Research (NIDR) heard about jaborandi from some ethnobotanists, they got all excited. (An ethnobotanist is a plant specialist who studies the medicinal uses of plants in other cultures.) Lots of people suffer from dry mouth syndrome, medically known as xerostoma, so the folks at NIDR are always on the lookout for new substances that stimulate salivation. Jaborandi sounded promising.

The ingredient in jaborandi (*Pilocarpus*, various species) that causes salivation is a compound called pilocarpine. Good studies have shown that pilocarpine increases production of saliva up to tenfold, easily relieving the uncomfortable sensation of oral dryness. Clearly jaborandi deserves more study.

Drooling over the Possibilities

Actually, when I learned about jaborandi, I got pretty excited myself. I imagined incorporating it into a chewing gum that could relieve dry mouth, providing easy relief for millions of people.

But there was a catch, both for me and for the NIDR. Brazil has a virtual monopoly on the supply of pilocarpine, which is also used to treat certain types of glaucoma, and they don't want any of their precious living source leaving the country. If they control the supply, they control the price. They are happy to export the pilocarpine they extract from jaborandi, but the government prohibits the export of living plants for fear that someone else will start extracting pilocarpine from them and sell it more cheaply. As a result, I was never able to get any jaborandi out of Brazil.

And Lord knows, I tried. I hooked up with a Johns Hopkins ophthalmologist and some of his friends, who had an interest in jaborandi's anti-glaucoma action, and we went chasing through the bush country of Brazil in search of the precious plants. But our efforts came to a halt when we were blocked by the authorities.

Some time later, I succeeded in obtaining a related species of *Pilocarpus* from Paraguay. But again there was a catch. Some of my colleagues at the U.S. Department of Agriculture (USDA) were concerned that my jaborandi citrus relative might harbor viruses that could decimate the U.S. citrus industry. They destroyed my plant.

A year later, I managed to get one jaborandi plant into the United States for research purposes. Again, the USDA got nervous about viruses, but this time I succeeded in persuading them not to destroy the precious plant. Instead they placed it under quarantine at the Beltsville Research Station where I worked. My jaborandi sat there for quite a while, and my hopes of ever retrieving it faded.

After I retired, I learned that the quarantine had been lifted. I picked up my jaborandi and transplanted it to my backyard. It's a nice plant.

Meanwhile, MGI Pharma of Minneapolis developed a pilocarpine-based mouth-moistening drug that it hopes to call Salagem; it's awaiting approval from the Food and Drug Administration (FDA). It looks like they'll get rich while a perfectly effective nondrug solution languishes in my backyard and in Brazil.

Caught High and Dry

Dry mouth is not only uncomfortable, it's also not good for you. Saliva helps control bacteria populations in the mouth, and in doing so it helps prevent tooth decay, gum disease and mouth infections.

An estimated 25 percent of older Americans complain of dry mouth. The condition is common among public speakers like me, hence the inevitable water glass at the podium. It is also related to aging and is a side effect of more than 400 widely used medications, including many prescribed for high blood pressure and depression.

In addition, dry mouth is a symptom of Sjögren's syndrome, a condition often associated with rheumatoid arthritis that also causes dry eyes.

Green Pharmacy for Dry Mouth

If you're ever caught with dry mouth in Brazil, you could try chewing some jaborandi. Here in the states, until the pilocarpine medication wins FDA approval, sip water frequently, especially when eating or speaking. Avoid coffee and sugary beverages, both of which can aggravate dry mouth. Also avoid alcohol, tobacco and salty foods. In addition, try these herbs.

❧ Echinacea (*Echinacea*, various species). One compound in echinacea, echinacein, is a proven saliva producer. I recommend taking a dropperful of tincture in juice. If you have access to the fresh plant, you can also chew the root. In addition to stimulating salivation, echinacea tends to numb the mouth, but this effect is temporary and harmless.

❧ Evening primrose (*Oenothera biennis*). Oil from the evening primrose (EPO) is a rich source of a compound known as gamma-linolenic acid (GLA). Few reviewing the medical literature can have any doubts that GLA is a potent treatment for autoimmune disorders, which are caused by a confused immune system attacking the body itself. Sjögren's syndrome is thought to be an autoimmune disorder.

If I had dry mouth caused by Sjögren's, I would try EPO. You can buy capsules of EPO in natural food stores. Simply follow the package directions.

❧ Multiflora rose (*Rosa multiflora*). In China, people simmer two to four teaspoons of the dried flower per cup of boiling water to make a tea for treating dry mouth.

❧ Red pepper (*Capsicum*, various species). Capsaicin, the fiery compound in hot pepper, stimulates not only salivation but also other watery discharges—sweat and tears. The hotter the pepper, the more capsaicin it contains. You can add red pepper to food or stir it into juice or tea.

❧ Yohimbe (*Pausinystalia yohimbe*). This herb is an African folk aphrodisiac that stimulates both erection and salivation. Currently, many American men are taking yohimbine, an extract of yohimbe, to treat erection impairment, so it's readily available. If you want to try this herb to treat dry mouth, I recommend asking your doctor for a prescription for yohimbine. Using the herb itself—a dried bark—can be hazardous.

Earache

There I was on Kelley's Island in Lake Erie on a beautiful spring day, leading a workshop on medicinal herbs. At our feet were mullein plants, an age-old remedy for earache. It was early June, too early for the mullein to be in flower. But the fuzzy leaves were everywhere, and the previous year's tall flower stalks were abundant as well.

Down in southern Ohio, there's an herbalist who is producing an earache salve based on mullein flowers and goldenseal. More than half of the participants in my workshop had tried this salve on their children after doctors had failed to cure their ear infections with antibiotics and even surgery. Several swore that it worked. Because of what I know about mullein and goldenseal, I'm inclined to trust their reports.

Earache has many possible causes. In children, the most common by far is an infection that invades the middle ear— what doctors call otitis media. But earache can also be caused by excess earwax, a perforated eardrum and other conditions in the head and neck. There's also an outer ear infection called otitis externa.

The actual infection may be bacterial, viral or fungal. An estimated 80 percent of children have at least one middle ear infection during their first five years. Breastfeeding apparently offers some protection. Compared with bottle-fed babies, breastfed infants develop fewer ear infections, and the longer the baby nurses, the lower the risk.

Often, pediatricians have prescribed antibiotics to help stop ear infections. But recently, more and more physicians are advising against being trigger-happy with antibiotics.

Problems with Aspirin

Earache treatment begins with pain relief and then proceeds to dealing with the cause. Physicians treat the pain with acetaminophen (or aspirin for adults), then give antibiotics and decongestants to treat the infection itself.

There are also some good herbs that can help adults deal

with the pain even before they see the doctor. For adult earaches, I'd try relieving the pain with a tea made of willow bark and wintergreen. These herbs contain salicin and salicylates, which are natural precursors of pharmaceutical aspirin. (If you are allergic to aspirin, however, you probably shouldn't take herbal aspirin either.)

But do not give either aspirin or its natural herbal alternatives to children who develop ear infections along with colds. When children take aspirin-like drugs for viral infections (especially colds, flu and chicken pox), there's a chance that they might get Reye's syndrome, a potentially fatal condition that damages the liver and brain. This herbalist hates to say it, but if my grandkids developed ear infections from colds, I'd treat their ear pain with acetaminophen rather than herbal relatives of aspirin.

Once you've treated the pain, it's time to consider the cause. A doctor can look in the affected ear and decide if you have an external or an internal problem.

Green Pharmacy for Earache

There are a number of herbs that can help alleviate the pain of earache or treat the causes.

✤ **Echinacea (*Echinacea*, various species).** Echinacea, also known as coneflower, has both antibiotic and immune-boosting effects. You can try using a teaspoon of dried herb in tea or a dropperful of echinacea tincture in juice or tea. Drink either three times a day. I use echinacea to treat all sorts of infections, and I would probably try it if I had an earache. (Although echinacea can cause your tongue to tingle or go numb temporarily, this effect is harmless.)

✤ **Ephedra (*Ephedra sinica*).** Also known as *ma huang* or Chinese ephedra, this herb contains two powerful decongestants, ephedrine and pseudoephedrine. They can help drain the fluid in the middle ear that is associated with middle ear infections. Pseudoephedrine is the active ingredient in many over-the-counter decongestants. One of these products, Sudafed, even takes its name from this compound. In a study of fliers with recurrent ear pain, 70 percent of those who took pseudoephedrine experienced relief.

❧❦

Be Gentle with Eardrops

Warning: The essential oils of several of the herbs described in this chapter can be dripped into the ears to help heal the infections that cause earache. If a doctor has told you that your eardrum has been perforated or you have any reason to suspect that it has, do not use herbal eardrops.

❧❦

Be careful to stick to the recommended doses when using this herb. Adults shouldn't use more than one teaspoon of dried herb to make a tea or take more than one teaspoon of tincture. Although the herb can be taken up to three times a day, you should be cautious because ephedra is a stimulant and might cause insomnia or raise blood pressure. Some people have died from overdosing on this herb in an attempt to get high, and the Food and Drug Administration has taken steps to stop the sale of ephedrine supplements.

Ephedra could be great for treating some children's problems, but because of the controversy surrounding it, you should consult your pediatrician before using it. Children should be given less than half of the amount appropriate for adults.

❧ **Garlic (*Allium sativum*).** Like echinacea, garlic and its extracts have antibiotic and immune-boosting benefits. In studies, dripping garlic oil directly into the ear canal has been shown to treat fungal infections as well as or better than pharmaceutical drugs.

Taken internally, garlic can help cure a middle ear infection. If you have an earache, I suggest adding more garlic to your cooking. You might also try putting a few drops of garlic oil in the painful ear.

❧ **Goldenseal (*Hydrastis canadensis*).** This is another potent natural antibiotic. Some naturopaths suggest using a mixture of echinacea, goldenseal and licorice root (this just for flavor). You can make a tea using either a teaspoon of each herb or a dropperful of each tincture per cup of boiling water. Enjoy a cup three times a day.

Although I don't have proof that this mixture is superior to either echinacea or goldenseal alone, I suspect that the combination of herbs is a better treatment.

❧ **Forsythia (*Forsythia suspensa*), gentian (*Gentiana officinalis*) and honeysuckle (*Lonicera japonica*).** All three of these herbs produce antibiotic activity. Practitioners of traditional Chinese medicine often prescribe them in powdered form, sprinkled on applesauce to treat children's ear infections. I've had such good success with this approach for colds and flu that I would also try it for earache. They are easily used to make tea.

❧ **Mullein (*Verbascum thapsus*).** Mullein flowers have many fans, and I've decided that these people must be on to something. One British herbalist suggests putting mullein flower oil drops in the affected ear.

❧ **Peppermint (*Mentha piperita*).** A number of herbalists suggest using mints, which are antiseptic, to relieve earache. To me, peppermint sounds most promising, because it contains menthol. I would suggest using it as a tea.

❧ **Teatree (*Melaleuca*, various species).** Aromatherapists and many herbalists consider teatree oil a significant antiseptic when applied to the skin. Try mixing a few drops in vegetable oil to make eardrops. Just don't use the drops if there is a possibility that the eardrum has been perforated, and don't take teatree oil, or any essential oil, internally. The oils are extremely concentrated, and even small quantities of many of them can be poisonous. I've also heard one anecdotal reference to problems arising from using teatree oil in the ear, so just to be on the safe side, discontinue use if you experience any irritation.

Emphysema

It's not unusual for me to get desperate calls from people who know about my herbal expertise and want help for one serious disease or another. One such call came from a distant relative of mine. Her mother, age 72, had emphysema.

A friend of the family had recommended "food-grade hydrogen peroxide" as a way of "getting more oxygen to the lungs." The sick woman's doctor hit the ceiling when he heard of this. My relative wanted to know what I thought of food-grade hydrogen peroxide, and I had to tell her that I had no idea what it was. I knew only that the liquid was a topical antiseptic and hair lightener.

I had a strong gut feeling that the doctor was right and that food-grade hydrogen peroxide, whatever it was, was a bad idea. I felt I had good reason for concern. I've been impressed with all the research showing that antioxidants, which abound in fruits, vegetables and herbs, can help heal many conditions, including many problems common in the elderly.

Antioxidants are substances that neutralize highly reactive free radical oxygen molecules, which cause cell damage throughout the body. But hydrogen peroxide is the opposite of an antioxidant. It's a pro-oxidant, meaning that it increases the number of free radicals in the body and might well increase cell damage. I weighed in on the side of the physician and told my relative that I wouldn't touch hydrogen peroxide, except for use as a topical antiseptic.

Still, that inquiry got me interested in antioxidants and emphysema. I checked my trusty database, and wouldn't you know that there's some intriguing research that antioxidants just might help? It appears that they help protect lung tissue from damage caused by smoking, which is the underlying cause of emphysema.

The Disease That Leaves You Breathless

Emphysema is slow suffocation. The tiny air sacs in the lungs (alveoli) become damaged and lose their ability to transfer oxygen into the blood and carbon dioxide out of it. As a result, the lungs function poorly.

The main symptom of emphysema is shortness of breath, which becomes worse as the condition becomes more severe. Because of the constant struggle to breathe, the chest becomes barrel-shaped. In advanced emphysema, an individual may require supplemental oxygen and be unable to tolerate even small amounts of physical activity. The condition is difficult to treat and is often fatal.

Emphysema results from chronic respiratory irritation. Smoking causes just about every case, although long-term exposure to dust, air pollutants and chemical vapors may also play a role.

Smoking also causes the vast majority of cases of a closely related condition, chronic bronchitis. In chronic bronchitis, the tiny hairs (cilia) that line the respiratory tract lose their ability to sweep out mucus. Uncleared mucus becomes thick and sticky, and it accumulates, becoming an emphysema-aggravating respiratory irritant. The combination of emphysema and chronic bronchitis is known as chronic obstructive pulmonary disease (COPD).

Green Pharmacy for Emphysema

Clearly, the best way to deal with emphysema, chronic bronchitis and COPD is to quit smoking. Once diagnosed, emphysema is not reversible. Still, remaining lung function can be maximized by avoiding respiratory irritants and by using supplemental oxygen. In addition, herbs that can help thin mucus or clear it from the lungs are particularly helpful.

🌺🌺🌺 **Mullein (*Verbascum thapsus*).** Herbal pharmacologist Daniel Mowrey, Ph.D., author of *The Scientific Validation of Herbal Medicine* and *Herbal Tonic Therapies*, praises velvety mullein for its ability to treat respiratory conditions, including emphysema. Mullein is rich in soothing mucilage. I've had such impressive results with using mullein to treat colds, flu and bronchitis that if I had emphysema, I would try it.

You can make a tea with one to two teaspoons of dried, crushed mullein leaves or flowers per cup of boiling water. Strain it carefully before drinking it. Dr. Mowrey also recommends a combination of mullein, red pepper and licorice (discussed below).

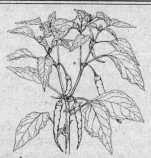

Red Pepper

American Indians used this medicinal spice, and it has changed the cuisines and medicine of the world since Columbus.

🌿🌿🌿 **Red pepper (*Capsicum*, various species).** British physician Irwin Ziment, M.D., urges his emphysema patients to eat a hot, spicy meal every day or down a glass of water spiked with 10 to 20 drops of hot-pepper sauce. There are two reasons for this. First, red pepper is a rich source of antioxidants that help protect lung tissue from damage at the cellular level. Second, it helps thin mucus and move it out of the respiratory tract.

Red pepper is far from the only spicy plant with expectorant value. The ancients used all of the hot spices to thin mucus and help propel it out of the lungs, particularly garlic, onions, ginger, mustard and horseradish. I'd recommend any or all of them. In fact, I've included most of them in my Mucokinetic Mule, the tea with a kick. (See page 223.)

🌿🌿 **Camu-camu (*Myrciaria dubia*) and other herbs rich in vitamin C.** A good deal of research demonstrates that vitamin C has mucus-thinning properties and helps treat all manner of respiratory conditions. In that case, I must put in a good word for camu-camu, the Amazonian fruit with the world's highest vitamin C content. On a dry-weight basis, it is nearly 4 percent vitamin C. That may not sound like much, but lemons have only 0.56 percent, and no other high-C fruit or vegetable comes close to camu-camu.

That said, I must add that camu-camu is not readily available in the United States, although I'm working on it and expect it will be available sometime within the next few years. Until your neighborhood grocer carries it, feel free to use citrus fruits, bell peppers, guava, watercress and all the other high-C fruits and vegetables. Rosehips are also a good source.

❦❦

Mucokinetic Mule

This emphysema tea kicks like a mule, so be careful how much of the ingredients you use. A mucokinetic herb, by the way, is one that has the ability to move mucus up and out of the lungs. Most of the herbs in this tea are mucokinetic.

Start with small amounts of herbs and add more only if your sinuses and taste buds can handle it. The herbs to use are garlic, ginger, hot pepper, horseradish and mustard; steep them in two cups of boiling water for ten minutes. You can add a bit of fruit that contains vitamin C, such as lemon or orange.

Drink this tea slowly and with caution! It will be *very* hot and could trigger gagging. If you can tolerate it, however, it will help unplug that mucus and get it flowing. If you just can't get it down, don't force it. Instead, try some of the other herbs mentioned in this chapter.

❦❦

❦❦ **Cardamom (*Elettaria cardamomum*).** This herb is very high in cineole, a potent expectorant compound. If I had emphysema, I'd add a teaspoon or two of powdered cardamom to fruit juice or tea.

Other herbs high in cineole (in descending order of potency) include spearmint, rosemary, sweet Annie, ginger, lavender, nutmeg, bee balm, peppermint, tansy, yarrow, cinnamon, basil, turmeric, lemon leaf, hyssop, tarragon, lemon verbena and fennel. Eucalyptus should really be at the top of this list, but I want to discuss this herb separately.

❦❦ **Eucalyptus (*Eucalyptus globulus*).** Eucalyptus oil is very high in cineole. This herb, a potent expectorant, is an ingredient in several sore throat lozenges and in commercial chest rubs.

Studies suggest that the benefits of a eucalyptus chest rub are an illusion. When inhaled, eucalyptus stimulates cold receptors in the nose, producing a feeling of increased air flow but no demonstrable decongestant activity.

Other studies, however, show that cineole has both expectorant and decongestant activity when ingested. Personally, I'd forget the chest rubs and go with a tea made with one to two teaspoons of dried, crushed leaves per cup of boiling water. Drink up to three cups a day.

Licorice (*Glycyrrhiza glabra*). Licorice contains nine expectorant compounds plus ten antioxidant compounds. If I had emphysema, I'd add an occasional teaspoon of sweet, powdered licorice root to herbal beverage teas. (While licorice and its extracts are safe for normal use in moderate amounts—up to about three cups of tea a day—long-term use or ingestion of larger amounts can produce headache, lethargy, sodium and water retention, excessive loss of potassium and high blood pressure.)

Peppermint (*Mentha piperita*). Peppermint contains nine expectorant compounds. In addition, its main active component, menthol, reportedly has mucus-thinning properties. You can take peppermint as a tea, tincture or capsule, but do not ingest the oil, which is for external use only.

Seneca snakeroot (*Polygala senega*). Commission E, the German expert panel that judges the safety and effectiveness of herbal medicines for the German counterpart of the FDA, recommends one to two teaspoons of seneca snakeroot tincture as an expectorant. This herb is useful in treating emphysema and bronchitis, according to Norman Bisset, Ph.D., professor of pharmacy at King's College at the University of London and author of *Herbal Drugs and Phytopharmaceuticals*.

Basil (*Ocimum basilicum*). Although basil is not widely known as an expectorant, it does contain six compounds that are useful for this purpose. I personally like pesto so much that I thought I'd mention this herb. Pesto is that wonderfully flavorful pasta sauce made with garlic and fresh basil, and in my opinion it's a particularly nice way to get a medicinal dose of both herbs.

Elecampane (*Inula helenium*). With respected British

herbalist David Hoffmann, author of *The Herbal Handbook*, reporting expectorant and lung-protective benefits for this herb, I would probably use it if I had emphysema. Try one to two teaspoons of dried, crushed herb per cup of boiling water. Drink up to two cups a day. Elecampane is bitter, so you can add lemon, licorice and honey to taste, or make a tea of mixed herbs with any of the other herbs mentioned in this chapter.

❧ **Oregano (*Origanum vulgare*).** Oregano contains six compounds that are expectorants. Like basil, it's not widely known as an expectorant, but also like basil, it's a wonderful culinary herb.

❧ **Tea (*Camellia sinensis*).** Speaking of expectorant teas, regular old green or black tea contains six expectorant compounds and one, theophylline, that can help mucus move up from deeper in the lungs. It also contains some caffeine, which studies have shown has some antidepressant value. That and its stimulant effect might help people with emphysema feel better.

Endometriosis

In women who have endometriosis, tissue closely resembling the uterine lining (the endometrium) grows outside the uterus in various locations in the pelvic cavity. This tissue swells and bleeds in conjunction with a woman's monthly menstrual cycle. Endometriosis may cause pain, nausea, heavy menstrual bleeding, pain during intercourse and in some cases, infertility.

Estimates vary about the prevalence of endometriosis, but most authorities suggest that 2 to 5 percent of women may have this condition. It's most likely to show up between the ages of 25 and 40.

As far as I can tell, neither mainstream nor naturopathic doctors can claim much success in treating endometriosis. Mainstream doctors often prescribe synthetic estrogen, usually in the form of birth control pills. And naturopaths have favored herbs and foods with natural plant hormones (phytoestrogens) that are related to the estrogens. Phytoestrogens are much less potent than the body's own estrogens. They actually block the body's estrogen receptor sites, thereby reducing the effect of a woman's own hormones.

There are many theories about the possible causes of endometriosis. According to some sources, evidence links it with immune system damage caused by estrogen-like environmental pollutants, such as certain pesticides. Other immune-suppressing drugs and toxins may be equally suspect. Some experts also speculate that using tampons, IUDs or the contraceptive cap might contribute to the risk of developing endometriosis. Apparently no one knows for sure.

Green Pharmacy for Endometriosis

If you're battling endometriosis, various authorities suggest avoiding alcohol, caffeine, whole-milk dairy products, eggs, fried foods, red meat, salt and sugar. I can't swear that any of these dietary changes will help, but they make good sense even if you don't have endometriosis.

And although I don't promise that any natural herbal alternatives will cure endometriosis, I believe that the ones described below may help. They are safe, and I believe they are worth a try.

✖✖✖ **Soybean (*Glycine max*) and other beans.** Many in the natural medicine camp have embraced soy products for treating endometriosis and other ailments, notably breast cancer, that are related to estrogen.

The soy supporters tout soybeans because they are high in two estrogen-like plant compounds, genistein and daidzein. Both of these phytoestrogens prevent your body from taking up the more harmful forms of estrogen circulating in your blood. They take the place of that estrogen, binding to your cells' estrogen receptor sites and preventing more harmful estrogens from binding to the same receptors. Significantly, they also protect the body from pollutants that chemically mimic estrogen.

The soy supporters are right. Soy *is* high in genistein and daidzein, but lots of other beans are also quite high in genistein, which appears to be the more active of the two phytoestrogens.

I predict that in the near future, the scientists who have been claiming that soy is a unique source of genistein will stop doing so. I also predict that there will be more emphasis on bean sprouts. As beans germinate, their genistein content (and the total phytoestrogen content) increases. And if the sprouts have fungi (as many home-grown sprouts do), the genistein content may increase as much as a hundredfold.

Pinto beans have almost as much genistein and daidzein as soybeans. Also, consider that some beans that don't have as much daidzein as soybeans have quite a bit more genistein. These include yellow split peas, black turtle beans, lima beans, anasazi beans, red kidney beans and red lentils. Also quite high in genistein are black-eyed peas, mung beans, adzuki beans and fava beans. Our analysis of scurfy peas showed that they have 50 times more genistein than soybeans.

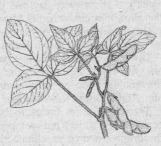

Soybeans

Soybeans share great medicinal potential with other edible legumes.

If you have endometriosis, I'd suggest eating as many edible beans as possible as often as possible. Also use generous amounts of bean sprouts in your salads and be sure to eat lots of bean soups, baked beans and Mexican bean foods like burritos. I enjoy all of these more than tofu.

🌿🌿 **Flax (*Linum usitatissimum*).** Flaxseed contains generous amounts of compounds called lignans, which help control endometrial (and maybe breast) cancer. Endometriosis is not the same as endometrial cancer, but because both involve uncontrolled growth of endometrial tissue, I'd suggest that you try flaxseed for preventing or treating endometriosis.

Flaxseed might be particularly helpful for anyone who is not a vegetarian. Vegetarians have high blood and urine levels of lignans, while eating meat suppresses lignans substantially. So if you're accustomed to meat in your diet, you may need an extra supply of lignan to compensate for this suppressant effect.

Some breads contain ground flaxseed; check labels. I've also ground the seed myself and added it to cornbread batter. I suggest you experiment with finding ways to get flaxseed into your diet on a regular basis.

❧❧ **Peanut (*Arachis hypogaea*).** I love peanuts. I munch some just about every day, and I'm always looking for studies that show they confer health advantages. When peanuts are analyzed, it turns out that they contain many of the same healthful substances as soybeans and other beans.

Given two foods with equal potential for health benefits, the one you enjoy should be better for you. That's assuming, as immunologists claim, that pleasure is good for the immune system. And let's face it, who doesn't prefer peanuts to soybeans?

There's an extra bonus to be had if you select Spanish peanuts. The papery red membrane around Spanish peanuts is the original source of oligomeric procyanidins (OPCs), substances that also may help control hormone-dependent cancers and possibly endometriosis.

❧ **Alfalfa (*Medicago sativa*).** Alfalfa sprouts contain phytoestrogens, so use them liberally on salads. Even if they don't relieve endometriosis symptoms, they are green vegetables, and eating more vegetables lowers cancer risk. If you have lupus or a family history of lupus, however, steer clear of alfalfa sprouts. There's some evidence that they may trigger lupus in sensitive individuals.

❧ **Evening primrose (*Oenothera biennis*).** I think of evening primrose oil (EPO) more as a treatment for the symptoms of premenstrual syndrome (PMS) than for endometriosis. (For more information on EPO and PMS, see page 441.) But the natural medicine guides I trust mention it almost as often as flaxseed and soy for treating this condition. EPO contains gamma-linolenic acid and tryptophan, both substances that seem to promote general good health in women.

Erection Problems

Not long ago, doctors and psychologists believed that 90 percent of erection difficulties were psychological and that a stimulating partner was all a man needed. Now authorities agree that most erection impairment has a physical cause: clogged arteries, alcohol or other drugs, diabetes, pelvic injuries, sleep deprivation, smoking or prostate surgery.

But how can a man know if his erection problem is physical or psychological? I like the postage-stamp test mentioned by herb advocate Andrew Weil, M.D., professor at the University of Arizona College of Medicine in Tucson and author of *Natural Health, Natural Medicine*. It is based on the fact that a normally functioning man has spontaneous erections in his sleep every night.

To take this test, fasten a strip of postage stamps around the shaft of your penis before you go to bed. If the strip is intact in the morning, you have not had any erections during sleep, and there is probably something wrong physically. If, on the other hand, a nighttime erection broke the stamps as you slept, your penis is working okay, and the problem may well be psychological.

This test is not foolproof, but it's a good place to start. The next logical step, of course, is to discuss the results with your doctor.

Impotence is the inability to raise or sustain an erection that is adequate for intercourse and ejaculation. Some 30 million American men experience some form of impotence, with more than a million currently being treated. Some take prescription medication. Others get penile implants. The newest approach involves self-injecting a hormone known as prostaglandin E. Within a few minutes, it produces a 90-minute erection.

Green Pharmacy for Erection Problems

But before you go sticking needles into your penis, you might try some of these herbal approaches.

🌿🌿🌿 **Fava bean (*Vicia faba*).** Alleged to have incited the ancient Roman poet Cicero to passion, the fava bean is our best food source of the compound L-dopa, which is often used to treat Parkinson's disease. Large amounts of L-dopa may cause priapism, a painful, persistent erection that has nothing to do with sexual arousal.

I wouldn't advocate doses of L-dopa large enough to cause priapism, but you'd be hard put to eat enough fava beans to ever cause a problem. Fava beans have an age-old reputation as an aphrodisiac. I suspect that a big serving—8 to 16 ounces—just might contain enough L-dopa to give erection a nice boost.

If fava beans seem to help, try sprouting them. The sprouts contain even more L-dopa.

❧❦

Stiff Drinks for Better Performance

I do a lot of traveling in Latin America, and the herbal formulas I find there—and people's faith in them—never cease to amaze me.

When it comes to enhancing men's sexual potency, there is a very long list of herbs with a reputation for delivering. I find a couple of alcoholic beverages made from herbal formulas added to a wine or rum base to be particularly intriguing.

One is *siete raices*. In English this translates to "seven roots," which is rather odd, because the drink is made from seven dried barks. The other is *rompe calzon*—"bust your britches." The name comes from its folklore reputation for producing erections large enough to strain trouser material. (I'm not making this up.)

There is only anecdotal evidence that *rompe calzon* stimulates erotic interest, but those anecdotes sure sell a lot of this brew in Latin American countries. I confess that I've tried it myself and haven't found it all that stimulating.

You won't be able to buy either of these formulas in the states, but one ingredient common to both may be available here. Clavohuasca (*Tynnanthus panurensis*) is an aromatic vine that is often found climbing to the forest canopy in Amazonian Peru, where I lead my Rainforest Pharmacy Workshops.

One traveler in my first Physician's Workshop, an acclaimed herbalist himself, says he has empirical evidence that tincture of clavohuasca, a rather pleasant and warming liqueur, sexually excites both the male and female of the human species—namely him and his wife.

I know of only one herb shop in the United States that carries tincture of clavohuasca, Smile Herb Shop in College Park, Maryland, so I'm assuming that it's imported and can be found in other herb shops. If you're anxious to give it a try, you might have to search for it—but you'd have to work a whole lot harder to get your hands on either siete raices or rompe calzon.

❧❧

❧❧❧ Ginkgo (*Ginkgo biloba*). Ginkgo is best known for improving blood flow through the brain. But it also seems to boost blood flow into the penis, thus aiding iffy erections.

In several small studies, physicians have obtained very good results with 60 to 240 milligrams daily of a standardized ginkgo extract. In one nine-month study, 78 percent of men with impotence due to atherosclerotic clogging of the penile artery reported significant improvement without side effects.

People normally think of atherosclerosis as a disease that clogs the blood vessels that supply the heart, thereby leading to heart attacks. This same disease can also clog the blood vessels that supply the penis and lead to erection problems.

In another six-month study, half of the men being treated with ginkgo regained their erections. The active compounds are too dilute in ginkgo leaves to do much good, so standardized extracts concentrate it: A 50:1 extract means that 50 pounds of leaves were used to produce 1 pound of extract. These extracts are available at many health food stores and herb shops.

You can try 60 to 240 milligrams a day, but don't go any higher than that. In large amounts, ginkgo may cause diarrhea, irritability and restlessness. And do give it time to work. In about six months, you'll know whether it's going to do the trick.

❧❧❧ Velvet bean (*Mucuna*, various species). Years ago, while working in Panama, I was told by more than one informant that the seeds of the velvet or ox-eye bean (in Spanish, *ojo de buey*) were aphrodisiac. That was before I knew that these seeds can contain as much L-dopa as fava beans, and perhaps more.

❧❧❧ Yohimbe (*Pausinystalia yohimbe*). For at least ten years, I have maintained that if there is a real herbal erection enhancer, yohimbe is it. I based this on centuries of folklore about the African tree bark and a few small clinical trials that showed that the herb produced erections in about half of men with psychological impotence and about 40 percent with physical erection problems.

Unfortunately, the side effects were a little unnerving, including anxiety, increased heart rate, elevated blood pressure, flushing, hallucinations and headache. This is not an herb that you want to mess around with.

But then the drug companies got into the act. They figured out how to extract the active compound and eventually won approval for yohimbine hydrochloride (Yocon, Yohimex) as a prescription medication. After one month, 14 percent of men taking it reported restoration of full and sustained erections, 20 percent reported partial responses, and 65 percent reported no improvement. Still, one-third improved, which isn't bad.

Generally, I advocate taking a whole herb rather than a pharmaceutical derivative, but this is an exception to my rule. Compared with the raw herb, the prescription drug causes fewer side effects, and those are generally benign. If I had erection difficulties, I might ask my doctor to put me on yohimbine.

❧❧ Anise (*Pimpinella anisum*). Anise contains several compounds that are estrogenic, so it might seem an unlikely herb for erection problems. Estrogen is a female hormone, and a number of plants contain substances that act like this hormone in the body. That's why they're called estrogenic. Oddly enough, though, some people who have used estrogenic herbs report androgenic (male sex hormone) effects as well. And anise has a reputation for increasing male libido.

I think anise is worth a try, which is why it's an ingredient in my Erector Set Tea: Combine to taste a dash or two of anise, cardamom, epimedium, ginger and ginseng. Sweeten with licorice root.

❧❧ Cardamom (*Elettaria cardamomum*). This herb contains at least two androgenic compounds. For centuries, Arab cultures have held this spice in high esteem as an aphrodisiac, thus Arab coffee houses often mix some into coffee.

What could account for cardamom's aphrodisiac reputation? In my database, cardamom shows up as the best source of the compound cineole. Cineole is a central nervous system stimulant, and people have a way of thinking that any stimulation is sexual stimulation. It probably can't hurt to spike your coffee or tea with a little cardamom, though, and this herb tastes good, too.

Cinnamon (*Cinnamomum*, various species). Alan Hirsch, M.D., director of the Smell and Taste Research Foundation in Chicago, attached measurement devices to the penises of medical students to test their reactions to various aromas. The smell of hot cinnamon buns generated the most blood flow, hence suggesting the most help for erections. A combination of the aromas of pumpkin pie (pumpkin plus nutmeg) and lavender also stimulated penile blood flow.

Okay, I know that all of this sounds somewhat far-fetched, but these are valid scientific studies we're talking about. How do you take advantage of this research? Well, if the way to a man's heart really is through his stomach—and you want to get somewhere else as well—why not give him cinnamon buns and pumpkin pie?

Ginger (*Zingiber officinale*). In an article titled "Studies on Herbal Aphrodisiacs Used in the Arab System of Medicine" published in the *American Journal of Chinese Medicine*, some Saudi scientists asserted that ginger extracts significantly increase sperm motility and quantity.

Ginger, a botanically close relative of cardamom, certainly has a piquant taste, and maybe it stirs enough sexual interest to help a flagging erection. I make no promises, but I have great respect for folk medical traditions, which is why I include both ginger and cardamom in my Erector Set Tea.

Ginseng (*Panax*, various species). American gin-

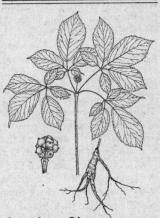

American Ginseng

First discovered in southern Canada by a French explorer, American ginseng is an expensive, rare herb that was said to "invigorate the virile powers."

seng (*P. quinquefolius*) is probably North America's most famous—and perhaps most overrated—aphrodisiac. Even though studies have shown that animals increase their sexual activity when they eat ginseng, I'm not entirely convinced that this herb will spark anyone's fire.

Still, I grow several varieties—American, Asian (*P. ginseng*) and Siberian (*Eleutherococcus senticosus*), which is also known as eleuthero. I'm not currently using any of these herbs, however, as they are expensive. But I am preparing for old age by holding some in reserve just in case the Chinese are correct in saying that ginseng makes an old man young again. America, by the way, exports close to $100 million worth of ginseng annually, mostly to Asians who have great faith in American ginseng and regard it as the herbal fountain of youth.

❧❧ **Muira puama (*Ptychopetalum*, various species).** There is one study showing that this little-known Amazonian tree "may be effective in restoring libido and treating erectile dysfunction," according to Melvin Werbach, M.D., assistant clinical professor of psychiatry at the University of California, Los Angeles, School of Medicine, and naturopathic physician Michael Murray, N.D., who cited the study in their book *Botanical Influences on Illness*. Of 262 men taking 1 to 2.5 grams (½ to 1¼ teaspoons) of muira puama extract a day for two weeks, 51 percent of those with erection problems reported improvement, as did 62 percent of those with loss of libido. I confess I haven't reviewed the original study, but if I had an erection problem, I might try this herb. You can find it in some herb stores. So far I have seen no reports of side effects. (Some men find the Amazonian ladies so attractive as to render the muira puama superfluous.)

❧❧ **Oat (*Avena sativa*).** Stallions that are fed wild oats supposedly become friskier and libidinous, which is where we got the phrase "sowing wild oats." Some studies suggest that oats are a sexual stimulant for the human male as well. Esteemed California herbalist Kathi Keville, author of *The Illustrated Herb Encyclopedia* and *Herbs for Health and Healing*, includes the herb in the tea she recommends to men: a half-ounce each of wild oats, ginkgo leaves, ginseng root, yohimbe bark and damiana leaves. I'd recommend the same, but leave out the yohimbe bark, for the reasons I've given previously. (If you want the effects of yohimbe bark, ask your doctor for a prescription for yohimbine instead.) Steep this mixture in a pint or two of boiling water, then let it cool before drinking.

☙☙ **Quebracho** (*Aspidosperma quebracho-blanco*). In South America, this herb, which the Food and Drug Administration includes on its list of herbs generally recognized as safe, is considered a male aphrodisiac. It does contain the proven erection-raising compound yohimbine, but I'm leery of the herb yohimbe for the reasons I've given previously. If you do use it, make a tea by steeping about five teaspoons of bark per cup of boiling water and sweeten it with licorice root. But don't try this herb if you have high blood pressure, and if you experience any side effects, such as dizziness, don't use it again.

☙☙ **Wolfberry** (*Lycium chinese*). Can the wolfberry make a young wolf out of an old man? In one study, men over age 59 ate about two ounces (50 grams) of wolfberries a day for ten days and came away with significantly raised testosterone levels. Raising testosterone boosts male sexuality only in cases of a deficiency of this male hormone, but some elderly men do become deficient. Perhaps that's why the Chinese consider wolfberries to have anti-aging properties.

☙ **Ashwaganda** (*Withania somnifera*). Practitioners of Ayurvedic medicine, the traditional medicine of India, regard this root as the Indian answer to ginseng for the male libido. Ashwaganda, they claim, can help treat impotence and male infertility. But I wouldn't recommend taking this particular herb every day—just occasionally. Try a cup or two of tea made with five teaspoons of dried herb per cup of boiling water.

☙ **Country mallow** (*Sida cordifolia*). Here's another stimulant herb with a folk reputation as an erection-enhancing aphrodisiac. Its stimulant compound is ephedrine, the same one found in Chinese ephedra, the decongestant, anti-asthma herb. Country mallow contains some 850 parts per million of ephedrine, which probably explains its use for impotence. As with caffeine, ephedrine can get you wired, and some men experience that as sexual arousal.

☙ **Guarana** (*Paullinia cupana*). Brazilians drink gallons of guarana tea and guarana soft drinks and often mention it as an aphrodisiac. The reason is that this herb contains a fair amount of caffeine, and traditionally, any stimulant eventually came to be viewed as a sexual stimulant. Drink guarana if you like, try a few teaspoons per cup of boiling water, then see how amorous you feel. (You could simply drink some coffee, tea, Coke or Pepsi, but that's not going to have the same exotic appeal.

When it comes to sexual enhancement, anything that engages your mind in the process can prove helpful.)

✿ **Saw palmetto (*Serenoa repens*).** This small palm tree native to the Southeast has been shown to help shrink enlarged prostate tissue. But a century ago, it was also considered useful for treating impotence and loss of libido. The main effect of saw palmetto is that it shrinks the prostate, allowing older men to urinate more freely. Prostate enlargement does not necessarily interfere with sexual function, but relieving the condition can only help men feel better about their sexual equipment, which just might be of some help with erection.

✿ **Assorted essential oils.** For erection problems, aromatherapists often recommend whole-body massage with a combination of a few drops of the essential oils of clary sage, jasmine and rose mixed into a vegetable oil base. (Remember not to ingest the oil, however, as even a small amount can be toxic.) Personally, I've found massage to be a wonderful aphrodisiac, even without the aromatic oils.

Fainting

Herbs for fainting? The picture that comes to mind is definitely turn-of-the-century—a scented handkerchief being waved under the nose of a fainting woman. And it's true that women fainted a lot in the days of Queen Victoria's reign. Often it was because they wore their corsets too tight.

Folk medicine does, in fact, offer a number of different "smelling salts," strong-scented substances that can wake up the slumbering and jar them back to full consciousness.

Fainting, or swooning, is simply sudden loss of consciousness as a result of decreased blood flow to the brain. Among the causes are hunger, exhaustion, severe emotional upset and pain. A hot, stuffy environment can do it, too.

If you feel faint, standard first-aid advice is to lie on your back and elevate your legs to coax more blood into your brain. Or sit with your head lowered between your knees to accomplish the same thing.

A number of medical conditions can cause fainting, and

some of them are fairly serious. If you have a tendency to faint easily, or if you faint for no apparent reason, a doctor's visit is usually in order.

Green Pharmacy for Fainting

Herbalists no longer recommend routinely carrying smelling salts. But if you have a tendency to faint, there are a couple of herbs that act like smelling salts that you can have on hand. There are also a number of stimulant herbs that might prove helpful in preventing fainting.

✦✦ **Broomweed (*Sida rhombifolia*).** Canary Islanders brew the leaves of this herb into a tea. I'm not surprised, because it contains ephedrine, the potent central nervous system stimulant and decongestant. I'd try a strong tea made with about five teaspoons of dried herb per cup of boiling water. Steep until cool.

✦✦ **Cardamom (*Elettaria cardamomum*).** For centuries, Arabs have added cardamom to their coffee in the belief that it was an aphrodisiac. I can't swear that it stimulates the libido, but it certainly stimulates the nervous system.

According to my database, cardamom is the best source of the stimulant compound cineole, which is present in most of the herbs that aromatherapists recommend for fainting. For a little extra kick, I frequently add one or two cardamom seeds to coffee or tea. It tastes really good.

✦✦ **Coffee (*Coffea*, various species) and other caffeine-containing beverages.** Coffee contains that famous stimulant, caffeine. It's an old favorite for getting rid of that faint feeling. But other caffeine-containing beverages have also been used to treat fainting, including tea, colas and the South American drinks mate, guarana and cacao. Hot chocolate works, too, since it also contains caffeine.

✦✦ **Country mallow (*Sida cordifolia*).** Here's an herb that's generously endowed with the stimulant compound ephedrine. The seeds have the most. Because of its stimulant action, country mallow has even been used to treat narcolepsy, a condition that gives people the overwhelming urge to fall asleep.

Try making a strong tea using five teaspoons of this herb per cup of boiling water. Steep until cool.

✦✦ **Ephedra (*Ephedra sinica*).** Also known as *ma huang* or Chinese ephedra, this herb is the best source of ephedrine.

The big problem with whole ephedra, as well as its chemical components ephedrine and pseudoephedrine, is its side effects: insomnia, anxiety, restlessness and possibly aggravation of high blood pressure. So you have to be careful with this herb. In fact, if you take really high doses, very strange things can happen. The medical literature contains 20 case reports of ephedrine psychosis.

Over the past couple of years, several people have died as a result of abusing this herb. They took large overdoses of commercial products containing ephedra in an attempt to get high. Unfortunately, because of these incidents, the Food and Drug Administration has decided it's too much of a stimulant, and they have taken steps to remove ephedrine supplements from the market.

When I use ephedra, I brew a tea using a half-teaspoon or so of dried herb (or a half-teaspoon to one teaspoon of tincture) per cup of boiling water. I steep it until it's cool enough to drink. These forms of the herb are safe to use at the recommended doses.

Eucalyptus (*Eucalyptus globulus*). This herb has a sharp, pungent aroma that is familiar to anyone who has ever sniffed Vicks Vapo-Rub. It comes about as close as we get in modern times to smelling salts. Aromatherapists suggest placing a drop or two of eucalyptus essential oil on a cloth and holding it under the nose to revive someone who has fainted. (Eucalyptus oil should never be ingested, however.)

Eucalyptus is also high in the stimulant compound cineole, so after the person is more or less revived, try giving some eucalyptus tea made with one to two teaspoons of crushed leaves per cup of boiling water.

Rosemary (*Rosmarinus officinalis*). The oil that gives rosemary its unique aroma is well-endowed with cineole, which has been shown to be active whether it's inhaled, ingested or applied directly to the skin.

Use rosemary as you would eucalyptus: If someone faints, place a drop or two of rosemary essential oil on a tissue and hold it under the person's nostrils. (Again, though, the oil should not be ingested.) Or crush a handful of rosemary's needlelike leaves into a ball and hold that under the person's nose.

Once the person has revived, brew up some rosemary tea using one to two teaspoons of crushed leaves per cup of boiling water.

Other herbs with good amounts of cineole include sweet
Annie and ginger. You can use them the same way.

❧ **Lavender (*Lavandula*, various species).** My good friend,
respected California herbalist Kathi Keville, who wrote *The
Illustrated Herb Encyclopedia* and *Herbs for Health and
Healing*, notes that the Victorians were clearly prepared for
swooning. The ladies carried little aromatherapeutic "swooning
pillows" filled with stimulating lavender and camphor. She offers
a good recipe for smelling salts: Fill a small vial with table salt
and add a dozen drops of lavender, rosemary or eucalyptus oil.

❧ **Soursop (*Annona muricata*).** The leaves of this tropical
member of the pawpaw family contain aromatic compounds. In
the Caribbean, people crush the leaves and use them as
smelling salts when someone feels faint. In a pinch, I'd try
seeds from any of our North American pawpaws, but don't get
the juices in your eyes—they may cause eye problems.

Fever

The worst fever I ever had laid me low in Darien, Panama, in
1961. I was part of a team that included a geographer, a
hydrologist and a world-renowned tropical ecologist, Les
Holdridge, Ph.D.

In between forays into the bush to study the vegetation in that
wild, frontier area, we stayed in a modest yellow house rented
from a German oil man. Sometimes there was pure rainwater to
drink, and rarely, when the town generator ran in El Real, we
had electricity. Returning to the house one day, I suddenly developed alternating chills and fever. My buddies told me I was
delirious for hours.

In my lucid moments, I assumed that I had malaria, since
alternating fever and chills are a hallmark of that tropical
scourge. But there was no doctor around, so I couldn't be sure.
I took some antimalaria medication, figuring that the pills that
suppress the malaria bug might also get rid of all sorts of other
microorganisms, any number of which might have found their
way into my body. Whatever was causing my fever, the antimalaria pills knocked it out before it knocked me off.

Now it's 35 years later, and I've just retired from the U.S. Department of Agriculture and the job that took me to so many exotic locales. But my beloved database will remain on the Internet, accessible to anyone who's interested. There you can find hundreds of plants that are said to reduce fever. But to save you a hunt in the wild frontier of the Internet (which could *give* you a fever), I'll review the highlights here.

Cooling the Fevered Brow

Around the world, an extraordinary number of plants have been used to treat fever. In Indonesia alone, 256 plants are folkloric fever fighters. Many of them I've never seen, and I've spent a lifetime in this field.

In my experience, more than half of folkloric medicinal plants live up to their reputations. But I suspect that for fever, the figure is higher. It's fairly easy to tell if an herb actually reduces fever, so the ones that don't work would rarely if ever have developed a reputation for efficacy.

If I developed a serious fever in any other out-of-the-way place and had no access to a physician, you can bet I'd consult the locals, in sign language, and let them feel the heat on my forehead. And I'm sure I could find someone who could lead me to fever-cooling plant medicine, probably growing close at hand.

Bitter Bounty

The world's best-known fever medicine is aspirin, derived from the salicylates in willow bark and many other plants. I've seen willow growing almost everywhere, all the way from Maine, where I give my summer ethnobotany class, to the Amazon, where I hold my winter classes. Willow trees grow from the arctic to the tropics and were used by thousands of ethnic groups long before Bayer decided to turn Nature's aspirin into a pharmaceutical pill.

While salicylates are very familiar to me as a botanist, I must admit that they are also unfathomable. Salicylic acid lowers my temperature, but the very same chemical causes plants to warm up by as much as 20 degrees above the temperature of their surroundings. Salicylates are the reason that snow melts around skunk cabbage in February. Don't ask me to explain it; I'm just telling it like it is.

Salicylates have a bitter taste, as do the vast majority of fever-reducing plant chemicals. It seems to go with the healing territory. My database contains a list of 25 plants used in Oaxaca, Mexico, to treat malaria, and all but one is bitter. So if you're treating fever with herbs, you'll have to brace yourself for a bitter natural pill.

While people rightly regard fever as a sign of infection, attempting to bring it down is sometimes a mistake. Up to a point, fever is a friend. Most microorganisms that cause disease die when exposed to high temperatures, so fever is one of the ways in which the immune system tries to kill them. The trouble is that prolonged high fevers can kill us, too.

A good rule of thumb is: Don't treat every fever right away. Treat it when it starts making you feel uncomfortable. For high fever—above 103°—you'll want to consult a doctor as soon as possible, of course. For milder high temperature—99° to 101°—you may choose to take aspirin, acetaminophen or ibuprofen (Motrin or Advil). One word of caution: Most benign fevers start to let up within a day or two. If any fever, even a mild one, persists for more than 48 hours, see your doctor.

Green Pharmacy for Fever

There are a number of herbs that can help reduce a fever. As a general rule, however, remember that it's not a good idea to give aspirin or aspirin-like herbs to children who have fevers with viral infections such as colds, flu and chicken pox. There is a chance that they could develop Reye's syndrome, a potentially fatal condition that causes liver and brain damage. And if you are allergic to aspirin, you probably shouldn't use aspirin-like herbs.

🌿🌿🌿 Willow (*Salix*, various species). When the eighteenth-century British minister Edward Stone set out to find a cheap substitute for expensive imported cinchona bark, which was used to treat malaria and other fevers, he noticed that willow bark tasted just as bitter and decided to try it.

Willow proved to be a good pain reliever and fever fighter, and its use spread around England, Europe and the Americas. The active compound salicin was isolated in 1830, and the

Bayer company tinkered with salicin to create aspirin. The new Bayer Aspirin was released in the 1890s, and it quickly became one of the world's most popular drugs. But you can still use willow bark. I do.

Try making a tea with one to two teaspoons of dried bark steeped in a cup of boiling water for about 20 minutes. You can mask the bitter taste with cinnamon, ginger, camomile or other flavorful herbs.

Meadowsweet (*Filipendula ulmaria*). This is another excellent source of salicin, the chemical in willow bark that fights fever. Commission E, the body of experts that advises the German government about herbs, suggests making a tea with one to two teaspoons of meadowsweet flowers. Try up to three cups a day.

Elder (*Sambucus nigra*). Commission E endorses using two to three teaspoons of elder flowers a day in tea for feverish chills.

Ginger (*Zingiber officinale*). In studies with animals, several compounds in ginger have been shown to have anti-fever value, according to Varro Tyler, Ph.D., dean and professor emeritus of pharmacognosy (natural product pharmacy) at Purdue University in West Lafayette, Indiana. Neither he nor I know of any human studies of ginger for fever, but it's a safe herb, so it probably shouldn't hurt if you want to brew ginger tea, eat candied ginger or sip ginger ale. Also, ginger's flavor can help make other fever-reducing herb teas more palatable. And it just might help fight fever.

Peppermint (*Mentha piperita*). Many herbalists recommend peppermint for relieving fever, suggesting such combinations as elder and peppermint or willow and peppermint. If I had a fever, I would add peppermint to fever-fighting teas. It would certainly enhance the flavor.

Red pepper (*Capsicum*, various species), cinnamon (*Cinnamomum*, various species) and cranberry (*Vaccinium macrocarpon*). In my database, red pepper is a fair source of salicylates. Cinnamon and cranberry also have anti-fever reputations. The next time I have a fever, I think I'll try cranberry sauce topped with cayenne and cinnamon.

Flatulence

Recently, my wife and I tried fava beans, also known as faba beans. These are similar to, although bulkier than, big lima beans. We expected that like all other beans, they would generate a lot of gas. Imagine our surprise when gas was not a problem.

Perhaps the reason was that I had resorted to folklore in an effort to eliminate bean-induced flatulence. I soaked dry beans in water overnight, then discarded the water and cooked the soaked beans in new water. It's an age-old anti-gas strategy.

In addition, I used an old Chinese approach that I got from *Chinese Healing Foods and Herbs*, a book by pharmacognosist (natural product pharmacist) Albert Leung, Ph.D. The Chinese soak their beans in water to which they add the annual wormwood (*Artemisia annua*).

Finally, for added protection, I also followed an Appalachian anti-flatulence suggestion and cooked my beans with a small, whole carrot.

If I'd had any wormseed, or *epazote* (*Chenopodium ambrosioides*), I would have added a dash of that as well. Mexicans cook their beans with this herb to reduce flatus.

What with overnight soaking, wormwood and a carrot to help us, Peggy and I experienced no significant flatulence from our fava beans.

Bacteria at Work

Most flatus is produced in the intestine by undigested carbohydrates. Instead of being broken down in the stomach, some starches enter the small intestine intact. The intestine does not produce the enzymes necessary to digest two specific carbohydrates, raffinose and stachyose, so they just sit there until the bacteria that normally inhabit the bowel ferment them, a process that releases gas.

Guess which foods are highest in raffinose and stachyose? You guessed it—beans. And among beans, the three that are highest in that pair of carbohydrates are English peas, soybeans and black-eyed peas. But those aren't the only ones: Limas, pintos, black beans and other legumes also contain enough of these indigestible carbohydrates to produce gas.

If you think that you're producing more gas than you used to, you may be right. If you've evolved your diet in a healthier direction recently and are eating less meat, fewer fats and more carbohydrates (especially beans), the chances are that you've been eating more of the foods that are most likely to produce gas.

Most people who complain of "excess gas," on the other hand, actually produce amounts that digestive system specialists (gastroenterologists) would call perfectly normal. Studies show that the average adult passes gas from 8 to 20 times every waking hour of the day. In other words, there's nothing unusual about releasing gas more than once an hour.

Green Pharmacy for Flatulence

Just because flatulence is normal doesn't mean it's welcome. Flatus cannot be banished from the body, but you can significantly reduce the likelihood of unwanted exclamations. A number of herbs can help.

❦❦❦ **Assorted carminative herbs.** Any herb that soothes the digestive tract and has a reputation for minimizing flatus is known as a carminative.

Dozens of herbs fall into this category, so it's hard to highlight just a few. The most helpful are those containing the most gas-relieving chemicals, most notably the compounds camphor, carvone, eugenol, menthol and thymol. These compounds are especially concentrated in allspice, cloves, cornmint, caraway, dill, fennel, horsebalm, peppermint, sage and thyme.

❦❦

Banishing Gas

Besides taking herbs, you can try a number of other natural approaches to help shut off your body's gasworks.

One way is to stop eating beans, but I wouldn't recommend that. Beans are inexpensive sources of high-quality protein, fiber and other nutrients.

Or you could try Beano. This product, available at pharmacies, health food stores and some supermarkets, contains the enzymes that can digest the gas-causing carbohydrates raffinose and stachyose but which our bodies don't produce. A study has shown that it works.

It also helps to eat more slowly. Chew your food thoroughly. Make meals as relaxed as possible. If you eat quickly and wolf your food down, you swallow larger lumps, which are more likely to enter the intestine undigested.

Lactose intolerance is another major cause of flatulence. Try cutting down on or eliminating dairy products for a week or two and see if you experience less gas and stomach distress. If you do, you're probably one of the many people who have trouble digesting milk sugar (lactose). To deal with this, you have two choices: Either cut way back on dairy foods (although yogurt is usually okay) or try adding the commercial product Lactaid to milk. Lactaid contains the enzyme that digests lactose.

Some people notice an increase in flatulence when they eat foods that are artificially sweetened with sorbitol. Read food labels carefully and try avoiding sorbitol for a time. If you notice that you're passing less gas, you might want to permanently avoid this sweetener.

❧

In addition, most of the herbs in the mint and carrot families are good carminatives, including aniseed, basil, bergamot, camomile, cinnamon, coriander, garlic, ginger, hyssop, juniper, lavender, lemon, marjoram, nutmeg, onion, oregano, rosemary, savory and tarragon. Try using carminative herbs to flavor starchy dishes, especially those made with beans.

You can also deflate flatus with my Carminatea, made with camomile, caraway, dill, fennel, lemon balm (also known as melissa) and peppermint and sweetened with licorice.

Fungal Infections

Athlete's foot. Vaginal yeast infections. Jock itch. Fungal toenail infections. There is plenty of fungus among us. I've certainly had my own share of fungal infections.

While there are separate chapters in this book for athlete's foot and yeast infections, I thought it would be helpful to include this more generic look at herbs that can be used to treat *any* fungal infection. Whenever I get fungal infections at my Herbal Vineyard in Maryland, I often try mixtures of garlic and black walnut, both of which grow in profusion on my land, along with teatree oil, which I keep on hand. Each of these herbs is potently antifungal.

So why, you might ask, do I go to the trouble of mixing them? Why not just find a good one and stick to it, in the pharmaceutical tradition of isolating the magic bullet? One reason is that I love to work with herbs and have fun mixing them. Another is that the research is quite clear: Mixtures of antifungal herbs almost always work better than single herbs.

The synergy—the harmonious working together—of antifungal herbs has been demonstrated in several studies. In one test of ten plant species whose oils were antifungal, researchers noted that "combinations of the antifungal essential oils increased their activity remarkably." In a similar study, researchers noted that "in all the oil combinations, the antifungal potency was found to increase over individual oils."

We should not be surprised by this. After all, essential oils are complex combinations of compounds that evolved to protect plants against fungi and other diseases and pests. Synergy is the rule in nature, so it makes sense that combinations would work better than a single, isolated essential oil constituent.

Currently, many pharmaceutical "magic bullet" antifungals are more potent than herbal approaches, and sometimes when I have a bad fungal infection, I use them. But even then, I often combine them with herbs for an extra antifungal boost. If your doctor concurs, try this the next time you have a fungal infection and see how synergy works for you.

Green Pharmacy for Fungal Infections

Here are some antifungal herbs that can get the job done.

❧❧❧ Garlic (*Allium sativum*). I believe that garlic is among our best antiseptics in general and antifungals in particular, closely rivaling teatree oil.

At the Banaras Hindu University in India, scientists working with garlic compounds showed that one of its chemical constituents, ajoene, was almost as effective against mildew fungus as several pharmaceutical antifungals. Several other studies have shown similar results.

Clinical trials have also yielded impressive results. Among people taking 25 milliliters (five to six teaspoons) of garlic extract a day, their blood serum exhibited significant antifungal activity against several common fungi, including *Candida albicans*, which causes yeast infections.

Garlic extract is even more potent when applied externally. I know from both research and personal experience that it boosts the antifungal effectiveness of pharmaceutical antifungal drugs. Simply liquefy raw garlic in a blender and use a cotton ball or clean cloth to apply it directly to the affected area three times a day.

❧❧❧ Licorice (*Glycyrrhiza glabra*). Acording to my database, licorice contains at least 25 fungicidal compounds, more than any other herb listed. Oddly, I haven't found any good clinical trials on using licorice extracts to treat fungal infections, but based on this herb's antifungal content, I'm confident that it would help.

You can make a strong decoction by adding five to seven teaspoons of powdered licorice root to a cup of boiling water and simmering for about 20 minutes. Strain out the plant material. Using a cotton ball or clean cloth, apply the liquid to the affected area one to three times a day.

❧❧❧ Teatree (*Melaleuca*, various species). Teatree oil is a powerful antiseptic that is very useful against fungal skin infections, including athlete's foot and yeast infections. Australian chemists have determined that *C. albicans* is remarkably sensitive to teatree oil. This research led to the development of products to treat vaginitis caused by yeast. Several women I know have reported success using teatree oil for vaginal infections that could not be entirely eradicated by pharmaceuticals like nystatin and clotrimazole.

For skin infections, you can apply a few drops of oil directly to the affected area three times a day. You might want to dilute it with an equal amount of vegetable oil, as some people find it irritating to the skin. For vaginal infections, you can apply some diluted oil directly or mix a few drops of oil into a lukewarm douche or sitz bath. If you experience any discomfort, discontinue use. This is especially important if you use it on or around the vagina, as this is a particularly sensitive area. In fact, teatree oil is such a potent antiseptic that I would recommend using it on the vaginal area only as a last resort, and always in a diluted form. Try other, gentler herbal approaches first. Then, if you want to use this oil, discuss it with your doctor. And one final warning: Don't ingest the oil. Like so many other essential plant oils, small amounts of teatree oil, on the order of a few teaspoons, can be fatal.

❦❦ **Black walnut (*Juglans nigra*).** Kathi Keville, author of *The Illustrated Herb Encyclopedia* and *Herbs for Health and Healing*, a California herbalist whom I admire, recounts one impressive study showing that the fresh husk of the black walnut destroyed candida better than a commonly prescribed antifungal drug. Her Candida Tincture contains one ounce of tincture of fresh black walnut husk plus a few drops each of tinctures of lavender flowers, valerian root and pau-d'arco, with ten added drops of teatree oil. I'm partial to Keville's emphasis on black walnuts because at my place each autumn, these nuts are as common as golf balls at the driving range on a Sunday afternoon.

❦❦ **Camomile (*Matricaria recutita*).** Camomile is a fungicidal that's especially good against candida. It's also potently antibacterial and anti-inflammatory. Camomile is widely used in Europe, where it's incorporated into many over-the-counter antiseptics.

I suggest using camomile both internally and externally for fungal infections. You can make a strong tea using the dried herb and drink it several times a day. You can also apply the tea two to four times a day directly to the affected area with a cotton ball or clean cloth. Or simply use the spent tea bags. You might also apply a tincture purchased at a health food store or herb shop.

If you have hay fever, however, you should use camomile products cautiously. Camomile is a member of the ragweed family, and in some people, it might trigger allergic reactions.

The first time you try it, watch your reaction. If it seems to help, go ahead and use it. But if it seems to cause or aggravate itching or irritation, discontinue use.

☙☙ Goldenseal (*Hydrastis canadensis*) and other herbs containing berberine. Berberine is a powerful antifungal and antibacterial compound that's found in barberry, goldthread, Oregon grape and yellowroot as well as goldenseal. All have been used traditionally to treat yeast and other fungal infections.

If I had a fungal infection, I might buy some goldenseal tincture and, following the package directions, add it to juice three times a day. For skin application I would make a strong decoction using five to seven teaspoons of dried goldenseal to a cup of water. Bring it to a boil, then let it simmer for 20 minutes. After it cools, strain out the plant material. I'd apply it to the affected area one to three times a day with a cotton ball or clean cloth.

☙☙ Henna (*Lawsonia inermis*). This popular natural hair dye contains 5,500 to 10,000 parts per million of the compound lawsone, which is active against many fungi and bacteria. I would suggest making a strong decoction by simmering five to seven teaspoons of henna per cup of water for about 20 minutes. Allow it to cool and apply the liquid to the affected area one to three times a day with a cotton ball or clean cloth.

☙☙ Lemongrass

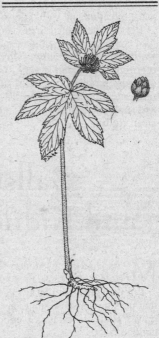

Goldenseal

Also known as golden root, goldenseal is a widely used and recommended antiseptic.

(*Cymbopogon*, **various species**). Scientists have demonstrated that lemongrass has significant fungicidal activity against several common infection-causing fungi. You can enjoy one to four cups of lemongrass tea a day. And for additional antifungal benefit, apply the spent tea bags directly to the affected area.

❦❦ **Pau-d'arco (*Tabebuia*, various species).** This herb contains three anti-yeast compounds—lapachol, beta-lapachone and xyloidine—that show activity against *C. albicans* and other common problem fungi. I have personally used a Latin American salve containing pau-d'arco extract to clear up a yeast infection and would do so again if I had another flare-up.

Here in the United States, however, I'd go with a standardized commercial preparation and follow the package directions.

❦ **Turmeric (*Curcuma longa*).** Pakistani studies show that oil of turmeric, even at very low concentrations, inhibits many common problem fungi. I'd suggest using commercial oil of turmeric, diluting it with water (one part oil to two parts water) and applying it directly to the affected area with a cotton ball or clean cloth.

Gallstones and Kidney Stones

My dad had kidney stones, but I've never had any. That surprises me, because they tend to run in families.

I'm very glad that I've avoided kidney stones so far. They say that passing a kidney stone, also known as bladder stones and gravel, is the closest men ever come to experiencing the pain of childbirth.

The fact that I've also never had gallstones is also good luck, especially since I'm at risk in this area, too. A key risk factor is being overweight, and I confess to being a tad on the heavy side.

So what has protected me so far? Well, I like to think that my near-vegetarian diet, heavy on herbs and liquids, has helped save me from both types.

Painful Passage for (Mostly) Men

Kidney stones form when certain substances, calcium oxalate, calcium phosphate, magnesium ammonium phosphate, uric acid or cystine—become so concentrated in the urine that they precipitate out as hard, solid lumps. The main symptom of kidney stones is pain in the left or right lower back or pelvic area that becomes excruciating as the stone attempts to leave the kidney through narrow tubes called ureters. Other symptoms are blood in the urine and a persistent urge to urinate.

Kidney stones affect mostly middle-aged and older men. You increase your risks if your diet is low in phosphates or protein or you eat a lot of food that's high in substances known as oxalates. Among the foods that have oxalates are coffee, black tea, rhubarb, sorrel, spinach, lamb's-quarters and purslane. Herbal formulas with rhubarb or sheep sorrel may contain more oxalates than would be beneficial.

Physicians usually don't treat kidney stones—they just medicate the pain until the stones pass on their own. Until recently, if a stone did not pass, surgery was necessary. Now a noninvasive procedure called lithotripsy usually breaks up the stones so that they can pass. During lithotripsy, which is done under anesthesia, shock waves are directed at the stone to pulverize it.

Back Pain in (Mostly) Women

Gallstones form when cholesterol and bile pigments become so concentrated that they form lumps inside the gallbladder. These lumps may be as small as a pinhead or as large as a golf ball. Gallstones that remain in the gallbladder rarely cause symptoms. But you can expect major problems if a stone blocks either the cystic duct (the tube that leads from the gallbladder to the bile duct) or the bile duct (the tube running from the liver and gallbladder into the intestine).

Gallstone symptoms include sudden, intense pain, usually in the upper right abdomen, accompanied by fever, nausea and sometimes vomiting. After attacks subside, usually in a half-hour to four hours, some soreness may linger for a day or so.

About 20 percent of women and 8 percent of men over 40 have

some gallstones, and these figures increase with age.

Physicians treat gallstones primarily with surgery, removing the gallbladder to eliminate the source of the problem. In the past few years, however, doctors have had promising results with a less invasive form of surgery called laparoscopy, which involves inserting a viewing device and tiny instruments through a small incision. In addition, some cholesterol gallstones can be dissolved with the use of bile acid drugs such as ursodeoxycholic acid (Actigall), given as tablets.

Green Pharmacy for Gallstones and Kidney Stones

The best way to prevent kidney stones is to drink six to eight glasses of water a day. That keeps the urine too dilute for stones to form. A vegetarian diet also helps because it's high in magnesium, and magnesium supplementation has been shown to reduce the likelihood of recurrent kidney stones.

To prevent gallstones, eat a low-fat, low-cholesterol diet, meaning one that's vegetarian or close to it.

If you have the bad luck to get either gallstones or kidney stones, I would urge you to follow your physician's advice. I would also suggest that some herbs can help.

Beggar-lice (*Desmodium styracifolium*). This vine got its name from its small, loose fruits, which cling to clothing. It has long been used by the Chinese for treating kidney stones, and Japanese researchers have discovered why it works. A compound in the plant works by decreasing the amount of calcium excreted in the urine and increasing the amount of citrate excreted, substantially decreasing the likelihood of kidney stone formation.

Celandine (*Chelidonium majus*). Celandine has traditionally been used for treating the liver, and with good reason. In one study, researchers gave tablets containing chelidonine, an active compound in celandine, to 60 people with symptoms of gallstones for six weeks. Doctors reported a significant reduction in symptoms.

Chelidonine and other compounds in celandine reportedly soothe the smooth muscles of the biliary tract, improving bile flow and curbing upper abdominal distress.

Couchgrass (*Agropyron repens* or *Elymus repens*). Commission E, the expert panel that judges the safety and effectiveness of herbal medicines for the German government, endorses using this herb, also known as quackgrass, for preventing kidney stones and inflammatory disorders of the urinary tract.

I'd try making a tea with two to ten teaspoons of the underground parts of the herb. Chop it and steep it for five to ten minutes in a cup or two of boiling water. Europeans drink up to four cups a day.

🌿🌿 **Ginger (*Zingiber officinale*).** Hot compresses made with concentrated ginger tea seem to help alleviate the pain of kidney stone attacks. The compresses act as counterirritants by causing superficial skin irritation, which takes the mind off the deeper kidney pain.

🌿🌿 **Horsetail (*Equisetum arvense*).** Commission E approves using horsetail for kidney stones and for the general health of the urinary tract. It increases urine output. (You should use this herb only in consultation with a holistic practitioner.)

🌿🌿 **Peppermint (*Mentha piperita*), spearmint (*M. spicata*) and other mints.** Mints have traditionally been used to treat gallstones. One stone-relieving mixture, a British over-the-counter "gallstone tea" preparation called Rowachol, contains chemicals from several members of the mint family. In one British study, this product helped a quarter of those who used it.

If I didn't have access to a doctor during a gallstone attack, I'd brew what I call Stone Tea from as many mints

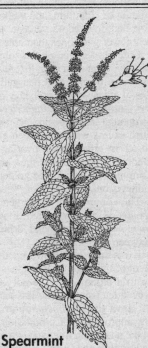

Spearmint

One of many members of the mint family, spearmint can help treat coughs and chest congestion as well as gallstones.

as I could gather from the garden or store, especially pepper-mint and spearmint, an old favorite. I'd add some cardamom, the richest source of borneol, another compound that is helpful.

❧❧ **Turmeric (*Curcuma longa*).** Turmeric is useful for pre-venting and treating gallstones, according to Commission E. This endorsement does not surprise me, since turmeric contains curcumin, a compound that has been tested for its effect on gallstones. In one study, mice with experimentally induced gallstones were placed on special feed containing a modest amount of cureumin, and within five weeks their gallstone vol-ume had dropped 45 percent. After ten weeks they had 80 per-cent fewer gallstones than untreated mice.

Curcumin increases the solubility of bile, which helps pre-vent the formation of gallstones and helps eliminate any stones that have formed. If I had gallstones, I would definitely cook lots of curries—and go heavy on the turmeric.

❧ **Goldenrod (*Solidago virgaurea*).** Goldenrod contains the compound leiocarposide—a potent diuretic that helps the body flush excess water. I've seen good clinical evidence that gold-enrod is effective in treating chronic kidney inflammation (nephritis). For both of these reasons, I wasn't surprised when Commission E endorsed goldenrod for preventing and treating kidney stones.

The commission recommends making a tea using five tea-spoons of chopped, dried flowering shoots per cup of boiling water. They recommend drinking three to four cups a day between meals.

I was surprised, however, to see Commission E's endorse-ment of this herb for gallstones as well. I'd suggest trying it for up to a month if you're not in serious pain. As a preventive, brew a tea using a little less herb.

❧ **Java tea (*Orthosiphon aristatus*).** The leaves of this herb are approved by Commission E for treating kidney stones. Make a tea with three to six teaspoons per cup of boiling water and drink it once a day. While it's not exactly clear how java tea works, the suspicion is that it helps open the ureters—the tubes leading from the kidneys to the bladder—allowing small stones to be passed.

❧ **Lovage (*Levisticum officinale*).** For treating kidney stones, Commission E suggests making a tea with two to four tea-spoons of dried herb per cup of boiling water and drinking it once a day. Lovage is a potent diuretic.

❧ **Milk thistle (*Silybum marianum*).** Rich in the compound silymarin, milk thistle is best known for the liver protection it offers. According to studies, silymarin also increases bile solubility, thus helping to prevent or alleviate gallstones.

❧ **Parsley (*Petroselinum crispum*).** Parsley is a diuretic that helps prevent and treat kidney stones. Commission E approves making the tea using one teaspoon of dried root and suggests drinking two to three cups a day. Steep the herb for 10 to 15 minutes, then strain.

❧ **Stinging nettle (*Urtica dioica*).** Finally, Commission E also recommends drinking several cups daily of stinging nettle tea to prevent and treat kidney stones. Steep a teaspoon of finely chopped dried herb in a cup of boiling water. Or boil up some nettle greens and enjoy the potlikker with a dash of vinegar, once a day. You will need to wear gloves when harvesting the leaves, but the stinging hairs lose their sting when the plant is cooked, and the greens are delicious.

Genital Herpes and Cold Sores

The phone rang. It was a woman who wanted to know if juice from mayapple roots would heal her genital herpes sores.

I get a lot of strange questions out of the blue, but there's usually a reason for them. This particular woman had heard me speak several months earlier at a seminar on shamanistic alternative medicine. At that time, I had mentioned four compounds in mayapple that together gang up on the *Herpes simplex* virus.

What's interesting here is that when you try each of these compounds individually, you get much less anti-herpes action. The "magic bullets" that the pharmaceutical industry so loves to extract from herbs simply aren't there. In other words, when it comes to mayapple, the whole is greater than the sum of its parts. That happens with a lot of herbs, which is why I'm a whole-herb herbalist.

I advised against using mayapple juice, as it can be caustic, and mayapple resin is downright dangerous. But I didn't leave her stranded. Instead I ended up settling on a different herb—lemon balm—to treat her problem. But before we get into discussing all the herbs that I recommend for this problem, let's take a closer look at this herpes bug.

Know Your Enemy

H. simplex comes in two forms, cold sores and genital herpes. This virus is a cousin to *H. zoster*, which causes another type of painful skin lesion called shingles. Cold sores develop around the mouth, generally on the lips. In women, genital herpes occurs in and around the vagina and cervix. In men, it shows up on and around the penis. In both sexes it also occurs around the anus.

Herpes is very contagious, and it shows pretty much the same pattern whether it develops on the mouth or the genitals.

Following initial contact with the virus, the first symptoms typically occur in four to seven days. These include tingling, burning or a persistent itch, followed a day or so later by pimple-like bumps over reddened skin. The pimples turn into painful blisters that burst and exude blood and yellowish pus. Five to seven days after the first tingling, scabs form and healing begins.

People with active lesions shed the virus and are contagious. But viral shedding also occurs during the tingling stage before any sore is visible. That's one reason that herpes affects so many people. People who have it can't always tell when they're contagious. Although most people develop sores within a week of infection, it's possible to be infected with the virus for quite some time before developing any sores.

Some 30 percent of American adults have had either oral or genital herpes. Sometimes the lesions recur periodically. Sometimes they appear once and never again. And sometimes they recur for a while and then stop. Probably everyone harbors the virus, but it remains dormant in most people.

Technically, there are two types of herpesvirus, one originally considered oral and the other genital. But oral sex can spread each type from the mouth to the genitalia and vice versa, so the distinction is increasingly meaningless. And in any case, both types respond to treatment with the same herbs.

Green Pharmacy for Genital Herpes and Cold Sores

Now to the anti-herpes herbal lineup. Here are the leaders of the virus-fighting pack.

❧❧

European Know-How

Think Americans have the best of everything? Guess again. When it comes to herbs, European commercial products are often better than our own.

An herbal ointment for treating herpes, which is widely available in Europe, has lemon balm as the active ingredient. The herbal content is quite concentrated—700 milligrams of dry leaf material per gram of ointment.

In a rigorous scientific test of 116 people with herpes, the ointment containing lemon balm was 2.5 times as effective as a similar cream without the herb (a placebo). The herbal product was especially effective when treatment was begun early, as the lesions were first erupting.

In another study involving 115 people using lemon balm, 96 percent had healed completely by day 8, with no significant side effects. Normally it takes anywhere from 10 to 14 days for herpes sores to heal. If I had herpes, and if European lemon balm cream were available here, I'd try it. Unfortunately, it is not, so I stick with my garden melissa.

❧❧

❧❧❧ **Lemon balm (*Melissa officinalis*).** Also known as melissa, lemon balm's demonstrated antiviral, anti-herpes properties seem to result from compounds in the herb, including tannins, that are known as polyphenols. Here's how these compounds work to tame herpes outbreaks.

The body's cells have receptors that viruses latch on to when they're trying to take over the cells. The polyphenol compounds have the ability to latch on to the cells' viral receptor sites. They take up those spaces and prevent the viruses from attaching to the cell, thus preventing the spread of infection.

This is a first-choice herbal treatment. In fact, I told the woman who was desperately seeking something to heal her herpes sores that I'd personally recommend making mixed mint tea, heavy with lemon balm. She could drink the tea, then apply the dregs from the tea bags directly to the lesions.

Mints, especially lemon balm, contain antioxidant vitamins and selenium, which strengthen the immune system. (Antioxidants are chemicals that mop up free radicals, the naturally occurring oxygen molecules that damage the body's cells.) All mints also contain at least four antiviral compounds that target the herpesvirus.

Not too long ago in Peru, naturopath Stephen Morris, N.D., taught our Amazonian Medicine Workshop how to make our own herpes ointment. We carefully heated some olive or palm oil, incorporating melted beeswax at a 1:4 ratio. To the cream, we added powdered lemon balm, mixed and strained it and then allowed it to cool. Our host, Socorro, smiled as we did all this over an open fire in her open-air, outdoor "kitchen."

You really don't need to get this elaborate, however. Varro Tyler, Ph.D., dean and professor emeritus of pharmacognosy (natural product pharmacy) at Purdue University in West Lafayette, Indiana, and author of *The Honest Herbal*, tends to be conservative when it comes to herbs. Dr. Tyler says that you can get results by using topical applications of lemon balm tea, which you can brew using two to four teaspoons of herb per cup of boiling water. Then apply it with a cotton ball several times a day.

"This treatment is probably as effective as any other self-selected remedy for cold sores," says Dr. Tyler.

∾∾ Echinacea (*Echinacea*, various species). Also known as coneflower, echinacea has been shown in many studies to have both antiviral and immune-stimulating properties.

Consider, for example, the following case report from the *British Journal of Phytotherapy*: After suffering for 12 years with recurrent genital herpes, a man took echinacea. He found that if he took it within an hour or two after he noticed the initial tingling, he had far less pain and the outbreak stopped.

Herbalists generally recommend taking echinacea in a tincture. Add about a half-teaspoon of the tincture to tea or juice and take it three times a day.

Some tinctures are a mixture of echinacea and goldenseal, which also has antimicrobial, immune-stimulating benefits. Although echinacea can cause the tongue to tingle or go numb temporarily, this effect is harmless. Some herbalists rely on this reaction to assure them that they have echinacea and not some adulterant. (Adulterants in commercial herb preparations are an ongoing problem.)

🌿🌿 **Mint family herbs.** Lemon balm is not the only mint with antiviral, anti-herpes activity. There are a whole bunch of other herbs in the mint family that are almost as effective.

Here's where I plug my Happy Herpicide Tea, which is made from several herbs that are members of the mint family: hyssop, lemon balm, oregano, rosemary, sage, self-heal (yes, this is the name of a widely available herb) and thyme.

To make the tea, fill a saucepan half full of water. Bring the water to a boil, then add fresh lemon balm leaves until the pan is about three-quarters full. If you don't have access to fresh leaves, you can use about a quarter-cup of dried lemon balm. (This is an unusually high amount of herb for brewing a tea, but you really need a lot of it to get the antiviral action that you want.) To the lemon balm and water, add two parts each of dried oregano and self-heal and one part each of hyssop, rosemary, sage and thyme.

Aside from the lemon balm, the actual amounts of the other herbs don't make much difference; just make sure you use twice as much of the oregano and self-heal as you do of the others. Finally, toss in a little licorice root to sweeten the tea and steep it for 20 minutes.

This mixture contains a dozen compounds that are active against herpes. The list of chemicals in this brew is rather imposing, but you should know what you get for going to all this trouble: caffeic acid, geraniin, glycyrrhizic acid, glycyrrhizin, lysine, protocatechuic acid, quercetin, rosmarinic acid, tannic acid, thymol, tocopherol and zinc.

🌿🌿 **Red pepper (*Capiscum*, various species).** The hot ingredient in red pepper is capsaicin. Tests on laboratory animals show that capsaicin can prevent outbreaks of herpes in the eye for up to two months, and topical capsaicin preparations

(Zostrix, Capzasin-P) are used to relieve the pain of shingles. (If you use capsaicin cream, always wash your hands thoroughly afterward to avoid the possibility of getting it in your eyes. Also, you should test it on a small area of skin before using it on a larger area. If you experience irritation, discontinue use.)

I wouldn't recommend sprinkling cayenne on any herpes lesions, especially those on the eye, since that could really hurt. But why not season your Happy Herpicide Tea with hot-pepper sauce? Although you drink it rather than dab it on, you'll still benefit from the active ingredients.

St.-John's-wort (*Hypericum perforatum*). One compound in St.-John's-wort, hypericin, helps kill *H. simplex* and several other viruses. Although ointments containing hypericin are effective against herpes sores, you don't need to buy one. Try brewing a strong tea, and after it cools, dab it on with cotton balls.

Garlic (*Allium sativum*). In test-tube studies, garlic has shown viricidal effects against both types of herpesvirus and many other viruses, including those that cause colds and flu. You can make garlic into a tea, but you will probably enjoy it a whole lot more if you just toss a few minced cloves onto a plate of pasta or add them to a mixed green salad.

Amino acids. Now let's wiggle a toe into nutritional waters. An amino acid, arginine, is considered necessary for viral replication. A preponderance of another amino acid, lysine, over arginine is supposed to suppress viral replication. Hence, those who value this theory seek foods with a high-lysine, low-arginine content. Several plants have high-lysine/low-arginine ratios, including star fruit (nearly 4:1), papaya (about 3:1) and grapefruit, apricot, pear, apple and fig (around 2:1).

Some people take a daily supplement of 1,300 milligrams of lysine at the first inkling of a herpes outbreak. It would take a little more than two pounds of fresh watercress to provide that amount, but only a half-cup of dried watercress. While you wouldn't want to eat this much watercress, there are a few other foods that will give you a fairly hefty dose of lysine.

A cup of black beans, lentils, soybeans or winged beans provides more than 2,500 milligrams of lysine. If you're making bean soup with these ingredients, spice it well with hot-pepper sauce for a little extra anti-herpes action.

❧ **Assorted essential oils.** Aromatherapists note that combinations of essential oils, such as lemon and geranium or eucalyptus and bergamot, can be helpful against herpes if applied at the first sign of an outbreak. Some aromatherapists say that rose oil and lemon balm oil have contributed, in some cases, to complete remission of *H. simplex* lesions, sometimes after only one application.

This approach seems worth a try. You can apply any of these oils topically using a cotton ball.

Warning: Essential oils are highly concentrated plant extracts. Make sure you never ingest them unless they've been prescribed by a reputable herbalist or aromatherapist. Small quantities of some oils, on the order of a single teaspoon, can be fatal.

❧ **Drug-herb combination.** I'll report news of a surprising study by Japanese scientists. They combined the pharmaceutical anti-herpes drug, acyclovir (Zovirax), with any one of four tannin-rich herbal extracts: Japanese avens (*Geum japonicum*), Javanese sumac (*Rhus javanica*), cloves (*Syzygium aromaticum*) and chebula (*Terminalia chebula*). The combination treatment worked significantly better than acyclovir alone or the herbs alone. Because acyclovir is a prescription drug, you'll have to ask your doctor about trying this one.

❧ **Healing beverages.** Tea and the juices of apple, cranberry, grape, pear, prune and strawberry all seem to help kill viruses. Tannins are usually the active components in these juices. Pear juice, which is rich in anti-herpes caffeic acid, might be your best juice choice.

Gingivitis

American Indians used bloodroot as an oral antiseptic. Modern research has shown that there is actually solid science to back up this ancient practice. The red root of this herb—from which the plant's name is derived—contains the antiseptic compound sanguinarine. This compound, which is now used in a few oral hygiene products, has the remarkable ability to prevent bacteria from forming plaque.

That's a powerful form of dental care, because when bacteria form gummy plaque on teeth, it causes the gum disease gingivitis. So anything that gets rid of plaque is really a way to head off gum problems.

These are the facts. But I got caught up in a controversy when I advocated wider use of bloodroot in toothpastes and mouthwashes. When I submitted a pro-bloodroot article for a conservationist wildflower journal, the editor sent the article out for review to a leading ethnodentist, someone who investigates the use of plant substances around the world for treating tooth and gum problems. The ethnodentist urged that the article be rejected.

Since this man's reaction was entirely unexpected, I did some checking on my own. It seems that this particular ethnodentist was busily promoting another herbal oral antiseptic, neem, and was dead set against bloodroot.

The ethnodentist maintained that bloodroot's active constituent, sanguinarine, caused cancer and glaucoma, which seemed to me to be a serious exaggeration. Sanguinarine is less toxic and presumably less carcinogenic than caffeine. Not only that, when it's used in toothpastes and mouthwashes, you spit it out rather than swallowing it. It's hard to believe that it could be very harmful, at least under these circumstances.

I have used toothpaste containing sanguinarine—without fear, I might add. I think both sanguinarine and neem should be available, but personally, I prefer the sanguinarine.

Gum Service

Gingivitis means "inflammation of the gums." It causes swelling, redness, a change in normal gum contours, watery discharge and bleeding. When it gets more serious, it becomes pyorrhea, degeneration of the gum tissue supporting the teeth. Together, gingivitis and pyorrhea are known as periodontal disease, a problem that all of us are more likely to have as we get older.

At age 10, about 15 percent of Americans have at least a mild form of gingivitis. At age 20, some 38 percent have it, and at 50, about half. People who don't brush, floss or get regular dental care are at greatest risk.

But you can get gingivitis even if you do brush and floss, because brushing and flossing don't clean out the deep, bacteria-harboring pockets between the teeth and gums. For those areas you need a little extra help.

Green Pharmacy for Gingivitis

Dentists treat gingivitis by irrigating the deep pockets with antiseptics. But if you want an alternative route to gum care, here are some herbs that can also help.

✿✿ **Bloodroot (*Sanguinaria canadensis*).** My advocacy of the compound sanguinarine, found in bloodroot, is backed up by many well-designed studies. Research shows that toothpaste containing sanguinarine is modestly effective against several types of oral bacteria and that it helps reduce the amount of dental plaque in the mouth in as little as eight days.

If you'd like to try this herb, look for sanguinarine in the list of ingredients on the labels of toothpastes and mouthwashes. The most widely available brand is Viadent.

In addition to their use in over-the-counter products, bloodroot extracts are used by dentists to treat periodontal disease.

✿✿ **Camomile (*Matricaria recutita*).** Commission E, the panel of experts that judges the safety and effectiveness of herbal medicines for the German government, considers camomile effective as a gargle or mouthwash for treating gingivitis. Camomile contains several anti-inflammatory and antiseptic compounds.

In addition to treating gum disease, you can use camomile to help prevent it. Try brewing a strong camomile tea using two to three teaspoons of herb per cup of boiling water. Steep for ten minutes, strain, and drink after meals. Or use it as a mouthwash. While ethnodentists caution that camomile, because it's kin to ragweed, may cause allergies, in my experience it is very rare. If you do notice an allergic reaction—itching or any discomfort—discontinue use of this herb.

✿✿ **Echinacea (*Echinacea*, various species).** In the *Handbook for Herbal Healing*, California herbalist and botanist Christopher Hobbs recommends echinacea for treating gingivitis, among many other conditions. The herb is antibacterial and immune-stimulating. Add a dropper or two of echinacea tincture to anti-gingivitis teas and mouthwashes. (Although echinacea can cause your tongue to tingle or go numb temporarily, this effect is harmless.)

❧❧ Licorice (*Glycyrrhiza glabra*). Licorice is a sweetener that won't cause cavities or gingivitis. Try it in teas instead of sugar or honey. In addition, licorice is high in magnesium and the compound glycyrrhizin, which some studies suggest help control gum inflammation and plaque formation.

While licorice and its extracts are safe for normal use in moderate amounts—up to about three cups of tea a day—long-term use or ingestion of larger amounts can produce headache, lethargy, sodium and water retention, excessive loss of potassium and high blood pressure.

❧❧ Purslane (*Portulaca oleracea*). Foods high in magnesium and vitamin C have often been recommended for treating gum disease. Because I am a big fan of spinachlike purslane, I can't help suggesting it as a good source of magnesium. Several other herbs, including coriander, cowpeas, dandelion, licorice root, lettuce leaf, poppy seeds, spinach, stinging nettle greens and string beans are high in magnesium as well.

Which brings me to my Magnesium Medley for keeping gingivitis at bay: Steam a mixed mess of dandelion, stinging nettle greens, purslane and spinach leaves. (Reminder: You'll need to wear gloves when harvesting nettle greens, but the stinging hairs lose their sting when the leaves are cooked.)

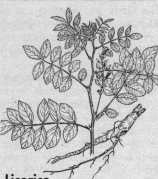

Licorice

Used by herbalists in the Middle Ages, licorice is now often suggested for relief of colds, sore throats and ulcers as well as gingivitis.

❧❧ Sage (*Salvia officinalis*). In the European herbal folk tradition, sage leaves, which are rather gritty, are rubbed on the gums and teeth as a stimulant dentifrice. I've done this, and it seems to help, thanks to sage's astringent tannin and several aromatic antiseptic compounds. I find sage leaves in my herb garden almost year-round, and collecting these leaves is a lot cheaper than buying products containing sanguinarine. Sage tea is perhaps as effective as a sanguinarine toothpaste.

Some modern research appears to support this folk medicine approach. Commission E endorses using two to three teaspoons of dried sage leaves per cup of boiling water to make an anti-gingivitis tea. It's best, though, to use sage in moderation, as it contains a fair amount of thujone, a compound that in very high doses may cause convulsions.

❧❧ **Tea** (*Camellia sinensis*). Like sage, tea is astringent, which helps fend off the bacteria responsible for tooth decay and gingivitis. Tea also contains at least five antibacterial compounds. Sweeten it with licorice.

❧ **Calendula** (*Calendula officinalis*). With antibacterial, antiviral and immune-stimulating properties, calendula extracts may be useful in treating gingivitis. Just beware if you have hay fever, though, because people who are allergic to ragweed might be allergic to this plant as well. And if you take it and have a reaction—itching or any other discomfort—discontinue use.

❧ **Peppermint** (*Mentha piperita*). You can't count on the "peppermint" in toothpastes to be of any help in preventing gingivitis, as most products are artificially flavored these days. But real peppermint fights the bacteria that cause tooth decay. You can make a tea using two teaspoons of crushed peppermint leaves per cup of boiling water. Steep for ten minutes, then sweeten it with licorice and drink the tea or use it as a mouthwash. You can also chew fresh mint leaves instead of sweetened mint candies and gums.

❧ **Rhatany** (*Krameria triandra*). Commission E approves of using rhatany bark to treat gingivitis. Like tea, this herb is rich in astringent, antiseptic tannin. To make a rhatany tea, steep a teaspoon of dried herb in a cup of boiling water. Drink it or use it as an astringent mouthwash.

❧ **Stinging nettle** (*Urtica dioica*). In addition to the magnesium in nettle greens, Russian studies show that nettle tea has antibacterial activity. Mouthwashes and toothpastes containing nettle reduce plaque and gingivitis. It's even more effective if you add juniper. Look for dental products containing these herbs at health food stores.

❧ **Teatree** (*Melaleuca*, **various species**). Teatree oil is a significant antiseptic, and many herbalists regard it as their first-choice disinfectant for external use. But if you're using teatree to treat gingivitis and canker sores, make sure you don't swallow it.

To combat gingivitis, add a couple of drops of teatree oil to a glass of water, then swish it in your mouth. As with any other essential oil, teatree should never be taken internally, as surprisingly small amounts—a teaspoon or so—can be fatal.

❧ **Watercress (*Nasturtium officinale*).** Pharmacognosist (natural product pharmacist) Albert Leung, Ph.D., author of *Chinese Herbal Remedies*, tells the story of how watercress was introduced into China a little over 100 years ago.

In nineteenth-century China, ancestral home of Dr. Leung's family, people used to call San Francisco *Gum San*, which means "golden mountain." Young men left China for Gum San, hoping to find fame and fortune.

Once in San Francisco, they were hauled off to work on the railroad, and many died from tuberculosis. Legend has it that they discovered through desperate experimentation that watercress helped treat tuberculosis. Some who recovered after eating it decided to take the secret home to China. With what money they had saved and the seeds of the lifesaving plant, they returned to their homeland.

Today southern Chinese chew watercress to treat sore gums. If you like the taste of watercress, you might try chewing it to treat gingivitis.

Glaucoma

Glaucoma is a leading cause of blindness. It typically develops after age 40 and becomes increasingly common with age. About 3 percent of Americans over age 65 have it—some two million people, about 60,000 of whom are legally blind.

Glaucoma is a group of eye diseases that involve an increase in fluid pressure in the eye (intraocular pressure) that develops when the drainage mechanism for this fluid becomes impaired. The increased pressure damages the optic nerve, causing blind spots in the field of vision.

In addition to blind spots, glaucoma symptoms include blurred vision, loss of peripheral vision, halos around lights, eye pain and redness. When diagnosed and treated, glaucoma is easily controlled. It's only when the disease goes undetected and untreated that it can lead to blindness. An estimated 500,000 Americans have undiagnosed glaucoma.

Glaucoma is a serious illness, and everyone, especially those with a family history of this disease, should have their intraocular pressure checked periodically. Anyone with glaucoma *must* be under a physician's care. The cause remains a mystery, but apparently a tendency toward glaucoma can be inherited.

Mainstream physicians typically treat glaucoma with a variety of drugs that reduce intraocular pressure, many of which are derived from herbal sources. In some people, the pressure must be reduced surgically by opening up the eyes' drainage tubes.

Green Pharmacy for Glaucoma

There are also a number of herbs that are likely to be helpful in treating glaucoma.

🌿🌿🌿 **Jaborandi (*Pilocarpus*, various species).** One standard glaucoma medicine, pilocarpine, is actually derived from jaborandi, a tropical tree that grows in South America. Jaborandi was widely used in folk medicine long before the Spanish explorers arrived. When they did, they quickly learned of its value.

As early as 1648, Spanish naturalists hinted at the ability of this herb to treat eye disease. Then in 1875, pilocarpine was first isolated from jaborandi. It was synthesized in 1930.

Since pilocarpine reduces intraocular pressure, it is often prescribed in the form of eyedrops to treat several types of glaucoma. One application takes effect in less than 15 minutes and continues to protect the eye for about 24 hours. Chances are that today people with glaucoma who use pilocarpine apply the synthetic version, but this standard medication is actually an herbal derivative.

🌿 **Fruits and vegetables containing vitamin C.** Many studies show that vitamin C lowers intraocular pressure. Good sources include bell peppers, broccoli, cabbage, citrus fruits, brussels sprouts, guava, kale, parsley and strawberries.

Nutritionists and naturopaths often recommend taking vitamin C supplements in amounts ranging anywhere from 2,000 to 35,000 milligrams a day. Since as little as 1,200 milligrams of vitamin C can cause diarrhea in some people, I'd suggest staying on the lower side. If you want to try higher doses, please discuss it with your doctor. If I had glaucoma or a family history of the disease, I'd take supplemental vitamin C.

❦

Smoke Gets in Your Eyes

People who advocate legalizing marijuana for medical uses typically mention it as a treatment for glaucoma. There's a good reason for this. Marijuana (*Cannabis sativa*) apparently does lower the pressure of fluids inside the eye, or intraocular pressure.

Of course, marijuana is currently illegal, and I wouldn't use it or recommend its use anywhere in the United States. Just how effective marijuana might be as a long-term treatment for glaucoma remains a mystery because there's been so little research on it.

Perhaps further research will be done, and marijuana will someday be "prescribed" by doctors. In fact, glaucoma treatment is not the only potential medicinal use of this herb. It also has the ability to reduce some of the side effects of cancer chemotherapy, especially nausea.

❦

❦❦ **Kaffir potato (*Coleus forskohlii*).** This herb contains a compound, forskolin, that lowers intraocular pressure. Studies have demonstrated that a forskolin preparation in the form of eyedrops significantly reduces intraocular pressure in just one hour. In the studies, the therapeutic effect reached its peak at two hours and remained significant for at least five.

This is not an herb that you would use on your own, but if you have glaucoma and use pharmaceutical forskolin, you might enjoy knowing that you're using a medicine that was derived from an herb.

🌿🌿 **Oregano (*Origanum vulgare*).** None of the scientific literature seems strong on preventive advice, so if glaucoma runs in your family, you might find this particularly interesting.

Naturopaths recommend getting plenty of foods containing antioxidants to prevent glaucoma. Antioxidants are substances that neutralize the naturally occurring, highly reactive oxygen molecules (free radicals) in the body that seem to contribute to the development of the disease.

My investigation of 60 mints suggested that wild oregano was among the richest in antioxidants. Since it's a weed at my place, fresh oregano is a standard ingredient in my Antioxidantea. You might try using one to two teaspoons of dried oregano per cup of boiling water. If you'd like to make some Antioxidantea, include some peppermint or rosemary.

🌿🌿 **Pansy (*Viola*, various species).** Pansy contains a compound called rutin, which naturopaths often recommend for the treatment of glaucoma. According to my database, wild pansy flowers can contain up to 23 percent rutin on a dry-weight basis. When used in combination with standard medications, rutin contributes to lowering the intraocular pressure of glaucoma.

Naturopaths suggest getting 20 milligrams of rutin three times a day. I once calculated that one edible pansy flower would give you about 20 milligrams. It's perfectly safe to munch on a few pansies, and they make spectacular additions to salads.

Rutin is also found in pagoda tree flower, violets, eucalyptus leaf and mulberry leaf. If I had glaucoma, I'd sprinkle my fruit cocktails with violets. I might also whip up some Rutinade by blending a couple of violets and a bit of eucalyptus leaf into fruit juice.

🌿 **Bilberry (*Vaccinium myrtillus*).** This berry has been recommended traditionally for almost every eye ailment, and glaucoma is no exception. It turns out that bilberries contain compounds called anthocyanosides that retard the breakdown of vitamin C. As a result, they help vitamin C do its job of protecting your eyes.

Joseph Pizzorno, N.D., president of Bastyr University in Seattle, and Michael Murray, N.D., co-authors of *A Textbook of Natural Medicine*, both recommend taking bilberry and its relative, blueberry, as a preventive and treatment.

People who advocate the healing properties of juices suggest mixing the juices of bilberry, blueberry, cranberry and huckle-berry, all of which are high in anthocyanosides.

━━━━━━━━━━━━━━━━━━━━━━━━━━━━━━━━━

❧

Watch That Toothpaste

Here's an herb to avoid if you have glaucoma or a family history of the disease. There is some evidence—not compelling, but worth noting—that consumption of sanguinarine, a compound found in bloodroot (*Sanguinaria canadensis*) may contribute to glaucoma.

The one place you're likely to encounter bloodroot is in toothpastes or mouthwashes, since the herb is an excellent preventive for gum disease. The products might have the compound sanguinarine rather than bloodroot itself listed on the label.

I don't think the risk is major; after all, you don't usually ingest either toothpaste or mouthwash. But if you're concerned about glaucoma, you should be aware of the concerns about bloodroot.

❧

━━━━━━━━━━━━━━━━━━━━━━━━━━━━━━━━━

❧ **Shepherd's purse (*Capsella bursa-pastoris*).** This antioxidant herb has been used traditionally "to brighten vision," according to pharmacognosist (natural product pharmacist) Albert Leung, Ph.D. I suggest adding a little shepherd's purse to your favorite herbal teas.

Gout

I have gout. I finally succumbed to my HMO doctor's pleading that I take allopurinol (Lopurin, Zyloprim). That would be one pill a day for the rest of my life to keep this condition under control.

Fortunately, I've now found an herbal alternative in celery seed extract, which I expect to continue taking as long as the threat of gout hangs over me. I know from experience that a gout attack involves such pain that I hope I never experience it again for the rest of my life.

My first gout attack came when I was just shy of age 50. One day I was out working in the garden, enjoying one of my favorite activities. And the next day, out of the blue, I woke up with classic gout pain and swelling in my big toe. The toe was so painful that, just as the books say, even the weight of a bedsheet on it seemed unbearable. I could hardly walk.

My doctor gave me a prescription drug that flushes pain-causing uric acid crystals from the body. I took the medicine like the good patient that I am whenever I'm faced with pain. And I quickly went from being an invalid who could barely walk to being back on my feet and puttering in my herb garden once again.

With all due respect for the prescription drug, however, I'm glad that I've found an herbal replacement that seems to do the trick.

Caused by Crystals

Gout is a form of arthritis because it causes pain in the joints, usually the big toe, although other joints can be affected. It's caused by a buildup of uric acid in the blood. When levels rise beyond a certain point, uric acid crystals form and collect in the affected joint or joints, causing excruciating pain. These crystals can also form in the body's major organs and do considerable damage, so avoiding pain is not the only reason to keep this serious condition under control.

Gout tends to run in families. Three hundred years ago, it

was associated with wealth, because gout attacks were thought to be provoked by eating a rich diet. Now we know that the disease afflicts rich and poor alike. More than 95 percent of people who have gout are men over 30. An estimated 10 to 20 percent of the population has elevated uric acid levels, but only 3 people in 1,000 experience gout.

Green Pharmacy for Gout

If you have gout, by all means take the medication that your doctor prescribes. But in addition, you might want to try some natural approaches to relieving this painful ailment.

🐝🐝🐝 **Celery (*Apium graveolens*).** Learning that celery extracts might help eliminate uric acid, I began taking two to four tablets of celery seed extracts daily instead of allopurinol. As I write, six months have gone by without a single gout crisis. For one week, I ate four celery stalks a day in lieu of the extracts.

These self-dosing anecdotal results lead me to believe the advertisement that led me to the celery seed. A skeptic then, I'm a believer now: Celery seed (or serendipity) has kept my uric acid below critical levels.

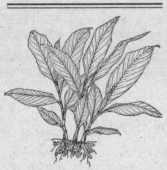

Turmeric

A spice related to ginger, this herb is native to India and Southeast Asia.

🐝🐝 **Chiso (*Perilla frutescens*).** This aromatic, weedy mint, imported accidentally or intentionally from Asia decades ago, is a popular food and medicine in the Orient. Here it's a rampant weed, but you'll find it grown intentionally behind some Japanese restaurants in the eastern United States.

Japanese researchers have touted compounds in chiso to relieve gout. It contains fairly high levels of four compounds known as xanthine oxidase (XO) inhibitors, which help prevent the synthesis of uric acid. I frequently add a little chiso to my mint teas, just as the Japanese add it to their sushi.

✿✿ Licorice (*Glycyrrhiza glabra*). Like chiso, licorice contains several XO inhibitors, but at fairly low levels. Still, a chiso-licorice combo could be interesting, and the two herbs might even work better together.

✿✿ Turmeric (*Curcuma longa*). One compound in turmeric (curcumin) inhibits the synthesis of substances called prostaglandins in the body that are involved in pain. The mechanism is similar to the one involved in the pain-relieving action of aspirin and ibuprofen, only weaker. Still, at high doses, curcumin stimulates the adrenal glands to release the body's own cortisone, a potent reliever of inflammation and the pain it often causes.

East Indians revere turmeric and use it liberally in curries. That's a particularly nice way to take your medicine, if you ask me. You can also make a tea using turmeric or simply take it in capsules.

✿ Avocado (*Persea americana*). My botanical friends in the Amazon believe that avocado is useful for treating gout. It reportedly lowers uric acid levels in the blood.

There's no scientific evidence that I'm aware of to support this assertion, but I have a lot of respect for the herbal wisdom of the Amazonian people, and avocados are certainly tasty. So here's a good reason to add an occasional avocado to your diet. Just don't go overboard, though, as avocados are high in calories.

✿ Cat's claw (*Uncaria*, various species). Once while I was on the Amazon, an attack of gout caught me without the prescription medication I usually take to alleviate the inflammation during a crisis. But I had some pills containing cat's claw (*uña de gato*), an herb with anti-inflammatory effects.

I took two pills. No relief. I tried four. Nothing. Then, at six, I began to notice some effect, but it took nearly a dozen to do as much as the drug. While I'm certainly not discarding my prescription medications in favor of cat's claw, in an emergency I'd use the herb again.

There are more than 30 brands of cat's claw on sale in health food stores and herb shops in the United States, and there's only one report in the scientific literature of an adverse reaction ever developing in anyone using the herb.

✿ Cherry (*Prunus*, various species). Many people claim to stave off gout attacks by eating eight ounces a day of canned or fresh cherries. I have one friend, for instance, who claims to have great luck in staving off gout when he eats black cherries. This therapy has never been scientifically demonstrated to work, but since so many people swear by it, I think it's probably worth trying. (One caveat, though: Buying this many cherries might be even more expensive than my allopurinol.) Other people favor strawberries.

I'm going to give my Cherry Cocktail a try. It's a mixture of cherry, pineapple, strawberry and blueberry juices spiced up with a little bit of licorice and a lot of ginger and turmeric.

❦ Devil's claw (*Harpagophytum procumbens*). Several reports indicate that this herb lowers uric acid levels and has anti-inflammatory action, both of which would be useful for treating gout. Other studies suggest that it may be useful for relieving arthritic conditions, and gout is a form of arthritis.

Unfortunately, studies rely on injections of an herbal extract of devil's claw, and an injection goes right into the bloodstream without passing through the stomach. This herb loses potency in the stomach, so I can't guess how effective (or ineffective) it might be in a tea or capsule. I think it's worth trying, however.

❦ Oat (*Avena sativa*). Teas made from the silica-rich green tops of the oat plant are said to have a diuretic effect that lowers blood levels of uric acid. (A diuretic is any substance that flushes excess water from the body.) If my other natural approaches failed, I'd be sure to try this one.

❦ Olive (*Olea europea*). Olive has a reputation as a diuretic dating back to biblical times. In 1993, a Japanese researcher showed that about four cups of olive leaf tea a day for three weeks increased daily urine output by 10 to 15 percent, lowering uric acid levels in the blood and increasing uric acid in the urine. I would not hesitate to try this one myself.

❦ Pineapple (*Ananas comosus*). Pineapple contains bromelain, an enzyme that helps break down protein. Naturopathic physicians often recommend pure bromelain, which can be purchased at health food stores, to reduce inflammation and swelling.

Bromelain clearly works if you inject it into swollen tissue, but the effectiveness of the ingested enzyme has been controversial. It's probably worth trying, however. My preferred way to get bromelain is in an occasional glass of pineapple juice.

❦ Stinging nettle (*Urtica dioica*). One scientific study showed that stinging nettle increases uric acid secretion, at least in ducks. These experimental animals exhibited lower blood levels of uric acid after they were given stinging nettle extract. The next time I have pain in my big toe, I intend to include stinging nettle tea in my own treatment program.

✦ **Willow (*Salix*, various species).** Willow bark is equivalent to herbal aspirin, as it contains compounds known as salicylates, from which aspirin is made.

Like aspirin, willow bark tea can help relieve pain and inflammation. In addition, some research suggests that salicylates can reduce levels of uric acid. Try two teaspoons of bark in a cup of boiling water and simmer for 20 minutes. (If you're allergic to aspirin, however, you probably shouldn't take aspirin-like herbs, either.)

Graves' Disease (Hyperthyroidism)

Perhaps we should start referring to Graves' disease as Bush disease. Both former President Bush and his wife, Barbara, had it during his term of office. Their condition was revealed in 1991, and they controlled it with medication.

Shortly after the Bushes' thyroid condition became known, a young lady told me that her Graves' disease medication was causing her some troublesome side effects, and she wanted to stop taking it. She asked me to check my database and other sources for herbal alternatives.

I warned her that her condition was nothing to toy with. Like all hormonal imbalances, Graves' disease is a complex condition that's not generally amenable to self-treatment with non-standardized medications, and herbs generally fall into that category. She countered that she was going to stop taking her drugs no matter what I said, so I figured the least I could do was see if any natural alternatives might help her.

Delving into the literature, I came up with bugleweed as one of the most promising alternatives. Months later, the young woman told me that she'd quit her medication and had been drinking mint teas containing plenty of bugleweed. After she'd been off her medication for a month, she dropped by my office, beaming. She'd just had a checkup, and her blood level of thyroid-stimulating hormone (TSH), one of the things that goes off-kilter in Graves' disease, was fine. The same was true a month later.

I honestly don't know why this woman got better. Maybe it *was* the bugleweed that did the trick, but I certainly wouldn't recommend that everyone with Graves' disease toss their medication and start drinking bugleweed tea.

Not being a medical doctor, I don't understand all that much about hormonal disorders. If you have Graves' disease, I'd say that you should see your doctor, not a botanist or herbalist, and do follow your doctor's advice. But in this case, a natural alternative succeeded in bringing Graves' disease under control, and we have her charts to verify her improvement.

Thyroid Set on High

With hyperthyroidism, there are abnormally high blood levels of thyroid hormones circulating in the body. These hormones are secreted by the thyroid gland, which is located in the neck just behind and below the Adam's apple. The disease was named after an Irish physician, Robert James Graves, who lived in the early 1800s and was the first to identify its telltale pattern of symptoms: enlarged thyroid gland, bulging eyes, rapid pulse, profuse sweating, fatigue, an increased metabolic rate leading to substantial weight loss and neurological symptoms such as restlessness, irritability and fine muscle tremors.

Levels of circulating thyroid hormones depend on several things: availability of the mineral iodine, levels of TSH released by the pituitary gland (located in the center of the brain) and the health of the thyroid gland itself. TSH levels are further regulated by yet another part of the brain, the hypothalamus. All of this translates into a simple formula in a healthy individual: As TSH levels increase, the levels of thyroid hormone also increase, until a balance is reached. If the thyroid is malfunctioning, its attempts to regulate hormone levels will throw the system further out of whack.

Thyroid diseases affect about 2.5 percent of Americans, or some 6.5 million people, most of whom are women. There are two types of thyroid hormone imbalance, hyperthyroidism (*hyper-* means "too much") and hypothyroidism (*hypo-* means "too little"). In this chapter, I deal with too much thyroid hormone; for more on hypothyroidism, see page 331.

Women are four times more likely than men to have Graves' disease. (They are also twice as likely as men to develop thyroid tumors.) There are several different kinds of hyperthyroidism, but Graves' disease is by far the most common. It's an autoimmune condition, meaning that it's thought to be caused by the immune system attacking the body, and it affects about one million Americans.

Doctors treat Graves' disease by trying to suppress thyroid hormone production. Any of several drugs may be prescribed, and sometimes, usually in drug-sensitive elderly people, radiation may be used to disable a portion of the thyroid gland itself.

Green Pharmacy for Graves' Disease

If you have symptoms of Graves' disease, see a doctor and take the prescribed medication. Do not attempt self-treatment, even though it worked for the young woman whose story began this chapter. In addition to following your doctor's advice, and with his permission, you might also try these herbs.

❦❦❦ **Bugleweed (*Lycopus*, various species).** Bugleweed has a considerable folk history for treating thyroid conditions, and modern research supports this use. This herb inhibits iodine metabolism and reduces the amount of hormone that's produced by thyroid cells.

Leaf extracts are more active than root extracts. The recommended oral preparation is a tincture (alcohol extract) rather than a tea. In one study using laboratory animals, bugleweed tincture resulted in a significant decrease in thyroid hormone levels.

Bugleweed is widely used in Europe as an herbal treatment for early-stage Graves' disease, often in combination with lemon balm. However, I must caution that bugleweed—and other herbal treatments for Graves' disease—have mild effects and are best used in early stages of the condition or in addition to synthetic pharmaceuticals.

❦❦❦ **Lemon balm (*Melissa officinalis*).** In Europe, lemon balm, also known as melissa, is often recommended along with bugleweed for treating Graves' disease. Studies show that lemon balm causes a decrease in blood and pituitary levels of TSH after a single injection, thus reducing thyroid hormone production. It's not clear if lemon balm has a similar effect when taken orally, but I believe the chances are good. It's probably worth a try.

❧·❧

Gravestea

To make a tasty mixed herb tea that combats Graves' disease, combine two teaspoons of lemon balm with one teaspoon of bugleweed and then add mint, rosemary, self-heal and verbena to taste. I think drinking this tea regularly just might help.

❧·❧

❧·❧·❧ Self-heal (*Prunella vulgaris*). A quarter-pound serving of self-heal greens with bugleweed tubers, spiced up with basil, oregano, rosemary and spearmint, should contain significant quantities of the compound rosmarinic acid, which helps suppress thyroid hormone production.

❧·❧ Kelp (*Laminaria*, various species). Herbal pharmacologist Daniel Mowrey, Ph.D., author of *The Scientific Validation of Herbal Medicine* and *Herbal Tonic Therapies*, notes that among the Japanese who consume a great deal of kelp, thyroid disease is practically unknown, but among the Japanese who have become Westernized and eat little or no kelp, thyroid disease is on the rise.

You can buy powdered kelp in health food stores to sprinkle on your food as a seasoning.

❧·❧ Verbena (*Verbena*, various species). Often called vervain, verbena seems to have properties similar to those of self-heal. Extracts have been shown to suppress thyroid hormone production by influencing levels of TSH in the body.

❧ Broccoli (*Brassica oleracea*). Remember how George Bush hated broccoli? His aversion to that wonderful vegetable deprived him of something that might have helped treat his

Graves' disease. Broccoli contains naturally occurring substances called isothiocyanates, which help restrain the thyroid from producing too much hormone. When Bush was diagnosed with Graves' disease, several alternative health authorities urged him to eat broccoli. One even published a book titled *Why George Should Eat Broccoli*.

❧ **Radish (*Raphanus sativus*).** All of the cruciferous vegetables gently and naturally suppress thyroid hormone production, but radishes do it best, according to medical anthropologist John Heinerman, Ph.D., author of *Heinerman's Encyclopedia of Fruits, Vegetables and Herbs*. Cruciferous vegetables include broccoli, brussels sprouts, cabbage, cauliflower, kale, mustard greens, radishes, rutabagas and turnips. Radishes are used in Russia precisely for this purpose.

Hangover

I'm what I call an antisocial drinker. I don't feel all that comfortable engaging in small talk, so I put a glass to my mouth, and occasionally I drink too much. I define "too much" as any amount that gives me the headache, stomach upset, thirst and general death-warmed-over feeling of a hangover. Conservatively, any more than two drinks a day is too much.

Maybe you've never had that kind of experience. But if you have, you may have occasion to use some natural hangover remedies.

Hangover is unfortunately quite common, because alcoholism is a major public health problem, affecting some ten million Americans. But you don't have to abuse alcohol to suffer an occasional hangover. You don't even have to get terribly drunk.

Why Hangovers Hurt So Much

Hangover is a mild version of alcohol withdrawal syndrome, which causes delirium tremens (DTs) in alcoholics. The headache is prompted in part by alcohol's relaxing effect on the blood vessels. As they open up, more blood flows through them, which causes the sensation of warmth we feel when drinking. But if the blood vessels of the head open too much, they trigger the pain nerves.

Alcohol is also a diuretic, so fluid loss contributes to morning-after thirst and can add to head pain.

The nausea and vomiting are a combination of alcohol's irritating effect on the stomach and its many effects on the central nervous system.

The fatigue and general lousy-all-over feeling result from alcohol's depressant effect and a buildup of acids in the blood (acidosis). The chemical acetaldehyde may also accumulate in the blood, leading to flushing.

Finally, additives and impurities in alcohol (congeners) contribute to hangovers. The general rule is that the darker the alcohol, the worse the hangover. Vodka and white wine contain few congeners, but bourbon, scotch and red wine are loaded with them.

Green Pharmacy for Hangover

I hate to state the obvious, but it needs to be said that a good basic approach to hangover is to prevent it by not drinking in the first place. Or you might try drinking clear liquor or white wine rather than the dark stuff. It also helps to drink lots of non-alcoholic beverages to stay well-hydrated and wash the acids out of your blood. All this helps head off both the headache and the upset stomach.

In addition, try these natural hangover aids.

❧ **Cinchona (*Cinchona*, various species).** The bitter bark that gives tonic water its flavor and is the source of quinine is used as a hangover remedy in China. Water in and of itself helps, but I suspect that bitter herbs like cinchona provide added benefit. Other bitter herbs often recommended for hangover include dandelion, gentian, mugwort and angostura, which is the same herb used in Angostura Bitters, a favorite hangover remedy among bartenders.

You can make an anti-hangover tea by adding a few drops of Angostura Bitters to a cup of boiling water. In fact, any of these herbs can be made into a very bitter tea. I'd suggest cutting the bitter flavor by adding the tasty herbs roselle and tamarind, both of which are also reputed to help banish hangover.

❧ **Ginkgo (*Ginkgo biloba*).** Ginkgo seeds are not approved as food by the Food and Drug Administration, but they are available here. The Japanese have long served ginkgo seeds at cocktail parties, based on folklore assertions that they prevent drunkenness and hangover. Scientific studies out of Japan have shown that there is good reason to suspect that ginkgo seeds really can get the job done. It turns out that the seeds contain an enzyme that speeds up the body's metabolism of alcohol.

In one study, the researchers gave laboratory animals enough alcohol to get them very drunk. When the animals were given ginkgo seed extracts in advance, they were better able to clear alcohol from their blood. I'm not sure that ginkgo seeds have a similar effect in humans, but I suspect they do, which calls for a little poem: "They say that you won't get real stinko/If you nibble the nuts of the ginkgo."

Not great poetry, I admit, but it will help you remember what you need to cure the day-after blues.

❧ **Kudzu (*Pueraria lobata*).** Some scientists finger a specific chemical (acetaldehyde) as the big culprit in hangover. Kudzu can cause acetaldehyde to accumulate in your blood faster, so you get your hangover—literally feeling headachy and nauseated—while you're drinking instead of the morning after. The trick is to take one or two capsules of dried kudzu with your first drink.

The advantage here, of course, is that as you start feeling lousy, you'll cut back on your drinking. Acetaldehyde accumulation makes drinking less pleasant and helps keep you from imbibing to excess. The Chinese use kudzu roots or flowers for this purpose.

You can also take kudzu as a tea the morning after, and experts say it can help provide some relief.

At this point, especially if you live in the South, you're probably wondering if I'm talking about that obnoxious vine that manages to drape itself over fields and forests for miles on end. Indeed I am. There *is* a valid use for this creeping green monster, after all!

❧ **Wintergreen (*Gaultheria procumbens*) and willow (*Salix*, various species).** I wouldn't recommend taking aspirin for a hangover, as it might aggravate your upset stomach. But I've always found herbal forms of aspirin gentler on the stomach, which is why I can recommend the attractive, aromatic wintergreen. It's loaded with an aspirin relative, methyl-salicylate, so it could help clear up a hangover headache. (If you are allergic to aspirin, however, it might be a good idea to avoid aspirin-like herbs as well.)

If you like, you might mix wintergreen with willow bark, which also contains salicylates. Both are available all year long where I live, and as far north as Maine. (Of course, if you can't pick 'em fresh, you can always buy these herbs in dried form.)

Cherry birch bark can also be used as a source of salicylates. I'd make a cherry birch bark tea and add as much hot-pepper sauce as my taste buds can bear. Hot-pepper sauce contains capsaicin, a superb painkiller.

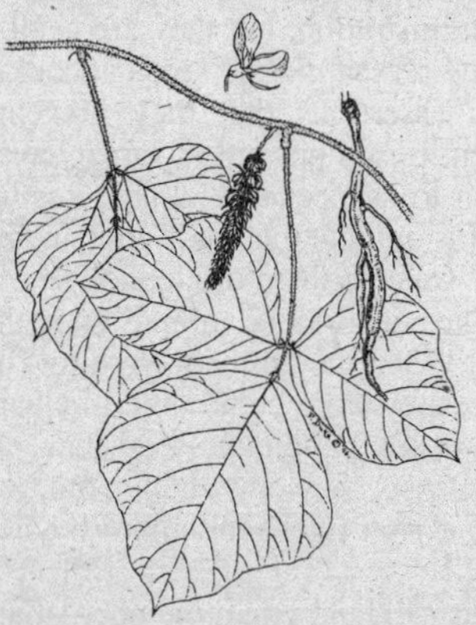

Kudzu

A notorious vine that sometimes completely smothers Southern pine trees, kudzu can be bought in medicinal capsules.

Or I'd try this aspirin-replacement herbal blend from Christopher Hobbs, distinguished fourth-generation Califor-nia herbalist and botanist and author of *Handbook for Herbal Healing*: Two parts each of passionflower, white willow and wood betony and one part lavender. Hobbs suggests steeping two teaspoons of the mixture in one cup of boiling water.

Folk herbs. Many herbs have been used folklorically for hangover. They might help, or perhaps it's simply the water in the tea that makes people feel better. I have great respect for medical folklore, so I'll share the herbs with you: basil, black pepper, caraway, cinnamon, coriander, forsythia, ginger, gotu kola, honeysuckle, lavender, lemongrass, onion, pennyroyal, peppermint, plantain, poppy seeds, rosemary, rue, tea and yarrow. The mints contain potent antioxidants, substances that can help prevent some of the cellular-level damage that alcohol causes.

Guatemalans use juices or teas of red roselle, while Latin Americans generally recommend a beverage made of the pulp of tamarind. Both of these are favorites of mine. We could mix them together, sweeten them with high-fructose honey, and call it the Red Hangover Zapper.

My own favorite remedy is vegetable juice cocktail with a bit of hot-pepper sauce. All those veggies that are used to make the juice contain antioxidants, and of course, hot-pepper sauce contains the painkiller capsaicin. I also like onion soup, another folk remedy for hangover and a surprisingly good source of fructose.

❧ **Fructose.** Fructose is fruit sugar. Korean scientists have suggested that fructose can speed up the body's metabolism of alcohol by about 25 percent.

Ginseng root is a favorite herb in Korea, and ginseng contains approximately 0.5 percent fructose. Perhaps that's why both Asian (*Panax ginseng*) and American (*P. quinquefolius*) ginseng have a long history of use for treating hangover. Personally, I rarely recommend ginseng because it costs so much.

Fortunately, there are cheaper and much better sources of fructose. Try putting some honey in your morning tea; it's more than 40 percent fructose. Maybe that's why one old-time hangover remedy among bartenders is simply honey in hot water.

Not far behind honey are dates, with 30 percent fructose. If you don't want tea in the morning, see if you can force down a couple of dates.

Headache

Everyone gets a headache now and then, but an estimated 15 percent of the population—some 40 million Americans—have at least one a week. There's a lot of pain out there.

An estimated 90 percent of headaches are tension headaches, which begin in the back of the neck or head and spread outward with a dull, nonthrobbing pain.

The other 10 percent, including migraines, cluster headaches and caffeine-withdrawal headaches, are caused by the opening and closing (dilation and constriction) of blood vessels in the head that set off pain nerves. Classic migraine is a severe and throbbing headache, usually on one side of the head and often preceded by visual disturbances. Nausea and vomiting often accompany the migraine.

Migraine headaches inflict misery on 25 million Americans. For unknown reasons, about three times as many women as men experience this painful condition. Women often develop migraines just prior to menstrual periods or during pregnancy, and the migraines disappear after menopause in about three-quarters of women.

Green Pharmacy for Headache

No single natural therapy—or pharmaceutical, for that matter—works for every type of headache. There are, however, several herbs that can help relieve the different types.

✿ ✿ ✿ Bay (*Laurus nobilis*). Bay contains compounds known as parthenolides that are extremely useful in preventing migraine. Although the mechanism of these headaches is not thoroughly understood, it appears that release of the neurotransmitter serotonin from blood cells known as platelets plays a causative role. Parthenolides inhibit serotonin release from platelets.

If I had frequent migraines, I might add bay leaves to feverfew, my top-choice herb for treating this condition.

✿ ✿ ✿ Feverfew (*Tanacetum parthenium*). It's been more than ten years now since feverfew helped my sister-in-law beat her migraines. This herb also helped my secretary's sister. I consider feverfew one of the most interesting herbs in modern herbalism.

In my own experience, and this is reflected in the medical literature, feverfew

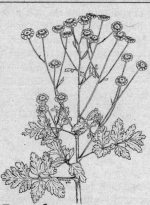

Feverfew

Feverfew, which is kin to dandelion and marigold, is most famous for preventing and even curing migraines and other headaches.

works for about two-thirds of those who use it consistently. My sister-in-law's experience is typical. Before she tried feverfew, she averaged about one migraine a week and spent about $200 a year trying to counteract the pain.

If we assume that the estimated 25 million Americans who suffer from migraines on a regular basis spend in the same way that my sister-in-law did, that would be an incredible $5 billion a year for migraine medication. I don't think the purveyors of modern pharmaceuticals would be pleased to see feverfew replace the many profitable drugs that are now prescribed for treating migraine. That's partly why I'm so interested in promoting this herbal alternative.

I'm not the only one. Studies published in the *British Medical Journal* agree that taking feverfew regularly prevents migraine attacks. And according to the *Harvard Medical School Health Letter*, "Eating feverfew leaves has become a popular method for preventing migraine attacks in England. Some people for whom conventional treatments for migraine have not worked have turned to feverfew with good results." It's nice to know that I'm in such good company on this one.

People who use feverfew often use fresh leaves, typically ingesting one to four leaves a day to prevent migraines. If you have access to the fresh herb, you might try this approach, but don't expect the leaves to taste good. And some 10 to 18 percent of the people who use fresh feverfew develop mouth sores and/or inflammation of the mouth and tongue.

The good news is that you don't have to eat the leaves to get the full benefits of this herb. You may be able to avoid the side effects by making a tea with about two to eight fresh leaves. Steep them in boiling water, but do not boil them, as boiling may break down the parthenolides.

You can also take this herb in capsules, which is really the easiest way to do it. Depending on the potency of the herb, doses may vary from one capsule a day (60 milligrams) to six capsules a day (about 380 milligrams) of fresh, powdered leaf or two daily 25-milligram capsules of freeze-dried leaf. Feverfew capsules are sold at many herb shops and health food stores. By all means discuss the herb with your doctor if you have a hard time arriving at an appropriate dose.

One caveat: Pregnant women should not take feverfew because of a remote possibility that it might trigger miscarriage. And women who are nursing should not use it because of the possibility of passing the herb to infants in breast milk. Finally, long-term users often report a mild tranquilizing or sedative effect, which may be welcome or unwelcome, depending on your temperament.

❦❦❦ Willow (*Salix*, various species). Commission E, the group of experts that advises the German government about herbs, endorses willow bark as an effective pain reliever for headache and anything else treated by willow's pharmaceutical derivative, aspirin.

When herbalists talk about willow bark as herbal aspirin, they usually mention white willow (*S. alba*). But this species is rather low in salicin, the aspirin-like chemical in the bark that relieves pain. If you want more headache relief per cup of tea, there are other willow species that are more potent: *S. daphnoides*, *S. fragilis* and *S. purpurea*.

Commission E recommends getting 60 to 120 milligrams of salicin to treat a headache, which works out to 1 teaspoon of the high-salicin barks or 1 to 1½ teaspoons of white willow. More than 86 percent of the salicin in willow is absorbed by the digestive tract, providing a good blood level of the chemical for several hours.

If you're allergic to aspirin, you probably shouldn't take aspirin-like herbs, either. And you should be aware that if aspirin upsets your stomach, willow bark may do the same. Then again, it might not. Leon Chaitow, a British naturopath and osteopath, says, "Unlike aspirin, which is an isolated, concentrated chemical, willow bark acts gently and without aspirin's potential for irritating the stomach." Also, do not give either aspirin or its natural herbal alternatives to children who have headaches with viral infections such as colds or flu, as there's a chance that they might develop Reye's syndrome, a potentially fatal condition that damages the liver and brain.

❦❦ Evening primrose (*Oenothera biennis*). This is one of the best sources of the pain-relieving compound phenylalanine. For those with chronic headaches, nutritionists may recommend a daily dose of six to eight capsules of evening primrose oil.

Sunflower seeds are also well-endowed with phenylalanine, with 4.8 percent on a dry-weight basis. Other good sources of phenylalanine, in descending order of potency, include watercress, bean sprouts, soybeans, pigeonpeas, swamp cabbage, lupines, pigweed greens, peanuts, lentils, yard-long beans, spinach, carob and butternut squash.

❦❦ Garlic (*Allium sativum*) and onion (*A. cepa*). The platelet cells that are involved in blood clotting are also involved in triggering migraines. Of course, you don't want to knock out your platelets entirely, because then you'd bleed to death from minor cuts. Making the platelets a little less active, however, apparently helps prevent migraines. Naturopaths suggest eating lots of garlic and onions, because these blood-thinning herbs interfere somewhat with platelet activity. (That's also why they're recommended for preventing heart attack.)

❦❦ Ginger (*Zingiber officinale*). People in Asian cultures often use ginger to prevent migraines. I don't know of any good studies on this, but I am aware of an intriguing anecdote: One 42-year-old woman who had regular migraines stopped taking all other migraine medicines and instead took 500 to 600 milligrams of dry ginger mixed in water at the onset of the visual disturbances associated with migraine. She'd then take the same dose every four hours for four days. Starting within about 30 minutes, her migraine episode was much less painful and disconcerting. Later she switched from dried ginger to fresh ginger. Migraines rarely recurred, and when they did, they were less frequent.

Since ginger is good for you in so many different ways, it seems like this approach is certainly worth a try. If you opt for ginger powder, try 500 milligrams of dry ginger in capsules. If you prefer fresh ginger, the equivalent amount is five grams (about 2½ teaspoons) of fresh, grated root.

For greater effect, you might also want to combine ginger with another herb. Naturopaths sometimes suggest taking turmeric, which is an anti-inflammatory and shares many of ginger's medicinal activities. If I had a migraine, I think I'd try a couple of teaspoons of each in a glass of lemonade, as needed.

❦❦ Ginkgo (*Ginkgo biloba*). A medical study found that headaches often clear up with increased cerebral blood flow. That's what ginkgo does—improve blood flow through the brain. If I had frequent headaches, I'd probably try this herb. I'd suggest taking 30 drops of a standardized extract containing at least 0.5 percent flavonoid glycosides three times a day for a day or two. You could also take capsules; follow the package directions. You can try 60 to 240 milligrams a day, but don't go any higher than that. In large amounts, ginkgo may cause diarrhea, irritability and restlessness.

❦❦ Red pepper (*Capsicum*, various species). The hot

ingredient in red pepper, capsaicin, is also a marvelous pain reliever. Eight studies I'm aware of show that external applications of capsaicin interfere with substance P, a chemical that scientists believe plays a key role in transmitting pain impulses.

Taken internally, red pepper looks good for treating headache. It is reportedly the richest food source of aspirin-like salicylates.

Capsaicin has been shown in studies to help prevent cluster headaches, which are painfully similar to migraines. In one small study of 12 people with this type of headache, 6 (50 percent) who inhaled one gram of capsaicin up their noses three times a day for several days got complete relief, 4 reported partial relief, and only 2 experienced no relief. Several other studies show similar results.

If I had either a migraine or a cluster headache, I'd try cayenne for relief. But you shouldn't inhale it; you can simply take capsules.

❧ Lemon balm (*Melissa officinalis*). This herb, also known as melissa, can be helpful in treating migraine, according to Norman G. Bisset, Ph.D., professor of pharmacy at King's College at the University of London and author of *Herbal Drugs and Phytopharmaceuticals*. Commission E endorses this herb for this use.

The recommended dose is a tea made with one to two teaspoons of dried herb per cup of boiling water and steeped until cool. If I had a headache, I'd spike my lemon balm tea with feverfew, ginger and turmeric.

❧ Peppermint (*Mentha piperita*). When mixed with a little alcohol and rubbed on the temples, peppermint oil helps alleviate headache pain. I'd mix my peppermint oil with lavender and add eucalyptus and rosemary if they were available. I believe that all of these healing oils can work together harmoniously. But remember, these oils are for external use only.

❧ Purslane (*Portulaca oleracea*) and other foods containing magnesium. Nutritionists suggest getting 600 milligrams of magnesium a day if you're prone to headaches. (The Daily Value is 400 milligrams.) I am particularly interested in magnesium's relationship to headache, because magnesium deficiency has been found in people who have frequent tension headaches or migraines.

Also, according to a Gallup survey, an estimated 72 percent of Americans report having a magnesium intake that would result in deficiency. Could there be a connection between the prevalence of low magnesium and headache? Perhaps. It certainly shouldn't hurt to get more of this vital mineral in your diet.

Besides leafy greens like purslane, legumes and whole grains are good food sources of magnesium. In my database, purslane is the clear leader in this nutrient with nearly 2 percent magnesium on a dry-weight basis, but green beans, poppy seeds, oats, cowpeas and spinach are close behind.

❧ **Tansy (*Tanacetum vulgare*).** Like feverfew, tansy contains parthenolides, which may help prevent migraines. (Pregnant women should not use tansy, though, as it has the potential to cause miscarriage.)

❧ **Thyme (*Thymus vulgaris*).** Medical anthropologist John Heinerman, Ph.D., author of *Heinerman's Encyclopedia of Fruits, Vegetables and Herbs*, suggests drinking thyme tea. Try one teaspoon of dried herb per cup of hot water. He also suggests using it in compresses to ease the aching muscles in the neck, shoulders and back that can contribute to tension headaches.

❧ **Turmeric (*Curcuma longa*).** As I've mentioned, you might want to try this anti-inflammatory, particularly in combination with another herb, like ginger.

❧ **Assorted herbs.** There are almost too many foods that are used as folk remedies for headache, and many have been shown to definitely contain pain-relieving compounds. One of my own favorite pain-relieving teas is a mixture of cinnamon, lemongrass, peppermint and rosemary.

Other herbs that are possibly worth a try include basil, black pepper, caraway, coriander, ginseng, lavender, pennyroyal, plantain, poppy seeds, rosemary, rue, tea and yarrow.

Heartburn

A colleague, who never struck me as herbally inclined, dropped by my office one morning and surprised me by asking what sort of herbal concoction I might recommend for heartburn. He said he'd had it on and off for several months.

But he'd started taking ginger about a week earlier, and he said he felt considerably better.

I was delighted that he'd tried an herb, but I was also a little surprised at his success. Studies show that ginger prevents nausea caused by motion sickness as well as morning sickness in pregnant women. That's how it has earned its well-deserved reputation as a stomach soother. But heartburn does not occur in the stomach.

Heartburn develops when the muscular opening from the esophagus into the stomach doesn't work properly. This set of muscles—the lower esophageal sphincter (LES)—opens to allow food into the stomach but then closes to keep stomach acids from washing up into the esophagus. In heartburn, the LES doesn't close completely, and the burning feeling in the chest is actually acid burning the esophagus.

I'd never heard of ginger for LES problems, but I didn't doubt him. I simply suggested that he add peppermint to his ginger tea. Peppermint has an age-old reputation for relieving upset stomach and heartburn, and a good deal of research validates the folklore.

Heartburn is very common. An estimated 30 percent of adults experience it at least once a month. Diet and lifestyle often contribute to it.

Heartburn is more likely to develop when you eat hurriedly, on the run, standing up or wolfing down your food without chewing it thoroughly. Fried foods, saturated fats, sugar, alcohol, cigarettes and coffee have all been associated with heartburn. To help prevent it, try to have meals and snacks when you're relaxed instead of on the go. It also helps to have a diet of fruits, vegetables and whole grains and avoid fried foods.

Green Pharmacy for Heartburn

In addition to avoiding aggravating foods and eating habits, here are some herbs that can help.

✺✺ **Angelica (*Angelica archangelica*) and relatives.** Aromatherapists wisely suggest oil of angelica as useful for heartburn in adults and colic and gas in children. Angelica is a member of the carrot family, and many members of that plant family seem to have a soothing action on the digestive tract, a quality that herbalists call carminative.

❦

Angelica for Angina

Angelica is good for treating heartburn, and although heartburn doesn't really have anything to do with the heart, angelica, curiously enough, is also good for the heart.

Angelica and other plants in the carrot family contain some 15 calcium channel blockers, chemicals that have been turned into pharmaceuticals to treat angina, the chronic chest pain that often accompanies heart disease. One of these natural calcium channel blockers is reportedly as strong as verapamil (Calan, Isoptin), an angina medication.

Vegetarians regularly eat lots of carrots, and perhaps this partially explains the lower incidence of heart problems that they enjoy as a group.

❦

If you have heartburn frequently, you should discuss it with your doctor. You might also wish to indulge in my Angelade, which contains six relatives of angelica, all carminative. You'll need a juicer to make this one, as Angelade consists of juiced angelica stalks, carrots, celery, fennel, garlic, parsley and parsnips. (You may have to add some water and spices to make it drinkable.)

If you don't have access to fresh angelica, it's okay to leave it out and go with just the other ingredients. In fact, it doesn't really make any difference how much of each you use. Simply pick your favorites, then mix and match until you create a juice that tickles your fancy.

❦❦ **Camomile (*Matricaria recutita*).** Joe and Terry Graedon, co-authors of *The People's Pharmacy* and *Graedon's Best Medicine*, share my opinion that camomile is the first-choice herb for heartburn and stomach distress.

❧❧ **Licorice (*Glycyrrhiza glabra*).** I agree with Michael Murray, N.D., co-author of *Encyclopedia of Natural Medicine* and several other scholarly books on nutritional and naturopathic healing, that deglycyrrhizinated licorice (DGL) successfully treats both heartburn and ulcers of the stomach and esophagus. Many studies show that licorice is an antispasmodic and that it reduces production of stomach acid, thereby decreasing heartburn.

The caveat is that while licorice and its extracts are safe for normal use in moderate amounts (up to about three cups of tea a day) long-term use (more than six weeks) or ingestion of larger amounts can produce headache, lethargy, sodium and water retention, excessive loss of potassium and high blood pressure. A cup of licorice tea now and then to relieve heartburn is safe.

❧❧

Don't Die from "Heartburn"

Sometimes heartburn hurts so much that people think they're having a heart attack, although actually they're not. But the reverse can be true as well: Sometimes what you think is heartburn is actually a heart attack or angina.

Heartburn typically develops during or shortly after a meal and produces pain or burning in the chest. Heart attack and angina can strike at any time. Frequently, the pain they produce is not limited to the chest but radiates up under the jaw or along an arm. Heart attack and angina may also produce faintness and sweating. When in doubt about chest pain, call 911 and describe your symptoms.

❧❧

✖✖ Peppermint (*Mentha piperita*). A while back, my daughter spent a vacation week with us, and we celebrated by grilling up big slabs of spareribs, which gave me heartburn. So I headed out to the garden and grabbed two handfuls of peppermint and one each of spearmint, lemon balm (also known as melissa) and bee balm, along with some basil, sage and oregano, and brewed up a tasty tea that helped. I know you might prefer a more specific recipe—one teaspoon of this, two teaspoons of that—but I never measure herbs that are generally regarded as safe.

There is a controversy about the use of peppermint for heartburn. I agree with herb advocate Andrew Weil, M.D., professor at the University of Arizona College of Medicine in Tucson and author of *Natural Health, Natural Medicine*, who strongly recommends this herb. Herbal lore certainly supports peppermint. Traditional cultures from ancient Egyptians to present-day Icelanders use peppermint for all sorts of digestive problems, including heartburn.

A few esteemed herbalists, however, contend that peppermint can aggravate heartburn. If that happens to you, don't use this herb, but personally, I doubt that you'll have problems. Many, if not most, mints have the ability to ease digestion, with peppermint and spearmint tops in my book.

✖ Cardamom (*Elettaria cardamomum*) and cinnamon (*Cinnamomum*, various species). Both of these herbs help eliminate gas. When Mrs. Duke suffers occasional heartburn or acid indigestion, one thing she does with my blessing is sprinkle one or the other of these two powdered herbs on her toast. (We rarely have cardamom around the house, though; it's too expensive.)

✖ Dill (*Anethum graveolens*). Dill has been used to soothe the digestive tract and treat heartburn for thousands of years. If I had heartburn, I'd try crushing a few teaspoons of seeds and making a tea with it. (If you are pregnant, using dill in medicinal amounts could cause problems. You should reserve it for occasional, moderate use.)

✖ Fennel (*Foeniculum vulgare*). Fennel has been used as long as dill, and for the same reasons. I'd use it, too.

✖ Gentian (*Gentiana officinalis*). Herbal pharmacologist Daniel Mowrey, Ph.D., author of *The Scientific Validation of Herbal Medicine* and *Herbal Tonic Therapies*, notes that gentian, especially when taken about 30 minutes before meals, is a remarkable heartburn preventive that also aids digestion. I agree. Gentian has a long history as a digestive herb. I would try simmering one teaspoon of gentian in a cup or two of water for about 30 minutes. Dr. Mowrey also suggests adding a sprinkle of cayenne and ginger to your gentian tea.

❧❧

Yeas and Nays on Comfrey

Comfrey has developed a bad reputation. Although many herbalists continue to recommend the herb, some authorities say that you shouldn't ingest any at all. That's because medical research has found that comfrey contains chemicals known as pyrrolizidine alkaloids (PAs). In sufficient amounts, PAs can cause liver damage and possibly cancer.

I don't think anyone should drink comfrey tea by the gallon every day, but I'm not afraid of a little comfrey now and then, even though the herb clearly contains these substances. I base my position on studies done by biochemist Bruce Ames, Ph.D., of the University of California at Berkeley.

Dr. Ames specializes in estimating the carcinogenicity (cancer-causing potential) of food items. According to his findings, a cup of comfrey leaf tea is less carcinogenic than a can of beer. And I'm not going to give that up, either!

❧❧

❧ **Papaya (*Carica papaya*) and pineapple (*Ananas comosus*).** These fruits are loaded with digestive enzymes and have been widely used to relieve heartburn and indigestion. Papaya with a little honey may even prevent it if eaten before a meal or between courses. Some nutritionists suggest that kiwifruit might help as well.

❧ **Herbal formulas.** I have a lot of respect for British herbalist David Hoffmann, author of a dozen or so books, including *The Herbal Handbook*. He recommends several combinations of herbs for digestive tract problems. Teas made from either of the following two formulas might be useful for heartburn.

Digestive formula: Two parts comfrey leaf, which soothes the digestive tract; two parts hollyhock (*Althaea officinalis*), another stomach soother; one part sweetflag (*Acorus calamus*), which has antacid and gas-relieving properties; and one part meadowsweet, which is both antacid and gas relieving.

Esophagitis formula: Two parts comfrey; two parts hollyhock; one part camomile, which is both a gas reliever and an anti-inflammatory; and one part marigold, which is also an anti-inflammatory.

❧ **Salad from the Bible.** Several plants mentioned in the Bible have folklore reputations for being helpful. These include almond, chicory, dandelion, garlic, lettuce, mustard, olives, onions and walnuts. If I suffered frequent heartburn, I'd try making a salad with several of these anti-heartburn ingredients.

Heart Disease

Dean Ornish, M.D., is a California doctor who astounded the medical world a few years ago by becoming the first researcher to actually reverse heart disease. Even more amazing, he did it with a low-tech combination of natural approaches: exercise, yoga, meditation, support groups and a very low fat vegetarian diet (10 percent of calories from fat).

I've always liked a story that Dr. Ornish tells about a group of rabbits that added an unexpected tidbit to the research on heart disease. Kept in a laboratory under research conditions, the rabbits were genetically similar, and all received the same food and got the same amount of exercise, yet one group had 60 percent fewer heart attacks than the others. What was the difference? It turned out that the healthier rabbits were the ones kept in the lower cages, and the short person who fed the rabbits could reach the lower animals and pet them when feeding them. Love, it seems, is a life preserver. I've always thought so.

Preventing Clogged Pipes

In heart disease—or more accurately, coronary artery disease—the arteries that nourish the heart become clogged. This disease is our number one cause of death. It affects approximately 7 million Americans and causes about 1.5 million heart attacks and 500,000 deaths each year.

Mainstream medicine hasn't yet adopted the safe, gentle, natural Ornish approach. Instead, our taxes and health insurance premiums go to finance approximately 300,000 coronary artery bypass operations each year at a cost of about $30,000 each, or $9 billion total.

Bypass surgery is only a temporary fix. The bypasses themselves usually clog up after a few months or years. If the $9 billion spent on bypasses went instead into natural therapies and preventive approaches, the U.S. health system would be better off.

Preventive therapies include treating high blood pressure and elevated cholesterol and doing everything possible to encourage Americans to quit smoking, lose weight, exercise more, manage their stress more effectively and cultivate more social support.

The National Institutes of Health (NIH) recognizes the value of prevention. In a 1994 report, the NIH said: "For health-care reform to succeed at reducing costs . . . disease prevention must be the *ultimate* focus of the primary health-care system, rather than disease treatment." I just wish doctors would embrace this concept.

Vegetable Power

One of my favorite approaches to preventing—and recovering from—heart attack is one you won't find in any medical texts. It's vegetable soup. Most people call it minestrone, but I call it Medistrone because it's as much a medicine as a food.

There is no recipe for this soup. You simply take the appropriate ingredients, which I'm about to describe, and combine them into any number of delicious soups. The idea is to concentrate on seasonal vegetables and make it a little different each time, so you never get tired of this healthful dish. It soon becomes a habit that you'll enjoy for the rest of your life.

Some of the vegetables and herbs I use in vegetable soup, notably garlic, onions, ginger and red pepper, make the blood less likely to clot, thus preventing the blood clots that trigger heart attack. Garlic and onion also help reduce cholesterol and blood pressure.

Other vegetables, particularly tomatoes, contain the compound gamma-amino butyric acid (GABA). Lately I've become fascinated by this compound. According to studies, the GABA in tomatoes and many other soup vegetables appears to reduce blood pressure and help strengthen the heart muscle. To Medistrone's tomato base we add other herbs, spices and vegetables that help reduce blood pressure, among them the aforementioned onions and garlic plus rice, celery and saffron.

Still other vegetables that you might add to Medistrone that help lower cholesterol are artichokes, barley, beans, carrots, eggplant and spinach.

In addition, my Medistrone contains vegetables high in glutathione, a powerful antioxidant. Antioxidants help prevent artery-clogging plaque from being deposited on coronary artery walls. You can find healthy amounts in asparagus, broccoli, cabbage, cauliflower, potatoes, purslane and tomatoes. (It's also found in avocados, grapefruit, oranges, peaches and watermelon, but I wouldn't use these in my soup.)

All of the vegetables that you might use in Medistrone are low in fat and have little or no cholesterol, so they can help control weight, blood pressure and cholesterol. Vegetables can even provide good exercise if you grow them yourself.

So if you're worried about heart attack, by all means have Medistrone as a meal once or twice a week—or more if you want. You can make a big pot early in the week, then freeze portion-size servings and have it whenever you want. I speculate that simply by replacing a few meat or cheese meals a week with Medistrone, you may reduce your risk of heart attack by about 20 percent.

More Reasons for Eating Your Veggies

Don't stop with Medistrone. There's such strong scientific evidence in favor of fruits and vegetables for preventing heart disease that you should make them part of every meal.

Fruits and vegetables are our main sources of potent antioxidants: vitamins C and E, the vitamin A–like carotenoids and folate, a B vitamin. Many studies show that as dietary consumption of these nutrients increases, risk of heart attack plummets by up to 40 percent. (And cancer risk drops about 50 percent as well).

No wonder the National Research Council, the National Cancer Institute and most nutritional health authorities urge all Americans to "strive for five." This means getting at least five servings of fruits and vegetables a day.

Keep in mind, though, that five is just the healthy minimum. Many nutritionists encourage eight or nine servings a day. That's a very tall order, considering that only about 10 percent of all Americans get even five, according to Gladys Block, Ph.D., a nutritional epidemiologist at the University of California at Berkeley. It's starting to sound as if a better slogan would be "tend toward ten." In 1997, I launched my own campaign called Strive for Five Times Five (fruits, herbs, legumes and grains, nuts and vegetables).

I have no doubt that if we put the $9 billion that goes for bypasses into a big advertising campaign to get Americans to eat more fruits and veggies, we'd see fewer heart attacks.

Green Pharmacy for Heart Disease

I've already said that garlic, onions, ginger and red pepper help prevent and treat heart disease by reducing blood pressure and that garlic and onions also cut cholesterol and discourage the blood from forming clots. If you know much about herbs, that information probably isn't news to you. But you may not know that many other herbs can help prevent and treat heart disease.

🌿🌿🌿 **Pigweed (*Amaranthus*, various species) and other plants containing calcium.** Pigweed leaves are one of our best plant sources of calcium (about 5.3 percent on a dry-weight basis). Studies suggest that calcium adds mineral density to bone, which can help prevent osteoporosis. But there's more: The mineral also significantly reduces heart attack risk.

Other high-calcium plants include lamb's-quarters, stinging nettle, broadbeans, watercress, licorice, marjoram, savory, red clover shoots and thyme.

In addition to calcium, pigweed is high in fiber. A six-year Harvard study of more than 40,000 men showed that compared with those who consumed the least fiber, those who ate the most had just one-third the risk of heart attack. You can add pigweed to salads, mixed vegetable dishes and Medistrone.

❧❧❧ **Willow (*Salix*, various species).** Willow bark contains salicin, the herbal precursor of aspirin. A great deal of research shows that low-dose aspirin—one-half to one standard tablet a day—can reduce heart attack risk substantially by preventing the blood clots that trigger it.

The body converts aspirin into salicylic acid, and it also converts the salicin in willow bark into salicylic acid. So if pharmaceutical aspirin helps prevent heart attack, herbal aspirin should, too. If you're allergic to aspirin, though, you probably shouldn't take herbal aspirin either.

Typically, people use the bark of the white willow (*S. alba*), but several other species are richer in salicin, including crack willow (*S. fragilis*) and purple osier (*S. purpurea*). If white willow is the only kind you can find at your health food store or herb shop, though, that's okay.

About a half-teaspoon to a teaspoon of white willow bark contains approximately 100,000 parts per million of salicin, or about 100 milligrams. After it's converted into salicylic acid, that should be about enough to provide aspirin's heart-protective effect.

I'd suggest brewing a tea with a teaspoon of so of bark to a cup of boiling water. Steep for 15 minutes and strain. You can try drinking one cup a day or one every other day.

❧❧ **Angelica (*Angelica archangelica*).** Doctors routinely prescribe calcium channel blockers such as verapamil (Calan, Isoptin) to prevent heart attack. This is a class of drugs that works by helping to reduce blood pressure.

Angelica contains 15 separate compounds that are calcium channel blockers. If you are taking a prescribed calcium channel blocker, I would not advise abandoning your medication in favor of angelica, but I do suspect that adding this herb to your regimen would improve the overall effect of your medication. You should discuss this herb with your doctor if you'd like to try it.

I make a concoction called Angelade, which consists of juiced angelica stalks, carrots, celery, fennel, garlic, parsley and parsnips, with some water and spices for drinkability. It's very tasty, and all of the ingredients contain either calcium channel blockers, antioxidants or compounds that lower cholesterol or blood pressure, thus helping to prevent heart disease in one way or another.

❧❧ Grape (*Vitis vinifera*). Some 30 long-term studies agree that moderate alcohol drinkers—those who have one or two drinks a day—reduce their heart attack risk by some 25 to 40 percent. Meanwhile, a debate rages about why.

Some researchers say that alcohol itself has a heart-protective effect, presumably by lowering LDL cholesterol (the "bad" kind). They say that any type of alcohol helps: beer, wine or distilled spirits.

Others insist that there's something extra in red wine, and I'm inclined to agree with them. Certain chemicals called phenolic compounds that are found in grape skin give red wine its color. They also protect the body from LDL cholesterol even better than powerful vitamin E.

You really don't need to drink red wine to get these compounds, though. They are also found in red grapes, red grape juice and many other fruits and vegetables, including bilberries, blackberries, blueberries, garlic and onions.

If you choose to get the benefits of these compounds by having a couple of glasses of red wine a day, fine. Just remember that imbibing more than two drinks a day damages the heart.

❧❧ Hawthorn (*Crataegus*, various species). Hawthorn has a well-established and well-deserved reputation as a mild heart tonic. It's especially useful in treating the heart fatigue known as congestive heart failure. But research shows that this herb also helps prevent heart attack. It improves blood circulation through the heart by opening (dilating) the coronary arteries. It also increases the heart's ability to cope with a loss of oxygen, which is what happens when clogged coronary arteries reduce the heart's blood supply.

Hawthorn also helps keep the heart beating properly and decreases what's known as peripheral vascular resistance. This means that it helps blood flow more easily, relieving strain on the heart and helping to reduce blood pressure.

In one study, people with heart disease who took 600 to 900

milligrams of hawthorn a day for two months reported that they felt significant improvement.

Hawthorn is a powerful heart medicine. If you want to take hawthorn to prevent heart attack, you should discuss it with your doctor and see a naturopath to get a standardized extract. Naturopaths do not recommend taking the raw herb to treat heart disease.

ᴇᴇ Purslane (*Portulaca oleracea*). I promote tasty, spinach-like purslane at every opportunity, and here's a good one. This easy-to-grow garden vegetable is our best leafy source of beneficial compounds known as omega-3 fatty acids. Omega-3's help prevent the blood clots that trigger heart attack. They're the reason that people who eat a lot of cold-water fish like salmon, which is a prime source of these oils, have low rates of heart disease.

In addition, purslane is extremely well-endowed with antioxidants, which also help prevent heart attack as well as cancer.

Finally, these greens contain calcium and magnesium in a one-to-one ratio. I've already mentioned that calcium is good for the heart, but calcium is most protective when you take it in a one-to-one combination with magnesium. That's a good argument for eating lots of fresh, leafy purslane. I eat it raw in salads or steam it, just like spinach.

ᴇᴇ Rosemary (*Rosmarinus officinalis*). Rosemary is one of the richer herbal sources of antioxidants, which is why it works so well as a food preservative. Its antioxidants help prevent the fats in meat from turning rancid. They do the same, in a manner of speaking, for your heart.

Rosemary makes a pleasant-tasting tea. You can also use generous amounts of rosemary in your cooking.

ᴇ Chicory (*Cichorium intybus*). According to California herbalist Kathi Keville, author of *The Illustrated Herb Encyclopedia* and *Herbs for Health and Healing*, whom I respect highly, Egyptian researchers have discovered that chicory root has two heart benefits. It slows a rapid heartbeat, and it also has a mild heart-stimulating effect, somewhat like the often-prescribed medication digitalis. And it's gentle enough to be safe.

Several commercial coffee substitutes contain roasted chicory. In France and Italy, the roots are not only consumed as a drink but are also considered a vegetable. Try some chicory coffee substitute and see how you like it. Follow the package directions.

❧ **Olive (*Olea europea*).** When taken daily, olive oil may have a significantly protective effect against heart disease. Certainly it is pivotal in the heart-healthy Mediterranean diet. In Mediterranean populations in which the main source of fat is monounsaturated olive oil, heart attacks are relatively rare, even when total fat consumption is fairly high.

If you haven't already done so, you should consider making olive oil the main oil that you use in the kitchen.

❧ **Peanut (*Arachis hypogaea*).** Leave the papery red skins on your peanuts, because that's where the heart-protective compounds called oligomeric procyanidins (OPCs) can be found. OPCs are potent antioxidants that help prevent not only heart attack but also cancer and stroke.

Since plants' OPC content has not yet been well-tabulated, I cannot tell you which ones have the most. I like to get my OPCs from peanut skins, red grapes and red wine.

Hemorrhoids

In August of 1990, the Food and Drug Administration (FDA) ruled which ingredients in over-the-counter hemorrhoid products were permissible and which were banned. Hemorrhoid products constitute a $150 million industry, and those rulings had an immediate impact on the kinds of products available at your local drugstore.

Permissible products included local anesthetics and analgesics to deal with the pain of hemorrhoids; vasoconstrictors to tighten the distended veins that lead to hemorrhoids; lubricants to help relieve constipation, the underlying cause of hemorrhoids; astringents, which help tighten anal tissue distended by hemorrhoids; and keratolytics, which help remove excess hemorrhoidal tissue. Some of the permissible products were herbal or derived from plant sources: benzyl alcohol, an anesthetic; cocoa butter, a lubricant; witch hazel water, an astringent; and menthol, camphor and juniper tar, for relief of pain and itching. That's the good news.

The bad news is that the FDA also banned several herbal hemorrhoid treatments with long histories of use for this common affliction, among them goldenseal, used for centuries as an anal antiseptic; mullein, a soothing, itch-relieving herb; tannins, well-documented astringents; and menthol and camphor as counterirritants, substances that produce minor irritation and thus relieve other pain.

But even though the FDA approves some herbal remedies and not others, I'd advise you to keep an open mind. Personally, I don't give much credence to the FDA's opinions about herbal remedies. Both folklore and scientific research suggest that the variety of usable remedies is much larger than the government agency attests.

The All-American Condition

Estimates vary, but it looks like hemorrhoids affect one-third of Americans—some 75 million people. All four people in my family have experienced them, more often when we get away from the high-fiber diet that we eat at home.

Hemorrhoids are varicose veins of the anus. Anal veins drain blood away from the area. They expand (dilate) during defecation and shrink back to normal size afterward. However, repeated straining during defecation, which is a common result of constipation, can interfere with the normal functioning of these veins. They may become permanently swollen, causing pain and itching.

In addition, defecation can rupture the swollen blood vessels, causing bleeding. This is a particular problem among pregnant women, because during pregnancy, the developing fetus places pressure on all the veins of the lower abdomen.

The best way to deal with hemorrhoids is to prevent them, and the best way to do that is to prevent constipation. You'll find several herbs that are good for relieving chronic constipation mentioned in this chapter. (For additional details, see page 171.)

A Regular Kind of Person

Basically, staying regular boils down to eating a high-fiber diet, with lots of fruits and vegetables, and drinking plenty of nonalcoholic fluids. I daresay that anyone who regularly eats five fibrous fruits and five fibrous veggies a day will not suffer from constipation. In other words, a preventive ounce of carrots or apples—and of course, prunes—is worth a pound of buck-thorn, an herbal laxative, taken later.

Another approach is to use an internal lubricant that allows stool to pass more easily. Mineral oil is the pharmaceutical approach, but you might try olive or linseed oil instead.

Finally, beyond preventing constipation, I'll offer a few more lifestyle suggestions. Never ignore "the urge" to go. When sitting on the toilet, don't bear down; try to relax. Straining leads to hemorrhoids. Don't sit on the toilet any longer than necessary. Adopt more of a squatting position and raise your feet on a small stool. This helps many people.

Green Pharmacy for Hemorrhoids

If you develop hemorrhoids, here are some herbs to try.

ℛℛ Comfrey (*Symphytum officinale*). Comfrey is rich in allantoin, a wound-healing chemical that is anti-inflammatory, stimulates the immune system and hastens the formation of new skin. You can moisten powdered comfrey with vegetable oil and apply the paste. Or you can pound the leaf to soften the fuzzy hairs it's covered with and apply the leaf itself, topically. You don't have to worry about washing it off, as the residue will come off the next time you shower.

ℛℛ

What's in a Name?

Just for the record, here's an herb you don't want to use but might be tempted to because of its name—pile-wort (*Ranunculus ficaria*). *Piles* is an old-fashioned word for hemorrhoids, and you can pretty much guess that an herb with that name would be good for hemorrhoids. In fact, this herb has an interesting history.

Early herbalists believed it was useful because they subscribed to the Doctrine of Signatures, the medieval idea that a plant's physical appearance hinted at its medicinal use. Pilewort tubers were thought to resemble hemorrhoids.

The Doctrine of Signatures obviously has problems, but people would not have kept using pilewort for hemorrhoids for thousands of years if it didn't help, at least a little.

Although there's some controversy about this herb, Rudolf Fritz Weiss, M.D., the dean of German medical herbalists and author of *Herbal Medicine*, concludes: "In my own trials and observations, pilewort has failed completely, both internally and as an ointment." But noted British herbalist David Hoffmann, author of *The Herbal Handbook*, whom I respect, is more positive, saying that it helps. Since many species of *Ranunculus* can cause blisters, and the benefits are elusive, you're probably well-advised to avoid.

❧❧

Plantain (*Plantago*, various species). Plantain has a strong folk reputation as a hemorrhoid remedy. This herb contains allantoin, the same soothing compound found in comfrey. If I were caught in the bush with a hemorrhoid and without my Tucks, I'd create a poultice and apply it to the afflicted area.

Psyllium (*Plantago ovata*). In one study, 51 people with hemorrhoids received a psyllium preparation. More than three-quarters (84 percent) reported improvement—less pain, itching, bleeding and discomfort on defecation. Commission E, the German herbal advisory panel, recommends taking anywhere from four to ten teaspoons of psyllium seeds a day for constipation. It's easy to get that much by using a commercial product such as Metamucil, which is made with psyllium seeds. Simply follow the directions on the package.

Psyllium works by absorbing water in the gut and swelling considerably, which adds bulk to stool and triggers the muscle contractions we experience as "the urge." If you use psyllium, make sure you drink enough fluids. You should get at least eight (eight-ounce) glasses of water or juice a day. And watch how you react to this herb if you have allergies. If allergic symptoms develop after you take it once, don't use it again.

Witch hazel (*Hamamelis virginiana*). For a long time, I thought the *H* in Preparation H stood for *Hamamelis*. This is the Latin name for witch hazel, the active ingredient in the popular Preparation H Cleansing Pads. (I guess I should have guessed that that the *H* actually stands for hemorrhoids.) Witch hazel is also the active ingredient in Tucks, the commercial pharmaceutical product often recommended for hemorrhoids.

Witch hazel is a soothing, cooling astringent that can help relieve hemorrhoidal pain and itching. But you really don't have to spend extra for a brand name. Simply make a compress using witch hazel, which is available at pharmacies for a much lower price. Just tuck a fresh compress in place whenever you feel the need for a little soothing. Then forget it's there and go about your business.

🐿 **Aloe (*Aloe vera*).** Aloe gel is astringent and helps heal wounds. You might try applying it topically to the anal area. When ingested, aloe juice is laxative. India's Ayurvedic physicians suggest drinking a half-cup of aloe juice three times a day until hemorrhoid flare-ups have cleared. You can buy aloe juice at most health food stores. (Don't try to prepare your own. The inner part of the leaf itself is such a powerful laxative that juicing that could cause problems.)

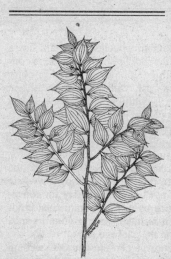

German physicians echo the Ayurvedics. Commission E suggests aloe as a stool softener for those with hemorrhoids or anal fissures or after anal or rectal surgery. The suggested dose is 0.05 to 0.2 gram of powdered aloes, also known as dry extract. This really isn't very much powder—a pinch thrown into a cup of tea would do it. (This remedy may turn the urine red.)

I wouldn't hesitate to apply the yellow gel from a

Butcher's Broom

You can get this herb in the form of powdered root or as a tincture.

kitchen aloe leaf to a hemorrhoid. I also might add a little gel (a spoonful or two) to some prune juice.

❦ **Butcher's broom** (*Ruscus aculeatus*). This woody herb has a long history as a treatment for venous problems like hemorrhoids and varicose veins. The plant contains chemicals called ruscogenins, which have anti-inflammatory and vasoconstricting properties. I'd try five rounded teaspoons of root in a cup of boiling water for internal consumption; you can sweeten the tea with honey. And for topical application, I'd use a tincture of the herb made with alcohol.

❦ **Horse chestnut** (*Aesculus hippocastanum*). The bark of this tree contains several chemicals that help treat hemorrhoids. Aesculin and aescin strengthen blood vessel walls, reducing the risk of further hemorrhoids. Other chemicals in this herb have anti-inflammatory benefits.

Some experiments have shown that horse chestnut does help relieve hemorrhoid symptoms. About 5 to 10 percent of the active chemicals are absorbed if you take this herb orally. There's just one problem: The herb contains tannins that tend to contribute to constipation if you drink it. But you can use a tea made from the herb to apply to the hemorrhoids or make a poultice by moistening powdered bark or seeds and apply the resulting paste directly.

❦ **Assorted essential oils.** Aromatherapists suggest adding one or two drops of any number of herbal essential oils to vegetable oil, then applying the ointment to the anal area. I'd suggest using an emollient oil such as almond as a base. For essential oils, I'd try cypress, juniper, lavender, lemon or rosemary. (Remember though, not to ingest essential oils, as even a small amount can be toxic.)

❦ **Assorted herbs.** I'll also share two hemorrhoid treatments recommended by herbalists I trust, both authors of good books on herbal medicine.

Herbal pharmacologist Daniel Mowrey, Ph.D., author of *The Scientific Validation of Herbal Medicine* and *Herbal Tonic Therapies*, suggests making a tea for topical application using alumroot (astringent), goldenseal (vasoconstricting), mullein (soothing), slippery elm bark (soothing) and witch hazel (astringent). You can use any amount of these ingredients.

David Hoffmann, noted British herbalist and author of *The Herbal Handbook*, recommends using a topical salve made from calendula, camomile, yarrow, plantain and St.-John's-wort after every bowel movement. Try mixing one teaspoon of each herb in powdered form with enough emollient oil (almond) to form a paste, then apply.

High Blood Pressure

Several years ago I spent three very long days filming what I hoped would be my first video about health food. But as fate would have it, the time was wasted because an equipment malfunction ruined the tape.

Correction: The time wasn't really wasted, because I got to know the cameraman. He had high blood pressure (hypertension), and I suggested some natural therapies. After we parted company, I didn't hear from him for quite a while, but later he wrote me: "I have been practicing what you preached for over a year now. I eliminated alcohol, pork and beef, now eat more plant foods and herbs and take supplements: beta-carotene, vitamin C, vitamin E, B complex. A recent physical was very revealing. My diastolic blood pressure was down almost 30 percent. My cholesterol dropped from 192 to 159."

Hearts Working Too Hard

Hypertension is generally defined as a blood pressure greater than 140/90. The first number (systolic) is the force that blood exerts on the artery walls when the heart is pumping. The second number (diastolic) is the residual force that remains when the heart relaxes between beats. Any blood pressure reading below "high"—say, a borderline 138/88—is safer, but you should still try getting it down closer to what's considered normal, 120/80. That's because any elevation in blood pressure raises your risk for heart attack and stroke.

About 50 million Americans have high blood pressure, which is often called the silent killer. While the condition itself causes no symptoms, it sets the stage for a heart attack or stroke. In the past few decades, doctors and other health professionals have made a big push to detect high blood pressure and treat it more aggressively, and the rate of heart attack has indeed gone down. But the problem, in my opinion, is that doctors are too quick to treat this condition with synthetic drugs. About half of the people diagnosed with high blood pressure have borderline to mildly high blood pressure. There's plenty of solid evidence that for them, diet and lifestyle changes, including regular exercise, stress management and self-monitoring with a home blood pressure device, work just as well as drugs, with no side effects.

Diet and lifestyle modifications all tend to provide a sense of control that in itself may be beneficial. But don't expect the pharmaceutical industry to encourage the natural way. It would cut into the $2.5 billion-a-year market for antihypertensive medication.

Green Pharmacy for High Blood Pressure

Eating hearty vegetable soups on a regular basis can do more than help normalize blood pressure and prevent heart disease. It can also help prevent cancer, obesity, diabetes and constipation. Vegetable soup is so good for health that I don't even call it minestrone anymore, but rather Medistrone.

What should you put in your Medistrone Soup? You can use just about any vegetables, especially the ones mentioned in this chapter.

There are also any number of herbs that can help control blood pressure, but you don't have to put those in a soup. They make rather nice teas.

✿-✿-✿ **Celery (*Apium graveolens*).** Celery has long been recommended in traditional Chinese medicine for lowering high blood pressure, and experimental evidence bears this out. In one study, injecting laboratory animals with celery extract significantly lowered their blood pressure. In humans, eating as few as four celery stalks has done the same.

✿-✿-✿ **Garlic (*Allium sativum*).** This wonder herb not only helps normalize blood pressure, it also reduces cholesterol. In a scientifically rigorous study, people with high blood pressure were given about one clove of garlic a day for 12 weeks. Afterward they exhibited significantly lower diastolic blood pressure and cholesterol levels.

"We now know that garlic can reduce hypertension, even in quantities as small as a half-ounce per week," says Varro Tyler,

Ph.D., dean and professor emeritus of pharmacognosy (natural product pharmacy) at Purdue University in West Lafayette, Indiana. A half-ounce per week works out to about one clove a day. If you cook with garlic and use it in your salads, getting that much should be a snap. If you haven't yet developed a taste for it, you can take garlic in capsule form. With so many health benefits associated with this herb, I'd recommend finding many ways to enjoy it in your food.

🌺🌺 **Hawthorn (*Crataegus*, various species).** Hawthorn extract can widen (dilate) blood vessels, especially the coronary arteries, according to a report published in the *Lawrence Review of Natural Products*, a respected newsletter. Hawthorn has been used as a heart tonic for centuries.

If you'd like to try this powerful heart medicine, discuss it with your doctor. You can try a tea made with one teaspoon of dried herb per cup of boiling water and drink up to two cups a day.

🌺🌺 **Kudzu (*Pueraria lobata*).** Chinese studies suggest that this weedy vine helps normalize blood pressure. In one study, a tea containing about eight teaspoons of kudzu root was given daily to 52 people for two to eight weeks. In 17 people, blood pressure declined markedly. Thirty others showed some benefit.

Kudzu contains a chemical (puerarin) that has decreased blood pressure by 15 percent in laboratory animals. With 100 times the antioxidant activity of vitamin E, puerarin also helps prevent heart disease and cancer. (Antioxidants are substances that neutralize cell-damaging oxygen molecules known as free radicals.)

🌺🌺 **Onion (*Allium cepa*).** In one study, two to three tablespoons of onion essential oil a day lowered blood pressure in 67 percent of people with moderate hypertension. Their systolic levels fell an average of 25 points and their diastolic readings fell 15 points.

The bad news is that you can't get this oil, and you wouldn't be able to eat enough onions to get this much of an effect. In my case, I'd have to ingest three times my body weight in onions. No thanks. But I do think that onions have enough going for them that you should definitely add more of them to your diet to help lower blood pressure.

🌺🌺 **Tomato (*Lycopersicon lycopersicum*).** A typical minestrone has a tomato base. That's also perfect for Medistrone

Soup, because tomatoes are high in gamma-amino butyric acid (GABA), a compound that can help bring down blood pressure. According to my database, tomatoes also contain six other compounds that do the same thing.

❦ **Broccoli (*Brassica oleracea*).** This vegetable has at least six chemicals that reduce blood pressure.

❦ **Carrot (*Daucus carota*).** According to my database, carrots contain eight compounds that lower blood pressure.

❦ **Purslane (*Portulaca oleracea*) and other foods containing magnesium.** Magnesium deficiency has been implicated in high blood pressure. Many Americans are deficient in this mineral and don't know it. A 1994 Gallup poll showed that about 72 percent of those surveyed reported inadequate magnesium intake.

To get magnesium, turn to leafy greens, legumes and whole grains. Purslane, poppy seeds and string beans are the best dietary sources, according to my database. Nutritionists suggest that a daily supplement of 400 milligrams of magnesium may also help, but I generally recommend getting nutrients from foods.

❦ **Saffron (*Crocus sativus*).** This expensive herb contains a blood pressure–lowering chemical called crocetin. Some authorities even speculate that the low incidence of heart dis-

Saffron

Saffron is a rare spice produced by the stigma of saffron flowers; the centers of about 75,000 flowers are required to make a pound of spice.

ease in Spain is due to that nation's high saffron consumption. You can use saffron in your cooking or make a tea with it.

❧ **Valerian (*Valeriana officinalis*).** Earlier in this chapter I mentioned that gamma-amino butyric acid helps control blood pressure. Well, the herb valerian contains a chemical called valerenic acid that inhibits an enzyme that breaks down GABA. So ingesting something containing valerenic acid would, in effect, ensure higher levels of GABA and lower blood pressure.

Valerian is also a tranquilizer/sedative, which also helps reduce blood pressure.

❧ **Assorted spices.** As for spices that you can add to your Medistrone, fennel contains at least ten compounds that lower blood pressure, oregano has seven, and black pepper, basil and tarragon each have six.

High Cholesterol

The cholesterol story began in 1951, when the Pentagon sent pathologists to Korea to study the bodies of servicemen lost in the war there. The pathologists autopsied some 2,000 soldiers.

Although almost no one under 35 dies of coronary heart disease, more than 75 percent of the soldiers, average age 21, had yellow deposits of atherosclerotic plaque on their artery walls. These artery-clogging deposits, doctors had wrongly assumed, were only prevalent in much older men. The reports of the Army pathologists shocked the medical community. Before the Korea autopsies, doctors didn't realize how early the process of heart disease begins.

Not long afterward, a waxy substance in the blood—cholesterol—was identified as a major contributor to the buildup of plaque and to heart disease risk. More recently, scientists have discovered that for every 1 percent drop in cholesterol levels, there is a 2 percent decrease in heart attack risk.

Understanding the Numbers

The total cholesterol level of the average American is higher than 200 milligrams per deciliter (mg/dl) of blood. Because heart attack risk rises sharply above that level, the American Heart Association urges everyone to take measures to reduce cholesterol if it's anywhere near that high.

How far below 200 should you go to feel that your risk is significantly less? That's not entirely clear, but research suggests that very low cholesterol levels, below 150 or so, increase risk of death from other causes, including liver cancer, lung disease and certain kinds of stroke. My reaction is that people should strive for a cholesterol range of 170 to 190.

To make matters more complicated, there are two kinds of cholesterol—low-density lipoproteins (LDL), which increase risk of heart attack, and high-density lipoproteins (HDL), which actually reduce it. You want to get your total cholesterol down below 190. But if you have high cholesterol, your doctor may focus specifically on your LDL levels and have you work to reduce those, since the "bad" kind is most clearly linked to heart disease.

An estimated 25 percent of Americans have cholesterol levels high enough to place them at risk for heart attack, and 10 percent have levels so high that doctors are quick to prescribe drug treatments. But they're far less likely to tell you the Green Pharmacy ways to reduce your heart disease risk.

Fiber Power

Any and probably all plant fibers can lower cholesterol. That means eating a diet that includes lots of fruits, vegetables and whole grains, hopefully one with a minimum of fats.

In one study, a high-fiber supplement (Fibercel) was added to the diets of laboratory hamsters, enough to comprise 5 percent of their daily calorie intake. The Fibercel lowered their total cholesterol by 42 percent and their "bad" LDL cholesterol by 69 percent. Beneficial HDL increased 16 percent.

Oat bran has gotten a lot of publicity as a cholesterol reducer, but it's just one of many high-fiber foods. Fruits, vegetables and grains have similar effects. In fact, oat bran is far from the best fiber for lowering cholesterol. Hamsters fed a diet with 5 percent oat bran showed reductions in total cholesterol and LDL of only 19 and 29 percent, respectively, a weak showing compared with that obtained with Fibercel.

The components of oat bran that lower cholesterol are beta-glucans. But here again, oat bran is not the richest source. Barley contains up to three times more beta-glucans than oats, and beans are also significant sources.

The good news is that often it isn't necessary to resort to drugs. There are plenty of foods and herbs that can help bring cholesterol levels down.

Green Pharmacy for High Cholesterol

Along with getting adequate fiber from the foods you eat, there are a number of individual foods and herbs that can prove helpful.

❧ ❧ ❧ **Carrot (*Daucus carota*) and other foods containing pectin.** Scottish studies showed that over a period of three weeks, a daily snack of two carrots lowered cholesterol levels by 10 to 20 percent in study participants. Carrots are high in the fiber pectin. Other good sources of pectin include apples and the white inner layer of citrus rinds. Enjoy these foods on a daily basis. (Yes, if you're eating an orange, nibble on a little of the white stuff.)

I know that juicing is really big these days, so I'd like to offer a little advice. If you want to take these fruits and vegetables in beverage form, fine. But don't use a juicer on them if you want to get the full benefit of their pectin content. Just whir them in a blender instead. If you use a juicer, you extract most of the fiber, and only about 10 percent of the cholesterol-lowering pectin remains.

You can also take supplements. University of Florida scientists reported that three tablespoons of grapefruit pectin daily, taken in capsules or as a food additive, can lower cholesterol by about 8 percent. If you go the supplement route, however, you should be aware that this type of fiber interferes with the uptake of certain important nutrients, including beta-carotene, boron, calcium, copper, iron and zinc. This is less of a problem when you consume the whole plant, because the plant itself supplies extra nutrients. But if you take pectin capsules, remember to eat your fruits and vegetables at a later meal to make sure you don't trigger any deficiencies.

☙☙ **Avocado (*Persea americana*).** Avocado is one of the highest-fat fruits, so people with heart disease often avoid it. But according to a report in the *Lawrence Review of Natural Products*, a respected newsletter, avocado can help reduce cholesterol. In one study, women were given a choice of a diet high in monounsaturated fats (olive oil) with avocado or a diet rich in complex carbohydrates (starches and sugars.) After six weeks, those on the olive oil-avocado diet showed an 8.2 percent reduction in cholesterol.

I'm not advocating that you should cut back on complex carbohydrates, which are important to a healthy diet, but I am suggesting that you enjoy an occasional avocado. It contains some unique chemicals that you may not be getting elsewhere.

☙☙ **Beans (*Phaseolus*, various species).** Beans are high in fiber and low in fat—just the ticket for lowering cholesterol. And they contain lecithin, a nutrient that also helps cut cholesterol. One study showed that a cup and a half of dried lentils or kidney beans a day, about the amount in a bowl of bean soup, can lower total cholesterol levels by 19 percent.

☙☙ **Celery (*Apium graveolens*).** In one study, researchers fed laboratory animals a high-fat diet for eight weeks, which raised their cholesterol levels. Then they gave some of them celery juice. The juice significantly lowered total cholesterol and LDL levels in the animals. It isn't clear whether eating celery would help reduce cholesterol levels in humans, but it certainly can't hurt to include more of this delicious vegetable in your diet.

☙☙ **Garlic (*Allium sativum*) and onion (*A. cepa*).** Many studies show that the equivalent of one clove of garlic a day (or half an onion) lowers total cholesterol levels by 10 to 15 percent in most people. In one study, people given 800 milligrams (about one clove) of garlic daily experienced lower cholesterol levels as well as lower blood pressure. Garlic is an approved remedy in Europe for cardiovascular conditions, especially high cholesterol.

In another study, two to three tablespoons of onion oil a day helped to lower cholesterol in about half of people with moderately high cholesterol. Their blood cholesterol levels fell 7 to 33 percent while they were taking the onion oil.

It sounds to me as if it would be a good idea to include generous amounts of both of these tasty herbs in your daily diet.

⭤⭤ **Ginger** (*Zingiber officinale*). Many studies show that ginger helps lower cholesterol. Why not add some ginger to spice up other cholesterol-lowering foods?

⭤•⭢

Dining for Low Cholesterol

There are many, many foods and herbs that lower cholesterol. Why not mix them all to create a tasty, healthy diet that gets those numbers down where you want them to be? Here are some suggestions.

For Breakfast

- Orange, grapefruit, apple and carrot whirred in a blender instead of plain orange juice
- Whole-grain muffins
- Fresh fruit as available
- Oatmeal with a touch of safflower oil (no butter or margarine)

For Lunch

- Cholesterol-cutting soup made with beans, barley, onions, carrots and garlic, plus other spices to taste
- Whole-wheat bread topped with any nut butter—even peanut butter (not butter or margarine)
- High-fiber salad
- Whole-fruit cocktail
- Oatmeal cookie or bran muffin

For Dinner

- Burrito made with refried beans, rice and salsa and wrapped in a whole-grain tortilla

OR

- Vegetarian chili made with tofu; cornmeal muffins slathered with nut butter

OR

- Hot Doggones: Hot dog buns filled with coleslaw, barbecue sauce, mustard and onions (if you just can't do without hot dogs, make them vegetarian); lentil or black bean and wild rice soup

OR

- New England Boiled Dinner: One cup each of diced cabbage, carrots, onions, celery and potatoes, with a dash of herbs

AND

- A big green salad
- Fruit cocktail

After a week or two on a diet like this one, I'll wager there'll be a cholesterol reduction of 10 to 20 percent in most people who have elevated levels.

🦋🦋

🦋 **Fenugreek** (*Trigonella foenum-graecum*). This herb is rich in a soothing fiber called mucilage. Its cholesterol-lowering activity has been demonstrated in laboratory experiments with animals and has also been demonstrated in humans.

🦋 **Nuts.** You might think that people with high cholesterol should avoid high-fat nuts, but a study of more than 25,000 Americans showed that those who eat the most nuts are the least likely to be obese. These subjects were all healthy, so I wouldn't recommend nuts to those with heart disease or high blood pressure. But for reasonably healthy folks, nuts don't seem to do much harm and are better than too much meat.

It's possible that the nuts help produce feelings of satiety. Walnuts, for example, contain the neurotransmitter serotonin, which is involved in the sensation of satiety.

High nut consumption, by the way, was also associated with lower incidence of fatal and nonfatal heart attacks. This should be of interest to anyone who is at risk because of high cholesterol levels.

🦋 **Safflower** (*Carthamus tinctorius*). One study showed that switching from other oils to safflower oil for eight weeks reduced total serum cholesterol levels by 9 to 15 percent and LDL cholesterol by 12 to 20 percent.

❧ Sesame (*Sesamum indicum*). All plants contain phytosterols, compounds that can be absorbed into the bloodstream, nudging out some of the cholesterol that's there. In my database, the food that shows up the highest in phytosterols (based on dry weight) is sesame seeds.

Other foods that contain high amounts of phytosterols, in descending order of potency, include lettuce, sunflower seeds, hazelnuts, cucumbers, asparagus, okra, cauliflower, spinach, figs, onions, strawberries, pumpkin or squash, radishes, apricots, tomatoes, celery and ginger.

You could easily use this information to concoct cholesterol-lowering salads and soups to replace cholesterol-raising meats. A high-phytosterol fruit salad, for example, would include figs, strawberries and apricots with ginger.

❧ Shiitake (*Lentinus edodes*). These delicious mushrooms contain the compound lentinan. According to the *Lawrence Review of Natural Products*, lentinan has cholesterol-lowering action, along with anti-tumor, antiviral and immune-stimulating effects. In experimental animals given a low dose of a compound related to lentinan, cholesterol levels fell 25 percent.

Hives

Many years ago, my son, John, now in his thirties, had a bout of hives. John had been digging in the garden, so his hives could have come from an allergy to one or more of the hundreds of plants in my garden. Or maybe he was allergic to one of the animals that called our place home—cats, chickens, goats, horses and rabbits, not to mention some rather social raccoons, deer, foxes, groundhogs and possums.

Hives bothered John on and off for about a year, then as he grew beyond his teens, his hives disappeared, never to return.

We never figured out what caused John's hives. They were never bad enough for us to consult an expensive allergy specialist, and it was probably just as well. Beyond a few common allergies, it's often very difficult for even the pros to determine what triggers hives.

Whenever the hives put in an appearance, we gave John some diphenhydramine (Benadryl), the synthetic over-the-counter antihistamine, instead of herbal antihistamines. Today I'd go the herbal route, but John had his hives before I became completely converted to natural medicines.

How Hives Happen

Hives are itchy red skin welts with whitish centers. Medically, they're known as urticaria or nettle rash, a name inspired by the fact that the stinging nettle plant can cause them.

Hives are a reaction to histamine, a substance secreted by special cells known as mast cells that are distributed throughout the body. Small amounts of histamine, incidentally, are also injected into you when you bump up against the tiny hairs that cover the stinging nettle plant.

The histamine made by your body plays a role in producing the symptoms of hay fever–type allergies, including sneezing and watery eyes. That's why *anti*histamines, substances that block the natural action of histamines, can help to treat so many allergy symptoms, including hives.

Some 15 to 20 percent of Americans experience hives at some point in their lives, most frequently as young adults.

Just about anything that can cause an allergic reaction can cause hives, including certain foods, aspirin and many other drugs. Sometimes unexpected things cause hives; about 3 percent of people who use sunscreen get hives, for example. But in many cases, the cause of hives remains a mystery.

Green Pharmacy for Hives

Prescription and over-the-counter antihistamines are the standard medical treatment for hives. There are also a number of herbal approaches.

❦❦❦ **Jewelweed (*Impatiens capensis*).** This is one of my favorite herbs for hives. It contains a compound called lawsone that works wonders.

I learned about lawsone's anti-hive action at the 1995 Annual Spring Wildflower Outing in Wintergreen, Virginia. My long-time friend, herbalist Jim Troy, slapped both of my wrists with nettle plant until both stung mightily. I had with me a bottled solution of lawsone which Robert Rosen, Ph.D., a chemist at Rutgers University in New Brunswick, New Jersey, had pro-vided. I rubbed the solution onto my right wrist and enjoyed instant relief. The hives on my left wrist kept right on itching. This mini-experiment convinced me that any plant containing the compound lawsone, such as jewelweed, is worth consider-ing as a treatment for hives.

In fact, several of the participants in that wildflower walk tried crushed jewelweed leaves on their nettle-produced hives with good results. Until something better comes along, I will heartily endorse jewelweed for the wheals induced by stinging nettle, and I'd recommend trying it on hives produced by other causes as well.

I'll never know whether a topical application of jewelweed would have helped my son's hives, but you can bet I'll try it on myself if I ever have the same problem.

If you'd like to try this remedy, you'll have to have access to fresh jewelweed, which is fairly common throughout the coun-try. If you aren't sure what jewelweed looks like, you should find someone in your area who can show you the plant—a local herbalist, perhaps, or an agricultural extension agent.

✴✴✴ **Stinging nettle (*Urtica dioica*).** Yes, I'm talking about the very same plant that will produce a wheal if its hairs inject their histamine into you. Andrew Weil, M.D., an herb advocate who teaches at the University of Arizona College of Medicine in Tucson and author of *Natural Health, Natural Medicine*, sug-gests using freeze-dried nettle leaf extract to treat hives and allergies. This might sound illogical, but the plant apparently doesn't contain enough histamine to be a problem when it's taken orally, and it does contain substances that help heal hives.

Stinging nettle is sold in capsules in health food stores. Dr. Weil suggests taking one or two every two to four hours, as needed.

I have a menacing stand of stinging nettle back behind the barn, so I'd personally opt for consumption of a tea made from the leaves or cooked greens. You'll need to wear gloves when harvesting the greens, but the stinging hairs lose their sting when the plant is cooked, and the greens are delicious. Stinging nettle is a fairly common "weed" throughout the country, so you may have access to the fresh herb.

More recent studies suggest that the root may be even more beneficial than the leaves. Capsules of root material are not yet available, but if you can get the fresh herb, try hanging some roots to dry, then making a tea from some dried, chopped root.

Natural antihistamines. What doctors don't say—because they generally don't know—is that many plants contain antihistamine compounds.

My database is full of these plants: Camomile and wild oregano have at least seven different antihistaminic chemicals, and rue has six. Weighing in with five we have basil, echinacea, fennel, fig, ginkgo, grapefruit, passionflower, tarragon, tea, thyme and yarrow.

Some herbal experts warn that camomile can *cause* histaminic allergic reactions. That may be so in some very sensitive people, but here are the antihistamine compounds in this herb: apigenin, isorhamnetin, kaempferol, luteolin, quercetin, rutin and umbelliferone. This set of compounds is a good reason to give this herb a try. If it doesn't help, or if it seems to make the hives worse, simply discontinue use.

For the greatest variety of antihistamine compounds, my computer suggests making a tea with a combination of several antihistamine herbs, including basil, camomile, fennel, oregano, tarragon and tea. (Just to clear up any possible confusion here, I'm talking about making a brew using the herbal method of preparing tea and including in it a typical beverage tea.)

I suggest pouring a few cups of tea made from this herbal mixture into your bath or dipping a clean cloth into it and applying it as a compress. You can also drink it as a beverage, because the antihistamines will work inside your body as well as on the outside.

If this tea helps, respect it and use it. If it doesn't seem to help, reject it. All of these herbs, however, are generally regarded as safe.

Parsley (*Petroselinum crispum*). One scientific study showed that parsley inhibits the secretion of histamine. If you have hives, try juicing some parsley and adding it to some other vegetable juice, such as carrot or tomato, to make it more palatable.

Amaranth (*Amaranthus*, various species). A tea made

with amaranth seeds makes a good wash for hives, eczema and psoriasis, according to the widely traveled medical anthropologist John Heinerman, Ph.D., author of *Heinerman's Encyclopedia of Fruits, Vegetables and Herbs* and many other books relating to healing with herbs and foods. To make this tea, add two teaspoons of amaranth seeds to three cups of boiling water and let it steep for 10 to 20 minutes. If I were treating my own hives, I'd add some jewelweed, too.

❧ **Ginger (*Zingiber officinale*).** When Canadian herbalist Terry Willard, president of the Canadian Association of Herbal Practitioners and author of *Textbook of Modern Herbology*, developed hives as a result of a food allergy, he simmered a half-pound of ginger in a gallon of water in a big pot for five minutes and added the resulting brew to a hot bath. After steeping himself for a while, he sponged off with camomile tea (one teaspoon in one cup of boiling water). "It worked every time," he says.

❧ **Assorted essential oils.** Aromatherapists suggest using camomile oil to treat hives, and I agree: Place a drop or two directly on your hives and massage it in. Speaking of essential oils, the oils of caraway, clove and lemon balm (also known as melissa) are all antihistaminic, according to pharmacognosist (natural product pharmacist) Albert Leung, Ph.D. Mixing a few drops of each of these oils into a couple of ounces of vegetable oil will result in a soothing ointment that might help relieve itching. Just remember not to ingest essential oils, as even a small amount may be toxic.

❧ **Assorted herbs.** Some herbalists suggest drinking valerian tea for relief of hives that are brought on by anxiety or stress, as valerian is a good natural sedative. Others suggest applying aloe gel to soothe the wheals.

For intensely itchy hives, try a few handfuls of oatmeal in a warm bath. It works surprisingly well.

Cornmint or peppermint, taken as a tea or a wash, might help in treating hives. Menthol, one of the ingredients in mints, has been shown to have itch-relieving action.

HIV Infection (AIDS)

He was a desperate man, dying of AIDS. His body was weak, his money was gone, and a friend had come to see me, asking, "What can we do?"

They had tried every standard medical treatment, but the AIDS patient's T-cell count was still going down. T-cells are part of the immune system. When a person has AIDS, the T-cells are eventually wiped out, leaving the person wide open to opportunistic infections.

I gave him my standard answer: "I am a botanist, not a doctor. I do not prescribe medicine."

"But Jim," the friend begged. "What would you do if you had AIDS? There must be something herbal you'd take."

The Herbal Approach

There were indeed several things, and I shared them with him. If I had AIDS, I said, I would brew a tea containing St.-John's-wort, oregano, self-heal and hyssop and generously sweeten it with licorice. I might still take the proven immune boosters, echinacea and astragalus, even though their use is not so widely recommended anymore. Finally, I'd eat a lot of garlic and onions.

I don't know if the man with AIDS tried any of my suggestions, as I never heard from his friend again. Maybe he and his "friend" were one and the same.

Herbs, of course, can't cure AIDS. Anyone infected with the human immunodeficiency virus (HIV) that causes it should certainly be under a doctor's care. The new combinations of antiviral medications now actually reduce the amount of virus in the body and help prolong life. And several of the opportunistic infections, particularly AIDS-related pneumonia, can be both prevented and treated.

But in addition to treatments prescribed by physicians, I'd

also suggest that people who are HIV-positive try certain immune-stimulating herbs. I believe that they help. You should be aware, however, that some researchers have suggested that boosting the immune system also increases the ferocity of the HIV attack on it. Based on what's now known, however, I don't find that view persuasive yet.

Personally, I would go the nutritional and immune-stimulant route, especially if my T-cell counts seemed to respond well. I would encourage anyone with HIV infection to keep abreast of the latest research and act according to the latest and best findings.

Green Pharmacy for HIV Infection

By all means, discuss with your doctor any herbs that you want to try. Here are several that might prove helpful.

❧ ❧ ❧ **Licorice (*Glycyrrhiza glabra*).** Licorice tea is active against many viruses. The active constituent in licorice (glycyrrhizin) can inhibit a number of processes involved in viral replication, such as a virus's ability to penetrate host cells and change their genetic material.

In studies, there are indications that glycyrrhizin inhibits the growth of HIV in the test tube. A few clinical trials have also produced intriguingly positive results.

In one study of people who were HIV-positive but without AIDS symptoms, Japanese scientists claim that glycyrrhizin delayed the appearance of symptoms related to HIV.

In another report, people with hemophilia who had gotten the HIV infection from blood transfusions were given glycyrrhizin for more than a month. During that time, the amount of virus in their blood decreased considerably, suggesting that the herbal compound might inhibit HIV replication in people.

Finally, glycyrrhizin seems to reduce side effects from AZT.

If I had HIV, I'd add a one-ounce piece of licorice root to a quart of any of my herbal teas, or I'd just chew on the root. Others might prefer taking standardized commercial preparations several times a day.

While licorice and its extracts are safe for normal use in moderate amounts—up to about three cups of tea a day—long-term use or ingestion of larger amounts can produce headache, lethargy, sodium and water retention, excessive loss of potassium and high blood pressure.

❦❀

Gobo Gumbo

All of the ingredients in this pungent vegetable dish contain compounds that help the immune system fight viruses, and researchers have found that burdock has properties that spectically fight HIV. (*Gobo* is Japanese for "burdock.")

    3   cups water
    1   cup fresh burdock stems, chopped
    1   onion, chopped
    5   cloves garlic, minced
    ½   cup fresh okra, diced
        Salt
        Pepper
        Turmeric

In a large saucepan over high heat, bring the water, burdock, onions, garlic and okra to a boil. Reduce the heat, cover and simmer until the vegetables are soft. Season to taste with the salt, pepper and turmeric.

Makes 2 servings

❦❀

❦❦❦ **Oregano** (*Origanum vulgaris*) **and self-heal** (*Prunella vulgaris*). Many AIDS deaths are fundamentally caused by a process known as oxidative stress, according to New York AIDS researcher Howard Greenspan, M.D. This kind of stress is the result of significant damage done to the body's cells by harmful oxygen molecules known as free radicals.

Dr. Greenspan suggests that increasing antioxidant intake can help maintain immune function in those who are HIV-positive. (Antioxidants are substances that mop up free radicals by neutralizing their ability to do damage.) His reasoning is persuasive. If I had HIV, I'd drink plenty of antioxidant teas, particularly those made from self-heal and oregano, the herbs with the most antioxidants among the 60 I've studied. Better yet, sweeten these teas with licorice to improve their flavor and get the additional benefits of glycyrrhizin.

❧❧❧ **St.-John's-wort (*Hypericum perforatum*).** This herb contains hypericin and pseudohypericin, compounds that are antiviral. These compounds have been shown to be active against HIV, at least in the test tube. In fact, a mixture of hypericin and several derivatives has been patented as a treatment for cytomegalovirus infection, one of the many opportunistic infections that can strike people with AIDS.

Researchers apparently still have a lot of work to do before they understand the full therapeutic value of these two compounds in treating HIV. In test-tube and animal studies, pseudohypericin has been shown to reduce the spread of HIV. While a few surveys of people with AIDS have suggested some value for hypericin, the data are iffy, and we'll have to wait and see.

Meanwhile, you can try taking St.-John's-wort. I'd use a tincture made from the whole herb and take 10 to 30 drops in juice several times a day.

St.-John's-wort contains MAO inhibitors. People who are taking MAO inhibitors, or using herbs that contain them, on a regular basis need to avoid certain foods (alcoholic beverages and smoked or pickled foods) and medications such as cold and hay fever remedies, amphetamines, narcotics, tryptophan and tyrosine. You should not take St.-John's-wort if you're pregnant, and you should avoid intense sun exposure while using it, since this herb can make the skin more sensitive to sunlight.

❧❧ **Aloe (*Aloe vera*).** There is some evidence that acemannan, a potent immune-stimulating compound found in aloe, may be beneficial in treating AIDS.

In test-tube studies, acemannan was shown to be active against HIV. Acemannan may also reduce requirements for AZT, thus minimizing the side effects of that potent drug.

The recommended amount of acemannan is up to 250 milligrams four times a day. Much higher doses (up to 1,000 milligrams per kilogram of body weight per day) have caused no toxic effects in dogs and rats. And according to the American Foundation for AIDS Research, "pilot trials have not revealed any toxic effects in man."

It takes about a liter of aloe juice (about a quart) to provide 1,600 milligrams of acemannan. I personally shudder at the thought of drinking almost a liter of aloe juice a day. But if I had HIV, I might feel differently. You can buy the juice at most health food stores, but don't try to prepare your own. The juice can have an overly powerful laxative effect if not prepared properly.

Astragalus (*Astragalus*, various species). Known as *huang qi* in China, this immune-boosting herb is the Asian answer to America's echinacea.

Astragalus has no demonstrated anti-HIV effect that I know of, but it's safe. If I had HIV, I would give it the benefit of the doubt based on its known potent antiviral activity against a wide range of other viruses.

In one study, ten people with serious viral infections showed low levels of natural killer cells (NKCs) in their bodies. NKCs are special white blood cells that attack disease-causing microorganisms. The study participants were given injections of astragalus extracts for four months. Compared with people who did not receive the extract, their NKC activity increased substantially, other components of their immune system perked up, and their symptoms improved. I believe that oral preparations have a similar effect.

Black-eyed Susan (*Rudbeckia*, various species). Based on its folkoric use, I suspected for years that the Maryland state flower, the black-eyed Susan, might be as strong an immune stimulant as the various species of echinacea. My hunch was confirmed by a research report saying that root extracts indeed do a better job of stimulating the immune system than do extracts of echinacea.

If I had AIDS, I'd make a tea with five teaspoons of dried herb per cup of boiling water and drink a cup two or three times a day.

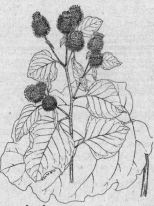

Burdock

Burdock contains compounds that may be active against HIV.

❧❧ **Blessed thistle (*Cnicus benedictus*).** Compounds found in this herb reportedly have anti-HIV activity. I would not hesitate to steep about five teaspoons of this herb in a cup of boiling water and drink it two or three times a day.

❧❧ **Burdock (*Arctium lappa*).** According to the *Lawrence Review of Natural Products*, a respected newsletter, burdock juice or extracts show test-tube activity against HIV. Not too long ago, I enjoyed a dish I called Gobo Gumbo (*gobo* is the Japanese name for burdock). The recipe is on page 325.

❧❧ **Echinacea (*Echinacea*, various species).** Also known as coneflower, this daisylike native of the Great Plains is one of the best immune-stimulant herbs. The active constituents appear to be caffeic acid, chicoric acid and echinacin, all of which have antiviral properties similar to those of interferon, the body's own antiviral compound. Recent evidence shows great promise for chicoric acid as a treatment for this disease.

Echinacea also increases the body's levels of a healing compound known as properdin. Properdin helps infection-fighting white blood cells reach infected areas in the body.

There is some disagreement over which of the three main echinacea species (*E. angustifolia*, *E. pallida* and *E. purpurea*) is best. Herbalist Paul Bergner, editor of *Medical Herbalism*, suggests mixing all three. I agree.

If I had HIV, I would not hesitate to make a tea with five teaspoons of dried herb per cup of boiling water and drink it two or three times a day. But for most people, it's easier to add a dropperful of tincture to juice a few times a day. (Although echinacea can cause your tongue to tingle or go numb temporarily, this effect is harmless.)

Most herbalists advise against taking echinacea daily. They maintain that the immune system eventually becomes accustomed to the herb and that the herb ceases to have a stimulating effect. If I had HIV, I'd probably take echinacea daily for a week or two, then stop taking it for several days, adopting this as an ongoing pattern.

❧❧ **Garlic (*Allium sativum*).** Clinical trials have shown garlic to be effective against several of the opportunistic infections of AIDS, including herpes and pneumocystis pneumonia. Researchers have also found evidence that the compound ajoene, found in garlic, may inhibit the spread of HIV within the body.

Eating three to five cloves of garlic a day is helpful in preventing opportunistic infections, according to herbalist Subhuti Dharmananda, Ph.D., director of the Immune Enhancement Project in Portland, Oregon, and author of *Garlic as the Central Herb Therapy for AIDS*.

✿✿ **Hyssop (*Hyssopus officinalis*).** Hyssop tea contains a compound called MAR-10. Studies have shown that in test tubes, this compound inhibits HIV replication with no toxicity to healthy cells. The researchers who discovered this effect speculate that hyssop might be useful in treating people with HIV.

It's too early to know for sure, but I've found no reports showing that hyssop causes any harm, even in large doses. If I were HIV-positive, I'd mix a few teaspoons of the dried herb into my herb teas.

✿✿ **Onion (*Allium cepa*).** Onion is one of our best sources of the antioxidant compound quercetin, which is most highly concentrated in onion skin. Onion is also a close relative of garlic and has many of the same antiviral effects.

If I had HIV, I would eat lots of onions. And whenever I made soups or stews using onions, I'd leave the skin on to get the full benefit of the quercetin. (You can fish out the skin just prior to serving.)

✿✿ **Pear (*Pyrus communis*).** If I had HIV, I'd eat a pear a day. This fruit is one of the better sources of caffeic and chlorogenic acids. Caffeic acid is an immune stimulant, and researchers have found that chlorogenic acid has activity against HIV. (These compounds can also be found in lesser amounts in apples.)

✿ **Elderberry (*Sambucus nigra*).** Elderberry has an age-old reputation as a remedy for

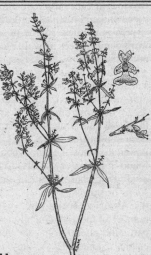

Hyssop

Another member of the extensive mint family, hyssop was commonly used as an air freshener in seventeenth-century Europe.

viral infections, and it is being studied for activity against HIV.
I suspect it has some.

If I had HIV, I'd eat lots of elderberries. Elderberry is a common
shrub in America, and the fruit is sometimes processed into jams
and jellies. Talk about a nice way to take your medicine!

❧ **Evening primrose (*Oenotherâ biennis*).** The oil of this
herb (EPO) is rich in gamma-linolenic acid (GLA). In studies
done by researchers in Tanzania, the life expectancies of people
who were HIV-positive were more than doubled by adding
GLA and beneficial oils known as omega-3 fatty acids to their
diets.

GLA can be obtained from four different food plants:
evening primrose, borage, currant and hops. Most people take
two to four capsules of EPO a day. What do I do? I grind up the
seeds and add them to cornbread or soup.

Fish is the best source of omega-3's, but you can get them
from plant sources as well, including flaxseed, purslane, butternut squash and walnuts. (Vegetarians take note.)

❧ **Iceland moss (*Cetraria islandica*).** University of Illinois
scientists have found that compounds isolated from Iceland
moss inhibit an enzyme that's essential to replication of HIV.
AZT and three other AIDS drugs that have been approved by
the Food and Drug Administration do the same thing, but it's
been shown that these drugs are toxic and do not completely
inhibit the virus. The moss constituents, on the other hand, were
found in laboratory studies to be nontoxic to cells. I feel this is
a safe food pharmaceutical and I would not hesitate to add it to
soups or salads.

❧ **Assorted fruits and vegetables.** In addition to taking a
number of the herbs mentioned in this chaper, I would also pay
particular attention to nutrition and eat lots of fruits and vegetables if I had HIV. A study by researchers at the University of
California at Berkeley showed that if people who are HIV-positive eat more fruits and vegetables, it takes them longer to
develop the opportunistic infections of full-blown AIDS.

❧ **Legume nodules.** If I were taking AZT, I would also consume a few legume nodules, the little "capsules" of bacteria
scattered along the roots of most legumes.

Legume nodules are reportedly the best vegetable source of
a compound called heme iron. Studies show that heme boosts
the anti-HIV activity of AZT. I have never seen legume nodules
for sale, but I grow a lot of beans, and I have uprooted them and

taken the nodules like capsules. There's no pleasure in this, as they don't taste good. But that's Nature's way of discouraging an overdose of these iron-rich nodules. Of course, if your doctor tells you that you have iron overload, you should avoid this therapy.

❧ Vitamins and minerals. Studies suggest that using nutrition to boost the immune system may prolong the lives of people with AIDS as effectively as some of the drugs used to treat it.

Antioxidants are especially recommended, including vitamins C and E, the vitamin A–like nutrients beta-carotene and lycopene and the mineral selenium. Selenium is plentiful in Brazil nuts, and the others can be found in fruits, vegetables, nuts and whole grains. Personally, I prefer foods to supplements, but these nutrients are certainly available in supplements. If I had HIV, I would definitely consult a clinical nutritionist.

Hypothyroidism

Thyroid hormones regulate the metabolism in every cell of your body. For that reason, having too little of the hormones, a condition known as hypothyroidism, can have a profound impact.

Symptoms include lethargy, depression, headaches, low body temperature, unusual sensitivity to cold, decreased libido, difficulty losing weight, dry skin, painful menstrual periods, slow reflexes, goiter and recurrent infections.

Hypothyroidism varies in intensity from very minor and almost unnoticeable symptoms to a severe and life-threatening condition known as myxedema. Many so-called allergic diseases may in fact be due to thyroid disorders.

The thyroid gland is located in the neck just behind and below the Adam's apple. Its hormone production depends on three things: the availability of the mineral iodine, the health of the gland itself and the amount of thyroid-stimulating hormone (TSH) circulating in the body. TSH is released by the pituitary gland, which is located in the center of the brain. Ordinarily, as

TSH levels increase, the levels of thyroid hormones in the body increase accordingly to reach a balance. If the thyroid is not functioning properly, the pituitary releases more TSH in a vain effort to correct the situation.

Thyroid disease affects more than six million Americans. Women are eight times more likely than men to have hypothyroidism, and it is especially prevalent among older women.

If your thyroid gland is not functioning properly, you need to have a doctor diagnose the problem and prescribe appropriate medication.

Green Pharmacy for Hypothyroidism

I do not recommend herbs as the primary treatment for any thyroid condition. Natural approaches, however, can be valuable supplements to medication. In addition to whatever your doctor recommends, you might consider several natural remedies.

My top herbal recommendations are bugleweed, lemon balm (also known as melissa), self-heal and verbena. Amazingly enough, these same herbs also help with Graves' disease, a condition that involves too much thyroid hormone, because they seem to have the ability to normalize thyroid hormone levels regardless of whether there's too much or too little. (For other details about these helpful herbs, see page 275.) Here are some other natural approaches for fighting hypothyroidism.

❧ **Gentian (*Gentiana officinalis*).** Herbal pharmacologist Daniel Mowrey, Ph.D., author of *The Scientific Validation of Herbal Medicine* and *Herbal Tonic Therapies* and an herbalist I respect, says that gentian "provides bitter principles known to normalize the functioning of the thyroid." He suggests gentian as the main ingredient in his own thyroid formula, a combination of gentian, red pepper (cayenne), Irish moss, kelp and saw palmetto. If I had hypothyroidism, I would not hesitate to take this combo.

❧ **Kelp (*Fucus vesiculosis*).** Kelp is high in iodine, a key mineral that the body must have in order to produce thyroid hormones. Urologist James Balch, M.D., and his wife, Phyllis, a certified nutritional consultant, strongly recommend sea kelp for treating hypothyroidism.

Working kelp into your daily diet isn't likely to hurt. You can buy powdered kelp in health food stores to sprinkle over your food as a seasoning. You might also try putting a little kelp in your soups, or go to a Japanese restaurant and order sushi, the veggie or raw fish and rice treat that's wrapped in kelp.

❧ **Mustard (*Brassica nigra, Sinapis alba* and others).** In addition to having a high iodine content, thyroid hormones are made from the compound tyrosine. Mustard greens are the best source of tyrosine I know, with 1.9 percent on a dry-weight basis. Several other foods that include tyrosine, in descending order of potency, are velvet bean seeds, carob, winged beans, bean sprouts, lupines, soybeans, oats, peanuts, spinach, watercress, sesame seeds, butternut squash, chaya, chives, fava beans, lamb's-quarters, pigweed, pumpkin seeds, snowpeas and cabbage.

Along with iodine from kelp, the tyrosine in any of these plants might contribute to increased production of the thyroid hormone thyroxine. I could see making a tasty soup with kelp, mustard greens, spinach, sesame seeds, squash and beans. Or try a salad with mustard greens, spinach, lamb's-quarters, bean sprouts, radishes, pumpkin seeds and sesame seeds.

❧ **Radish (*Raphanus sativus*).** Radishes have long been used in Russia for treating both types of thyroid problems, according to medical anthropologist John Heinerman, Ph.D., author of *Heinerman's Encyclopedia of Fruits, Vegetables and Herbs.* Russian researchers told him that one chemical in radishes, raphanin, helps keep levels of thyroid hormones in balance. With enough raphanin circulating in the blood, the gland is less likely to overproduce or underproduce these hormones.

❧ **St.-John's-wort (*Hypericum perforatum*).** Like many pharmaceutical antidepressants, this herb is a monoamine oxidase (MAO) inhibitor. Depression is a common symptom of hypothyroidism, and MAO inhibitors can help elevate mood. Although this herb addresses a common symptom of hypothyroidism, not the condition itself, it might help if you have depression. (For other helpful herbs for depression, see page 191.)

People who are taking MAO inhibitors or using herbs that contain MAO inhibitors on a regular basis need to avoid certain foods—alcoholic beverages and smoked or pickled foods—and some medications, including cold and hay fever remedies, amphetamines, narcotics, tryptophan and tyrosine. Also, pregnant women should not take St.-John's-wort, and everyone should avoid intense sun exposure while using it, since this herb can make the skin more sensitive to sunlight.

🍂 **Walnut (*Juglans*, various species).** In Turkish folk medicine, walnuts are used as remedies for various glandular disorders, including thyroid problems. It looks like there's something to it. In one study, the fresh juice of green walnuts doubled levels of thyroxine. A decoction of green walnuts, made by boiling them for about 20 minutes, boosted thyroxine at least 30 percent.

You might get some benefit from walnuts simply by enjoying them by the handful, and you could also use walnut oil as a flavorful addition to salad dressings. But it's the green husks that are more likely to be effective, even though they are not pleasing to the palate.

Indigestion

Some 30 years ago, my family and I spent a good deal of time in Panama. While they stayed in Panama City, I wandered about in the rain forest, sometimes living off the land.

When I emerged and returned to civilization, the late, great anthropologist Reina Torres de Araus had our family out to her Los Cumbres residence for wonderful dinners. Afterward, she never served coffee, just camomile tea. I confess that back then I didn't appreciate how much sense it made to end a meal with this wonderful beverage.

Now I know better. Camomile is what herbalists call a carminative, that is, a stomach soother, and it's especially good for indigestion. It's also sedative. In Latin America, some people drink camomile tea before bedtime to help them sleep.

Green Pharmacy for Indigestion

There are hundreds of herbs that can help soothe a troubled tummy. Here are several that I recommend.

🍂🍂🍂 **Camomile (*Matricaria recutita*).** Commission E, the German group of scientists that makes recommendations on herbal safety and effectiveness, considers camomile effective for relieving many gastrointestinal complaints, including indigestion. Andrew Weil, M.D., professor at the University of Arizona College of Medicine in Tucson and author of *Natural Health, Natural Medicine*, says that the best home remedies for upset stomach are camomile and peppermint tea. Personally, I prefer peppermint, but both are effective.

While drinking camomile tea is fine, the tincture is probably more effective. Camomile tea has only 10 to 15 percent of the herb's carminative essential oil, while tinctures prepared with 100-proof alcohol have much more.

✺✺✺ Peppermint (*Mentha piperita*). Most herbalists, myself included, have a special regard for peppermint's ability to relieve indigestion. I've needed peppermint more often since 1990, when the Food and Drug Administration (FDA) gave me a bad case of indigestion by ruling that peppermint is ineffective for stomach distress. This does not mean that peppermint is useless. Frankly, it means that the FDA's evaluation was useless.

Commission E endorses peppermint tea for treating indigestion. Given a choice between an FDA pronouncement and a Commission E endorsement, I'd go for the German decision. Those folks did some research and really know what they're about.

Peppermint tea works well, but being a native son of Alabama, I'm also partial to mint juleps, which, it turns out, work even better. Varro Tyler, Ph.D., dean and professor emeritus of pharmacognosy (natural product pharmacy) at Purdue University in West Lafayette, Indiana, notes that most of the carminative oils in peppermint and other mints are relatively insoluble in water. As a result, mint tea doesn't contain much of the plant's stomach-soothing constituents. It does contain enough to make it effective, but a peppermint tincture, which is made with alcohol, contains more. So if for some reason you don't want to drink a julep, you can use a tincture instead. Follow the package directions.

✺✺ Angelica (*Angelica archangelica*). Angelica root is good for treating indigestion, mild stomach cramps and lack of appetite, according to Commission E. The suggested daily dose is a tea made with two to three teaspoons of dried herb per cup of boiling water, or up to one teaspoon of tincture.

✺✺ Ginger (*Zingiber officinale*). Ginger's benefits for motion sickness and nausea have been amply proven, so it

❦❧

DyspepsiKola

If I had frequent bouts of indigestion, I'd mix up some of this tincture, which I guarantee tastes better than Mylanta. I have no recipe, so I just mix my herbs according to what I happen to have on hand. Here are the herbs I include: a dash each of angelica, anise, camomile, coriander, fennel, ginger, rosemary and turmeric with two dashes of any of the mints, especially marjoram and peppermint. It's okay to leave some out and to alter the mixture to suit your personal tastes.

Steep these herbs overnight in the refrigerator in a mixture of alcohol and water (one shot of vodka per cup of spring water). You can drink this as a tea or add some to pineapple juice.

❦❧

should come as no surprise that Commission E approves taking two grams (about a teaspoon) of ginger in tea for indigestion. Ginger contains certain chemicals (gingerols and shogaols) that not only soothe the gut but also aid digestion by increasing the wavelike muscle contractions (peristalsis) that move food through the intestine.

❦❦ **Marjoram (*Origanum onites*).** The British munch on marjoram sandwiches to treat indigestion and use dilute marjoram tea to relieve colic in infants. Marjoram is an aromatic mint, so it has digestion-soothing benefits that are similar to peppermint's.

❦ **Coriander (*Coriandrum sativum*).** No wonder coriander helps soothe indigestion: Its essential oil is carminative, antiseptic, bactericidal, fungicidal and a muscle relaxant. Traditional herbalists valued coriander, especially to counteract the stomach-upsetting properties of laxative herbs such as buckthorn, cascara, rhubarb and senna. In Amazonia, wild coriander (*Eryngium foetidum*), with nearly the same chemistry, is added to the daily bean ration, perhaps to alleviate the flatulence the beans could generate.

❧ **Papaya (*Carica papaya*) and pineapple (*Ananas comosus*).** Both of these fruits contain enzymes (proteolytics) that break down protein. Naturopaths and people who advocate juicing for health, among them medical anthropologist John Heinerman, Ph.D., author of *Heinerman's Encyclopedia of Fruits, Vegetables and Herbs*, maintain that papaya and pineapple juice are good for relieving indigestion. If they're right, you should also get benefits from eating other fruits that contain proteolytic enzymes, such as kiwifruit or some figs, after meals. If I had chronic indigestion, I might have these fruits for dessert more often.

❧ **Red pepper (*Capsicum*, various species).** Americans often believe that hot spices upset the stomach. But much of the rest of the world knows better—that hot spices like red pepper help soothe it. Red pepper also stimulates digestion.

❧ **Rooibos (*Aspalathus linearis*).** South African physicians recommend rooibos (pronounced *roo-ih-bus*) tea as an effective stomach soother that's gentle enough to treat infant colic, according to the late economic botanist Julia Morton, D.Sc. (Dr. Morton, author of some of the best books in the field, including *The Atlas of Medicinal Plants of Middle America*, was killed in a car crash in 1996. It is a great loss for everyone involved in the study of medicinal plants.) Unfortunately, rooibos is available in only a handful of stores in the United States.

❧ **Assorted carminative herbs.** If anything, there are too many herbal carminatives. In my database, I have more than 500 carminative entries, including all of the plants mentioned in this chapter. Most are supported by at least some research. Also included are agrimony, allspice, apples, basil, bay, beebalm, buckwheat, burdock, caraway, cardamom, catnip, celery, chervil, chives, cloves, coriander, cumin, dill, fennel, garlic, horehound, hyssop, lemon balm (also known as melissa), lemongrass, lovage, marjoram, nutmeg, onions, oregano, parsley, parsnips, pennyroyal, rosemary, sage, savory, tarragon, tea, thyme, turmeric, vanilla and yarrow. Feel free to try any of these herbs to relieve indigestion.

❧ **Assorted essential oils.** Aromatherapists often recommend a few whiffs of a number of different carminative oils to settle a troubled tummy, including aniseed, basil, bergamot, camomile, cinnamon, clove, coriander, fennel, garlic, ginger, hyssop, juniper, lavender, lemon, lemongrass, onion, peppermint, rosemary, sage, savory, tarragon and thyme. Do not ingest these oils, though, as some of them can be fatal in even small doses. They are meant to be used externally.

Infertility

In the early 1990s, there was a rash of articles reporting that sperm counts seem to have fallen significantly (about 40 percent) since the 1930s. We began seeing headlines like these:

"From Silent Spring to Barren Spring" (*Business Week*)

"What's Wrong with Our Sperm?" (*Time*)

"Downward Motility: When It Comes to Sperm, You're Half the Man Your Grandfather Was" (*Esquire*)

After these alarming articles appeared, however, some studies reported that all is well and the typical ejaculate still contains 100 million sperm, just as it did 60 years ago. But these studies have to be weighed against others reporting a sperm count closer to 60 million, a substantial decline.

In Search of Sperm

Among other responses to the studies, researchers began asking what could be causing the decline. Some evidence suggests that pesticides and other pollutants are estrogenic, meaning that they have chemical effects that mimic those of the female sex hormone. Expose the male of the species to enough estrogenic chemicals for long enough, and you get a feminization effect, including a lower sperm count.

Here's some of the evidence that feminization is, in fact, taking place: In Lake Opopka, Florida, there was a big spill of an estrogenic pesticide in 1988. Subsequently, male alligators developed abnormally short penises, reproductive impairment and female-like hormone levels.

In the lower Columbia River in the Northwest, juvenile male otters have testicles that are only one-seventh normal weight.

They, too, show evidence of exposure to estrogenic chemicals.

Florida panthers were exposed to the estrogenic pesticide DDT for years, and they ate other animals that were exposed. Panther fat has high levels of DDE, a DDT breakdown product. The panthers also have unusually high levels of abnormal sperm, low sperm counts, undescended testicles and thyroid dysfunction.

A growing number of scientists are calling for controls on all of these estrogen-like chemicals. I think we should listen to them. But guess who disagrees? The chemical industry.

No surprise there. I just hope that we figure out whether this falling sperm count is real, and if it is, what we're going to do about it to keep the human race reproducing.

Infertile Territory

Infertility is now generally defined as an inability to conceive after six months to one year of trying. An estimated 20 percent of couples have trouble conceiving. While it appears that falling sperm counts may be part of the problem, rising maternal age is certainly a factor, and as women are having babies later in life, the risk of infertility rises.

Treating infertility has become a huge medical industry during the past few decades, with doctors doing everything from prescribing fertility drugs to arranging for test-tube babies (in vitro fertilization). These well-publicized procedures can cost up to $10,000 apiece.

While some infertility problems in women can be addressed by having children earlier, men need to try some tactics to raise their sperm counts. The following section highlights primarily the natural alternatives that can be helpful for men.

Green Pharmacy for Infertility

Infertility is a major heartache, and it may require going the high-tech route. But before you try a high-tech solution, you'll want to thoroughly explore possible causes with your doctor to find out whether there are lifestyle or other changes that you can make to improve your chances of conception. And while you're at it, consider some natural alternatives.

🌿🌿 **Cauliflower** *(Brassica oleracea)* **and other foods con-**

taining vitamin B_6. People who advocate micronutrient supplementation often recommend vitamin B_6 for infertility. The best sources of this nutrient, in descending order of potency, are cauliflower, watercress, spinach, garden cress, bananas, okra, onions, broccoli, squash, kale, kohlrabi, brussels sprouts, peas and radishes.

✿✿ Ginger *(Zingiber officinale)*. According to reports of research with animals in Saudi Arabia, ginger significantly increased sperm count and motility. I hesitate to extrapolate one animal study to humans, but ginger is so safe and tasty that if I were troubled by a low sperm count or poor sperm motility, I wouldn't hesitate to reach for ginger tea, ginger ale, gingerbread and dishes spiced with this tangy herb.

✿✿ Ginseng *(Panax ginseng)*. California herbalist Kathi Keville, author of *The Illustrated Herb Encyclopedia* and *Herbs for Health and Healing*, tells two stories of infertile men who started taking ginseng, schisandra and saw palmetto to build up their physical stamina. Some time later, both of their wives became pregnant.

While I wouldn't hang my hat on this anecdote, ginseng has been revered in Asia for centuries as a male potency and longevity tonic. There is some research with animals suggesting that ginseng stimulates sexual activity, and of course, you need that to conceive.

✿✿ Guava *(Psidium*, **various species) and other foods containing vitamin C.** For treatment of male infertility caused by sperm abnormalities or clumping, vitamin C supplementation has been shown to be as effective as several fertility-enhancing drugs. Melvyn Werbach, M.D., assistant clinical professor of psychiatry at the University of California, Los Angeles, School of Medicine and author of *Nutritional Influences on Illness,* suggests taking 1,000 milligrams a day. (Although the Daily Value for vitamin C is only 60 milligrams, taking this much is considered safe.)

Besides guava, other good plant sources of vitamin C include bitter melon, emblic, rosehips, bell pepper, red peppers and watercress.

✿✿ Herbal formulas for men. The Chinese herb cangzhu *(Atractylodes lancea)* dominates two formulas widely prescribed in China for male infertility. One, called *hochu-ekki-to*, contains 4 grams each of cangzhu, astragalus and ginseng; 3 grams of Japanese angelica; 2 grams each of bupleurum root, jujube fruit, citrus unshiu peel (a Japanese citrus fruit); 1.5 grams of Chinese licorice root; 1 gram of black cohosh; and 0.5 gram of ginger. In one study, this formula boosted sperm concentrations and motility considerably after three months.

A similar formula called *ninjin-to* contains three grams each of cangzhu, ginger, ginseng and Chinese licorice.

If you'd like to try either of these formulas, I'd advise against attempting to mix them up yourself. Instead, consult a Chinese herbalist.

�✧ **Herbal formula for women.** For women, Maine herbalist Deb Soule, founder of Avena Botanicals and author of *The Roots of Healing*, offers several fertility formulas. Here's the one she suggests most often: two tablespoons each of chasteberry, Chinese angelica (also called *dang-quai*) and false unicorn root and one to two teaspoons of blessed thistle steeped in a quart of boiling water for 15 minutes. She suggests drinking two to three cups a day four or five days a week.

✧✧ **Jute (*Corchorus olitorius*) and other herbs containing folate.** For years, naturopaths have suggested folic acid, a B vitamin, for women who are infertile. And the Centers for Disease Control and Prevention in Atlanta have been urging pregnant women to get more folic acid because it prevents severe spinal birth defects.

Everybody's been touting folic acid supplements, but I generally recommend getting nutrients from foods whenever possible, and there are a number of foods that provide good amounts of folate, the naturally occurring form of folic acid. According to my trusty database, the food with the greatest amount of folate is edible jute, at 32 parts per million on a dry-weight basis. This is followed by spinach, endive, asparagus, parsley, okra, pigweed and cabbage.

Noting that many of these same plants are well-endowed with zinc, which is critical to male reproductive vitality, I suggest that this same assortment of vegetables might also help the man of the house.

✧✧ **Spinach (*Spinacia oleracea*) and other herbs containing zinc.** Several studies suggest that zinc deficiencies may be tied to male infertility and poor sperm quality. Good sources of zinc include spinach, parsley, collards, brussels sprouts, cucumbers, string beans, endive, cowpeas, prunes and asparagus. Simmer most of these together in a big pot, and you've got the makings of a good soup.

❧❧ **Sunflower (*Helianthus annuus*) and other herbs containing arginine.** Naturopaths often recommend supplementation with the amino acid arginine for men with low sperm counts. They call for getting four grams of arginine a day. That's the amount found in about two ounces of sunflower seeds.

Sunflower seeds are the highest entry for arginine in my database at 8.2 percent on a dry-weight basis. Other herbs rich in this vital nutrient include carob, butternuts, white lupines, peanuts, sesame seeds, soybeans, watercress, fenugreek, mustard, almonds, velvet beans, Brazil nuts, chives, broad beans and lentils.

❧ **Ashwaganda (*Withania somnifera*).** Ayurvedic physicians feel about this herb the way the Chinese do about ginseng, that it's a tonic for the male libido and sexual function, particularly erection problems.

❧ **Bottle gourd (*Lagenaria siceraria*) and other herbs containing choline.** Scientists at the University of North Carolina School of Medicine in Chapel Hill have found that in male rats, a deficiency of dietary choline, one of the B vitamins, is associated with infertility. I hesitate to make too much of a single study done with animals. But reproductive systems in mammals are more similar than different, and getting a little extra choline probably can't hurt.

In my database, fruits of the bottle gourd, a white-flowered vine suggestive of gourds, are highest in choline at 1.6 percent on a dry-weight basis. Other good herbal sources of choline include fenugreek leaves and shepherd's purse. The following run well behind in the amount of choline they contain but are still worth mentioning: ginseng, horehound, cowpeas, English peas, mung beans, sponge gourd, lentils and Chinese angelica.

❧ **Oat (*Avena sativa*).** Oats make horses frisky and have long been considered a male sexual energizer, hence our phrase "sowing his wild oats." Some herbalists suggest that oats boost male human fertility as well. You can get oats cheaply in oatmeal or more expensively in concentrated oat extracts found in many health food stores.

❧ **Raspberry (*Rubus idaeus*).** Raspberry leaf tea is usually recommended to pregnant women to calm uterine irritability. But animal breeders add raspberry leaves to male animal feed to increase their fertility. Keville suggests that infertile men try raspberry leaf tea. There's little or no harm in it, and the tea is quite tasty.

Inflammatory Bowel Disease

She was one of the smallest people on the plane, and clearly the sickest and weakest-looking. She wore the International Expedition badge, which meant that she was going to the Amazonian rain forest with me and several other instructors for one of our workshops. Quite frankly, I feared having someone so pale and frail-looking in the Amazonian heat, and I wondered how she would fare after enduring a cold winter up North.

It was a bad sign when she passed out on the flight from Miami to Iquitos, Peru, collapsing to the floor as she made her way down the aisle to the restroom. It turned out that this woman had Crohn's disease, a severe type of inflammatory bowel disease (IBD), which involves chronic inflammation of the intestines. (Another type of IBD is ulcerative colitis.)

This woman was trying to fit some meaningful experiences into her life. Not knowing what the future might bring, she felt as if this might be her only chance to see the Amazon before her condition made it impossible for her to travel.

She did get to take my workshop, and after we got back to the United States, she called to thank me for some natural healing recommendations for Crohn's disease that I gave her. She said that she felt better. I certainly hope she's better off now than she was on that flight.

Waste Disposal System Problems

Ulcerative colitis and Crohn's disease have similar symptoms, including chronic (possibly bloody) diarrhea, abdominal cramps, fatigue, weight loss and sometimes fever. But they have somewhat different origins. Simply put, colitis is inflammation of the colon, while the inflammation of Crohn's can occur anywhere in the intestinal tract.

Doctors generally treat any kind of serious IBD with corticosteroids, medications that sometimes suppress the inflammation but have side effects that can be hard to live with, including acne, blurred vision and weight gain. Corticosteroids can also cause gastrointestinal symptoms that may be hard to distinguish from those of IBD. You probably won't be surprised to learn that I'm not a big fan of corticosteroids. On the other hand, I haven't run across any sure-fire natural therapy that works, so I'll simply share some alternative approaches that make sense to me.

In the Grip of IBD

Most people with IBD become anxious and depressed over it. That's no surprise: It's an anxiety-provoking, depressing illness. But at the same time, anxiety, depression and other stress may intensify symptoms. I'd recommend getting involved in a stress-management program that appeals to you, such as meditation, biofeedback or yoga or some other form of moderate exercise. My personal stress-management technique is gardening among the herbs at my Herbal Vineyard.

❦

Juicing for Digestive Health

People who advocate juicing for health seem to have juice recipes for just about everything that ails you. Here are a few juicing suggestions that I think may be helpful in treating inflammatory bowel disease (IBD).

Naturopath Michael Murray, N.D., co-author of *The Complete Book of Juicing*, suggests that people with IBD try one or more of his fruit and vegetable drinks a day. These can be made in a blender or juicer. (I prefer to use a blender.)

Murray's Green Drink: Two apples, two kale leaves, a handful of spinach and some parsley and wheatgrass.

Murray's Cleansing Cocktail: One apple, one-half beet with tops, four carrots, two celery stalks and a half-cup of parsley or wheatgrass.

Murray's Enzymes Galore: One banana, one-half mango, two oranges, one-half papaya and a quarter of one fresh pineapple.

I have no problem with Murray's Green Drink and Cleansing Cocktail. I can't swear that they'll relieve IBD, but they're certainly loaded with fluids and vitamins and minerals, which can be depleted if you have chronic diarrhea.

In Enzymes Galore, I have no problem with the banana, mango, papaya and pineapple. All are used extensively in the tropics for digestive troubles. The special protein-digesting enzymes in pineapple and papaya (pancreatin and bromelain) have been shown in clinical studies to have anti-inflammatory action. They also have added value in fighting autoimmune diseases.

The Enzymes Galore ingredients that I'm not so sure about are the oranges. Some alternative medicine practitioners counsel avoiding citrus fruits if you have IBD. You can try Enzymes Galore with and without the oranges and see which works better for you.

ᑫᦞᑲ

Food sensitivities can definitely contribute to intestinal problems. An inability to digest milk and dairy products (lactose intolerance) is widespread, and many people with this problem don't know that they have it. I'd recommend avoiding all dairy foods for several weeks to see if it helps.

Other people have a similar, though rarer, intolerance to gluten, the protein in wheat that makes bread dough spongy. Most other grains, except rice and teff, a grain used in Ethiopia, contain gluten as well. It's not easy to eliminate grains from your diet, but if IBD is making you miserable, I'd say it's worth the adjustment for a few weeks to see if you feel better. Try substituting rice cakes for bread and rice noodles for pasta. Or go Ethiopian and enjoy some of their great teff pancakes, if you can find the grain in a natural food store.

Green Pharmacy for Inflammatory Bowel Disease

If you have IBD, you should be under a doctor's care, but feel free to discuss any of these herbal approaches with him. Here are several that can help relieve symptoms.

✷ Onion (*Allium cepa*). In my database, the top compound with anti-IBD effects is quercetin, and the best source of this compound is onion skins. We don't eat onion skins, but you can put the whole onion, skin and all, into soups and stews while they're cooking. Just remove the parchment-like skin at the last moment before serving.

Naturopaths suggest taking 400 milligrams of quercetin about 20 minutes before each meal. You can buy pure quercetin at many health food stores.

✷ Psyllium (*Plantago ovata*). You may never have heard of psyllium seeds, but I bet you've heard of Metamucil. Metamucil is a commercial fiber product that is basically ground psyllium seeds and husks with some flavoring added. Metamucil works as a laxative because in the intestine, the mucilage in psyllium seeds absorbs water and swells to many times its original size. It adds bulk to stool and helps stimulate the muscle contractions we experience as "the urge."

Psyllium's ability to absorb fluids also makes it useful for treating diarrhea, a common IBD symptom. In addition, as it travels through the digestive tract, the mucilage in psyllium exerts a soothing effect, which may help relieve the cramping of IBD. If you use psyllium, make sure that you also drink plenty of fluids. Also watch how you react to it if you have allergies. If allergic symptoms develop after you take it once, don't use it again.

✷ Tea (*Camellia sinensis*). Commission E, the body of experts that advises the German government about herbs, suggests using astringent herbs containing tannin, such as tea, for relieving gastrointestinal distress. Besides plain beverage tea, several common herbs are rich in tannin, including bayberry, bugleweed, bilberry, black walnut, English walnut, carob and raspberry.

✷ Valerian (*Valeriana officinalis*). An Italian study suggests that valerian is a useful addition to other medicines that relieve spasms in smooth muscles such as the intestine. Valerian also helps relieve stress, which apparently contributes to IBD.

✷ Assorted essential oils. Aromatherapists recommend massage with a few drops of any of the following essential oils diluted in a few tablespoons of vegetable oil: basil, bergamot, camomile, cinnamon, garlic, geranium, hyssop, lavender, lemongrass, rosemary, thyme and ylang-ylang. I can't vouch for them personally, but massage is relaxing, and using essential oils makes it even more relaxing. Relaxation helps relieve the stress of having IBD. I'd try this approach. (Remember, though, that essential oils are for external use only.)

❧ **Assorted herbs.** Herbalists I trust recommend camomile, peppermint and wild yam to help relieve muscle spasms, including those of the intestine.

Noted British herbalist David Hoffmann, author of *The Herbal Handbook*, suggests treating IBD with a combination herbal cocktail of two parts bayberry and one part each of camomile, mugwort, peppermint, valerian and wild yam.

Herbal pharmacologist Daniel Mowrey, Ph.D., author of *The Scientific Validation of Herbal Medicine* and *Herbal Tonic Therapies*, recommends several herbs for treating ulcerative colitis and Crohn's disease, including fenugreek, gentian, ginger, goldenseal, licorice root, myrrh gum and papaya leaf.

Inhibited Sexual Desire in Women

A certain physician, whom I don't care to name, has written a book about a great many herbs that are purported to be aphrodisiacs. This woman is a big fan of damiana, an herb of Mexico and the Southwest that has such a long and persistent folk history of use as a sex stimulant that one Latin name used for it is *Turnera aphrodisiaca*.

Here is some of what she says about it: "Mexican señoritas have long drunk damiana tea a couple of hours before bed to prime themselves for their men. It is also reported to induce erotic dreams when drunk at bedtime."

Love for Sale

This particular doctor is not the only authority to tout damiana for enhancing the sex drive. I've heard sex therapists talk it up as well, saying it is a mild mood enhancer that beckons lovers to the bedroom.

Statements like those should sell a lot of damiana, and that's part of the problem. You see, the doctor in question probably

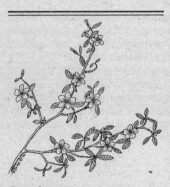

stands to gain from sales of this herb. In nearly every issue of one professional journal, her picture appears along with a picture of a damiana product. The ad says: "In my practice I have found damiana to be one of the most effective aphrodisiacs available to women. I've had great success with damiana in a number of cases. It's safe and effective."

Now, there's nothing inherently wrong with selling a product that you believe in. But when doctors tout controversial aphrodisiacs and also sell them, it makes you wonder.

And damiana is very controversial. Many pharmacognosists (natural product pharmacists), including Varro Tyler, Ph.D., dean and professor emeritus of pharmacognosy at Purdue University in West Lafayette, Indiana, insist that despite its Latin name, damiana's alleged sex-stimulating value is a hoax.

Damiana

This controversial herb from the Southwest has won a reputation as a sex stimulant.

Personally, I'm undecided on damiana. There's no real research to support its aphrodisiac reputation, but not so long ago I spoke with a young woman who mentioned that the herb had been very good for her. Her partner also praised the herb.

I've never come across any reports of damiana toxicity, so if you want to try it, go ahead. The young woman I spoke to was using a tea made with about a tablespoon of dried herb per cup of boiling water. It should be fine at that dose.

When You Lose the Inclination

Anyone, man or woman, can lose interest in sex. In women, the condition used to be called frigidity, but sex therapists have dropped that judgmental term in favor of the more neutral terms *loss of libido* or *inhibited sexual desire*.

Many factors can cause loss of desire, including illness, injury, emotional stress (especially because a relationship is on the rocks), alcohol and many prescription medications, particularly antidepressants. I suggest that before you go to a psychotherapist or write yourself off as asexual, make a list of all the medications that you take, both prescription and over-the-counter. Then take the list to your doctor or pharmacist and ask if any of these medications have side effects that could be affecting your sex life. If so, ask your doctor if you can substitute other medications that might have a less dastardly effect.

Green Pharmacy for Inhibited Sexual Desire

Once you've ruled out common causes of libido loss, then you might try some herbal approaches.

❧❧ **Chinese angelica (*Angelica sinensis*).** The Chinese say that this herb, also known as *dang-quai*, does for women what ginseng does for men—it's an all-purpose sexual and reproductive tonic.

Because of its reputation as a sex enhancer, Chinese angelica is one of the most widely used herbs in Chinese women's medicine. Typically, three to six teaspoons of powdered root are added to a pint of boiling water. Women drink up to three cups of the tea a day. (Do not take this herb if you are pregnant, however.)

❧❧ **Ginseng (*Panax*, various species).** Even though ginseng has long been considered an aphrodisiac for men, I've read reports of women who felt greater sexual responsiveness after consuming it.

Nowadays, several herbalists I know suggest ginseng for loss of sexual desire in women. This herb is very expensive, so few people take very much. The typical dose is a half-teaspoon or so of tincture in juice.

👟👟 **Quebracho (*Aspidosperma quebracho-blanco*).** This herb is one of the more famous aphrodisiacs in South America. It contains yohimbine, the active compound in the herb yohimbe. I've always thought of yohimbe and quebracho as male aphrodisiacs, but Atlanta sex therapist Roger Libby, Ph.D., author of *Sex from Aah to Zipper: A Delightful Glossary of Love, Lust and Laughter*, says he encourages women with low sexual desire to explore both of these herbs.

The biochemical properties of these plant medicines, according to Dr. Libby, contribute to the clitoris becoming engorged with blood, leading to increased sexual desire and more sustained arousal. But don't try this herb if you have high blood pressure, and if you experience any side effects, such as dizziness, don't use it again.

👟👟 **Yohimbe (*Pausinystalia yohimbe*).** If Dr. Libby is right, this herb does more than simply raise erections in men. The Food and Drug Administration has approved pharmaceuticals based on yohimbine for erection enhancement.

If this herb increases blood flow into the penis, and it reportedly does, I could imagine it doing the same for the clitoris.

Taking the herb yohimbe is problematic, as it can cause a number of side effects, including elevated blood pressure. This is one of the few cases in which I recommend taking the compound (yohimbine) that's derived from the herb instead. If you'd like to try yohimbine, you'll have to ask your doctor for a prescription. And you'll have to do a little explaining, because this compound is usually prescribed to men. It might help to take this book with you when you ask.

👟 **Anise (*Pimpinella anisum*).** Anise is high in anethole, a compound with effects similar to those of the female sex hormone estrogen. It has a folk reputation for increasing milk secretion, promoting menstruation, facilitating childbirth and increasing libido in women. Some scientists say that estrogen has nothing to do with sex drive, but I believe that plant estrogens (phytoestrogens) enhance lust for life—and plain old lust as well.

👟 **Chocolate (*Theobroma cacao*).** Chocolate really can boost levels of body chemicals that make you feel good, according to Debra Waterhouse, author of *Why Women Crave Chocolate*. These include the neurotransmitter serotonin and endorphins, which relieve pain and boost mood. The result, she believes, is that "all brain chemicals are positioned at optimal levels for positive moods and renewed energy." *Chemical and Engineering News* notes that "chocolate may mimic marijuana in the brain." I wouldn't push this too far, but there's nothing wrong with a little chocolate before sex. How sweet it is.

✥ **Cola** (*Cola nitida*). Cola is used as an aphrodisiac in Jamaica and traditional West African societies. The herb contains the stimulant compounds theobromine and kolanin as well as caffeine. Coffee—which is, of course, high in caffeine—has been considered a sex stimulant in the Arab world for centuries.

✥ **Epimedium** (*Epimedium*, **various species**). This delicate herb with narrow, heart-shaped leaves improved the sexual function of male animals in many experiments, according to pharmacognosist Albert Leung, Ph.D., and Arkansas herbalist Steven Foster. It has moderate androgen-like effects. Since androgens, which are sex hormones, are involved in sexual desire in both men and women, this herb might stimulate sexual desire in women who are androgen-deficient.

Maybe that's why the Chinese call it yin-yang—because it gives male hormones to women. I'd experiment with making a tea of one to five teaspoons of dried herb and drink no more than one cup a day. Few Americans, including myself, have first-hand experience with this herb, but the leaves are eaten as food in Asia.

Although the herb is imported into this country, it is not yet widely available, so you may have some difficulty locating it. I expect it to become much more popular over the next few years.

✥ **Fennel** (*Foeniculum vulgare*). Fennel increases the libido of both male and female rats, according to the *Lawrence Review of Natural Products*, a respected newsletter. Fennel has compounds that act like the female hormone estrogen and has been used for centuries to promote milk flow in nursing women. You might experiment with it as a libido enhancer. Don't use fennel oil, however. In pregnant women, the oil can cause miscarriage. And in doses greater than about a teaspoon, it can be toxic.

✥ **Fenugreek** (*Trigonella foenum-graecum*). Once fed to harem women to make them more buxom, fenugreek has estrogen-like (estrogenic) activity that may increase breast size and aid in milk production for nursing mothers. Lydia Pinkham's Compound—the nineteenth-century female reproductive tonic—contained fenugreek seeds along with several other herbs and alcohol.

Modern doctors may scoff at Lydia Pinkham's, but they do prescribe estrogen to women who are going through menopause. One of the things estrogen does is help with vaginal dryness, thus making sexual intercourse more comfortable. Let's face it, painful intercourse is bound to inhibit sexual desire. (It looks like Lydia Pinkham's was decades ahead of hormone replacement therapy.)

✷ **Ginger (*Zingiber officinale*).** On a trip to Peru, I found women in the marketplace selling "hot" ginger to warm up "cold" women. I can't make any scientific claims for this one, but ginger probably does no harm, and it's tasty, so you might want to give it a try.

✷ **Parsley (*Petroselinum crispum*).** Like fenugreek, parsley is estrogenic and has a folk history of use in promoting menstruation and milk production, facilitating childbirth and increasing the female libido.

✷ **Saw palmetto (*Serenoa repens*).** Nineteenth-century herbalists recommended saw palmetto to help restore libido in women. Today the herb is used primarily by men to shrink enlarged prostate glands.

Some research demonstrates that the compound beta-sitosterol, which is found in this herb, has aphrodisiac effects, according to the late Julia Morton, D.Sc., economic botanist and author of *The Atlas of Medicinal Plants of Middle America*. You can buy saw palmetto tincture and capsules at herb shops and health food stores.

✷ **Wild yam (*Dioscorea villosa*).** Susun Weed, an herbalist specializing in women's health and author of *Breast Cancer? Breast Health!*, makes salves out of the wild yam and gives them to women experiencing postmenopausal vaginal dryness. She and other herbalists say it helps. Wild yam contains estrogen precursors. You can make a salve by whirring the inner portion of the yam in a blender and adding it to a commercial vaginal lubricant.

✷ **Assorted essential oils.** Aromatherapists recommend whole-body massage with oils of clary, jasmine, rose or ylang-ylang in a vegetable oil base for loss of libido in both men and women. Even without aromatic oils, massage can be sexually stimulating. But I'm prepared to believe that adding an aromatic oil to a stimulating massage can be even more effective. (Remember, though, that essential oils are for external use only.)

Insect Bites and Stings

Say "insect repellent," and the brand names that jump into most people's minds all contain a chemical with a name that's so long, only a chemist could pronounce it. The rest of us call it DEET.

I confess I'm much opposed to DEET. It dissolves my plastic glasses, and once on the skin, it quickly passes through the skin into the bloodstream, where I don't want synthetic chemicals with tongue-twister names.

In some circumstances and in some places, DEET is banned altogether. At the Amazonian Center for Environmental Education and Research camp on the Napo River of Peru where I conduct some of my workshops, for example, they prohibit any use of DEET. This has nothing to do with its effect on people. They've banned the chemical because it speeds the deterioration of the synthetic fibers that hold up the canopy walkway that meanders through the tree branches, sometimes 100 feet above the forest floor.

Green Pharmacy for Repelling Insects

Of course, while I don't care much for DEET, I don't care much for bugs either. I've spent years trying out various herbal insect repellents, and I have reasonably good news to report.

🌿🌿🌿 **Mountain mint (*Pycnanthemum muticum*) and pennyroyal (*Mentha pulegium* or *Hedeoma pulegioides*).** Both of these herbs contain pulegone, a powerful insect repellent. Pennyroyal is the more popular of the two, and it has a long and honorable history. Pliny noticed in the first century A.D. that it was effective against fleas. In fact, this herb's insect-repelling action is incorporated into its scientific name: *Pulegium* means "flea" in Latin. You can find pennyroyal in many commercial herb-based insect repellents.

Based on my experience, however, mountain mint works

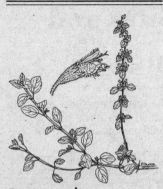

Pennyroyal

Pennyroyal has been called fleabane, tickweed and mosquito plant because of its power to repel insects.

better than pennyroyal. If you have access to fresh mountain mint, just pick some leaves and rub them on your skin and clothing. (But don't use pennyroyal or mountain mint if you're pregnant, as the ingredients in these herbs have been known to increase the risk of miscarriage.)

🌿🌿 **Basil (*Ocimum basilicum*).** Basil is mainly a spice in this country, but elsewhere it is used extensively in medicine, particularly in India. Indians rub the leaves on their skin as an insect repellent, and Africans do the same. If I were bothered by bugs in my garden and some of my culinary basil was close at hand, I might rub some on as an impromptu insect repellent.

🌿🌿 **Citronella (*Cymbopogon*, various species).** A lemon-scented plant from Asia, citronella has long been used as an insect repellent. It's often sold in candles that are burned to drive off mosquitoes. It's also the active ingredient in several non-DEET commercial insect repellents that you can apply to either your skin or your clothing.

As with many essential oils, pure citronella oil can be irritating to the skin (and it should never be ingested). If you want to use the oil, you'll have to dilute it by adding several drops to a vegetable oil base. You can rub the diluted oil directly on your skin.

The knock on citronella is that its protection wears off faster than DEET's. In one experiment, citronella oil repelled the mosquito that carries yellow fever for only a little over an hour, so maybe you should use DEET if you live in an exotic area where yellow fever is still a problem. But for American backyards, citronella works reasonably well.

A while ago, I received a most welcome letter from a high

school student, Rachel Smith. I had sent her some information about essential oils, including citronella, to help her with her science fair project, "Essential Oils as an Alternative Pesticide." She won a prize based on her demonstration that citronella oil, and, to a lesser degree, teatree oil, controlled aphids on her hibiscus plants. I was not surprised.

✢◦✣

Outwitting Bugs

Since I spend a lot of time in the jungle, I've always paid special attention to keeping creepy crawly-critters off me in the first place. Here are a few tips that I've found helpful.

Insect authorities always advise wearing long pants and long-sleeved shirts when you're out and about in bug and tick country. If you want to go that route, fine, but I confess that I do not wear long-limbed clothing. Instead I wear short pants so that I can easily spot any ticks on my legs.

When in bad tick country, I also sprinkle sulfur in my socks, having proved to myself that this works well on the related chiggers that haunted the blackberry patches where I grew up in the Carolinas.

I also learned in Panama to squat on my haunches, Indian-style, rather than sit on some inviting fallen log with its plethora of bugs and other vermin.

✢◦✣

✢◦ **Citrus essential oils.** Something about citrus, and plants with citruslike aromatic qualities, repels insects. The *Citrosa* geranium, for example, which has a strong citrus smell, has 30 to 40 percent of the repellent power of DEET. And crushed lemon thyme (*Thymus citriodora*) has 62 percent of DEET's repellency.

For this reason, it seems to me that any citrus-scented essential oils, including those of citrus leaves themselves, would be better for the user than DEET. After all, our ancestors were exposed to citrus fruits as they evolved. You sure can't say the same thing about DEET.

If you want to try citrus essential oils, you'll have to dilute them first by adding several drops to a vegetable oil base. You can experiment with using a couple of essential oils together. You might be able to customize an insect repellent that will also serve as a scent that is pleasing to you. I mean this for men, too; many men's colognes feature citrus scents.

❧ Lemongrass (*Cymbopogon*, various species). This is a close kin to citronella and has many of the same insect-repellent compounds. If you have access to the fresh herb, simply crush some and rub it directly on your skin.

❧ Assorted essential oils. I should also mention an herbal essential oil combination that I encountered on a 1995 trip to Amazonian Peru. I was amazed at the efficacy of a repellent given to me by North Hollywood herbalist John DuVall. It contained citronella, lavender and pennyroyal in a vegetable oil base, and it was the most effective repellent I've ever witnessed for the bugs down on the Napo River. A drop in the center of a sweaty red hat created a bull's-eye—a bright red, bug-free spot, surrounded by a solid brown horde of sweat bees. The shaman I was working with at the time, Antonio Montero, was more impressed with the aroma, saying that it contained "the spirits of the world."

Unfortunately, I don't have the complete recipe for this repellent, but you could experiment by mixing several drops of each of these oils into a vegetable oil base and see if you find a formula that works for you. Just remember never to ingest essential oils.

Green Pharmacy for Insect Bites and Stings

Doctors generally recommend pain relievers, ice packs and meat tenderizer to treat insect bites and stings. (Applying a dab of commercial meat tenderizer directly to a sting neutralizes venom.) These are all reasonable approaches. There are also a number of good herbal alternatives.

❧❧ Calendula (*Calendula officinalis*). I'm a fan of Maude Grieve, whose *Modern Herbal*, written in 1931, is now a classic in the field. Grieve writes picturesquely that calendula flower "rubbed on the affected part, is an admirable remedy for the pain and swelling caused by the sting of a wasp or bee." I believe her, and I would try it if I were stung and had some fresh calendula close at hand.

✖✖ Garlic (*Allium sativum*) and onion (*A. cepa*) Both garlic and onions contain enzymes that break down chemical substances known as prostaglandins that the body releases in response to pain.

Interestingly enough, garlic and onions work both internally and externally. You can make a poultice of these herbs and apply them directly to insect bites and stings. You can also get a measure of relief by eating foods that contain them.

One further note: Onion skin is an extremely good source of the anti-allergic chemical quercetin, which is especially good for relieving inflammation. You can get the added benefit of quercetin by leaving the skin on when you cook soups or stews. Fish out the skin just before serving; it will have released a good amount of quercetin into the dish, along with a rich, brown color.

✖✖ Plantain (*Plantago*, various species). Wherever I go— from the Appalachians to the Andes to the Rockies—plantain is one of the first herbs my botanical friends mention for bug bite. It's the first thing I apply at home, too, since it is a common weed in my lawn. (You need to rub on the fresh herb for this remedy to work.)

Edward E. Shook, author of *Advanced Treatise on Herbology*, tells a story about a woman who got a bee sting on her hand, and her entire arm began to swell. He told her to wash plantain leaves, make a poultice and apply it to the sting. The next day the woman returned, healed. I didn't see this happen, but I do know that plantain is many herbalists' herb of choice for bee stings.

✖ Assorted herbs. My database also lists a few other folk remedies for insect bites and stings: camomile, flanders poppy, indigo and St.-John's-wort. The typical approach is to rub the fresh herb on the site of the bite or sting. None of these would be my first choices, but if I were caught without the herbs discussed above, I'd try any one of these.

Insomnia

We live in a country that has a hard time getting enough sleep. About a third of Americans experience insomnia regularly, and up to ten million rely on sedative prescriptions to help them fall asleep. That's a whole lot of sleeping pills.

Insomnia is a broad term that encompasses any and all difficulties with sleep, including the inability to fall asleep or to stay asleep.

Green Pharmacy for Insomnia

Pharmaceutical sedatives work, but they can become addictive, and they interfere with natural sleep cycles. You won't be surprised to learn that I prefer natural alternatives, of which there are several.

Lemon balm (*Melissa officinalis*). Also known as melissa, lemon balm is endorsed as both a sedative and stomach soother by Commission E, the body of scientists that advises the German government about herb safety and effectiveness. The sedative action is attributed largely to a group of chemicals in the plant called terpenes. Several other herbs—juniper, ginger, basil and clove—are better endowed with some of these chemicals, but none of them has the combination that lemon balm contains, and none of them has its reputation as a bedtime herb.

I suggest trying a tea made with two to four teaspoons of dried herb per cup of boiling water.

Valerian (*Valeriana officinalis*). Drinking a tea made with one to two teaspoons of dried valerian root shortly before bedtime will promote sleepiness, according to Commission E. In fact, the commission considers the tea so safe that it also endorses drinking it up to several times a day to relieve restlessness, anxiety and nervousness.

Valerian has a fairly rank aroma and taste. If its earthiness is not to your liking, you can always opt for a tincture or capsules instead.

In the United Kingdom, there are more than 80 over-the-counter sleep aids containing valerian. Why? Because it works. In one study, a combination of 160 milligrams of valerian and

80 milligrams of lemon balm extracts brought on sleep as well as a standard dose of one of the drugs in the Valium family of pharmaceuticals (benzodiazepines).

I should mention here that Valium is not derived from the herb valerian. There's a common misconception that the two are related, probably because they both begin with a *V*.

Unlike prescription sleep or anxiety medications, valerian is not considered habit-forming, nor does it produce a "hangover," as do medications in the Valium group.

Some naturopaths I respect suggest that you treat insomnia by drinking valerian root tea about 30 minutes before retiring. Others suggest taking 150 to 300 milligrams of a standardized extract (0.8 percent valeric acid). Personally, I don't think it matters.

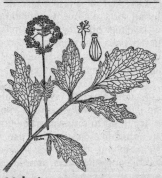

Valerian

The root of this herb has long been used as a sedative, and it's the active ingredient in more than 100 over-the-counter tranquilizers and sleep aids.

Valerian presents another opportunity for me to reiterate my belief that the whole herbal extracts used in natural medicines often make more sense than the "magic bullet" herbal derivatives that the drug industry favors. For years scientists believed that only two constituents in valerian, valepotriates and bornyl esters, produced its sedative effect. But one more recent Italian study notes that other chemicals in this herb, valeranone and kessyl esters, also contribute to its sleep-inducing effectiveness. The researchers concluded that the sedative effect of valerian comes from the actions of its many different constituents working in harmony with each other.

🌸🌸 **Lavender (*Lavandula*, various species).** It's nice to see lavender approved by Commission E for insomnia. I've seen accounts of British hospitals using lavender oil to help patients sleep at night. The hospitals administer the oil either in a warm bath or sprinkled onto bedclothes.

Lavender oil is also a favorite of aromatherapists, who use it for all sorts of ailments, including insomnia. Some components of lavender oil affect cell membranes, interrupting the interaction of cells with each other. Because the oil helps to slow nerve impulses, it can help reduce irritability and bring on sleep. It also has an anesthetic effect.

But beware: Not all lavender is tranquilizing. Some species, especially Spanish lavender, might have a stimulating action similar to rosemary's. When you buy lavender oil, be prepared to try it out to discover whether it's soothing. If you buy from an aromatherapist, specify that you're looking for an oil that can help you sleep. If you inadvertently buy a lavender oil that has the opposite effect, simply save it for other uses (you'll find many in this book). But remember that essential oils are intended for external use only.

🐟🐟 **Passionflower (*Passiflora incarnata*).** This is a mild sedative, according to Commission E. Respected herbalists around the world agree, among them Steven Foster, a distinguished Arkansas herbalist and photographer and co-author of *The Encyclopedia of Common Natural Ingredients*.

🐟🐟

Opium: History's Favorite Sleep Inducer

Do you have any pretty poppies growing in your backyard garden? If they're large red, purple or white annuals, it's just possible that you're harboring illegal plants. Because poppy plants are the source of both opium and heroin, the U.S. Drug Enforcement Agency has made it illegal to grow them.

If you're among the "guilty," however, you certainly have a lot of company. These poppies are grown as ornamentals throughout the nation. And opium poppies are so good at seeding themselves that they're hard to get rid of. (I've even seen them growing illegally in many state-run botanical gardens.)

If you do have an illegal poppy or two among your

petunias, you should also know that you're growing one of the world's oldest medicines. The sleep-inducing, pain-relieving powers of opium have been recognized for thousands of years. According to a manuscript sent to me by the famous Hungarian scientist Peter Tetenyi, people along the Rhine had fields of opium poppies as long ago as early Neolithic times, around 5000 B.C. Although the seeds were first used as food, the sedative effects of the pod and latex were recognized quite early.

By the middle of the second millennium B.C., the ancient Greeks used opium extensively as medicine. And by about 1000 B.C., the beautiful opium poppy was being used as an ornamental flower from Europe all the way to China.

I certainly don't recommend taking any of the narcotics derived from the opium poppy, except when they are prescribed by a doctor. But you might as well be aware that doctors still do make considerable use of drugs derived from this plant, including codeine and morphine. And just in case you're curious, the opium used for legal prescription drugs comes from poppy fields in Holland and Australia.

❧

In the United Kingdom, about 40 over-the-counter sedative preparations contain passionflower. But wouldn't you know that the Food and Drug Administration (FDA) banned the use of passionflower in over-the-counter sedatives because it has not been proven safe and effective? The problem here is not with the herb itself. The problem is with the FDA's unrealistic and exorbitantly expensive standard of proof.

Because of this, you may not be able to buy the kind of safe, gentle sleep-inducing preparations containing passionflower that are widely available in Britain or Germany. But you can buy the herb itself, as well as herbal tinctures, and these should be safe to use. Fresh or dried passionflower has been used successfully for centuries to treat nervous tension, anxiety and insomnia.

❧ **Camomile (*Matricaria recutita*).** Camomile tea has been used as a bedtime beverage for centuries. Although its reputed sedative effect was not scientifically proven until this decade, the folklore was right. Apigenin has proven to be one of the effective sedative compounds in camomile. I'd probably try it at bedtime, if I didn't have my valerian and lavender handy. It is a pleasant-tasting tea that you'll probably enjoy.

❧ **Catnip (*Nepeta cataria*).** The plant that intoxicates most cats also has mild tranquilizing-hypnotic-sedative effects on many people. Catnip contains chemicals (nepetalactone isomers) similar to the sedative constituents of valerian. And being a member of the mint family, catnip tastes much better than valerian. You can try a cup of tea about 45 minutes before bedtime.

❧ **Hops (*Humulus lupulus*).** Hops has been used to treat anxiety, insomnia and restlessness for more than 1,000 years, ever since the plant became a popular ingredient in beer. Hops' sedative ingredient is apparently the compound methyl-butenol, which has a sedating effect on the central nervous system. Smoking hops is said to have a sedative effect, and while I wouldn't recommend smoking it, it does make a pleasantly bitter-tasting tea.

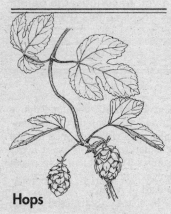

Hops

Hops comes from the female flowers of a grape-like, perennial vine.

❧ **Rooibos (*Aspalathus linearis*).** Although not usually grown in the United States, this shrubby African legume is available in selected herb stores. Tea made with this herb is a bedtime favorite among South African herbalists, consumers and even physicians. South Africans also use it to improve appetite, calm the digestive tract and reduce nervous tension. They regard it as safe enough to give infants.

❧ **Herbal formulas.** In searching my database for plants that are rich in sedative compounds, I turned up several surprises. Many plants

INTERMITTENT CLAUDICATION 363

that are rich in sleep-inducing chemicals have little or no folk-loric reputation as sleep aids. Among them are ginger, with 11 different sedative compounds; basil, thyme, tangerines and tomatoes with 9; cinnamon, spearmint, red pepper, pennyroyal and oranges, 8; and peppermint, 7. I can't prove that a tomato salad with basil and thyme or a cup of spearmint tea with ginger and cinnamon will bring on the Sandman, but if you have sleep problems, it might help to eat these foods and herbs more frequently.

In addition, California herbalist Christopher Hobbs, a fourth-generation botanist and author of about a dozen books I often refer to, suggests a number of combinations that can treat sleep-lessness and its close relatives, anxiety and stress. For insomnia Hobbs suggests treatment with passionflower, valerian and California poppy. To banish the anxiety that may cause insomnia, he recommends a combination of California poppy, hawthorn and hops. And to help cope with stressful situations that could contribute to insomnia, Hobbs recommends two parts each of camomile, lavender, lemon balm and linden with one part orange peel.

Intermittent Claudication

Having passed by the mature age of 67, I know I have to be careful about the many manifestations of cardiovascular disease. I like to keep active, so the last thing I want is chest pain or leg pain slowing me down.

When cholesterol-laden plaques substantially narrow the coronary arteries, the result is angina—chest pain brought on by exertion. When the same process occurs in the arteries of the legs, the result is intermittent claudication, which causes leg pain when you exercise. The pain tends to show up after you've walked a short distance.

Intermittent claudication is the most common symptom of what's known as peripheral vascular disease. The pain results from poor oxygenation of the leg muscles because of reduced blood flow in the narrowed leg arteries.

Among cardiovascular diseases, the ones we hear most about are heart attack, stroke, angina and congestive heart failure. Intermittent claudication doesn't get much press, but it's a leading cause of pain and loss of mobility in the elderly. About 750,000 Americans develop it annually.

Green Pharmacy for Intermittent Claudication

If you have intermittent claudication, you should be under the care of a doctor, who will usually prescribe medications to deal with the condition. I'm convinced that many people could get off the pharmaceuticals and feel better if they knew about herbal alternatives. You should discuss this possibility with your doctor, but do not stop taking your medications on your own. Here are the herbs that can help.

✺✺✺ Garlic (*Allium sativum*). In one rigorous 12-week study, a large number of people with intermittent claudication were given 800 milligrams of garlic a day. On average, they walked noticeably better by their fifth week of taking the herb. They also had lower blood pressure and cholesterol levels.

Garlic is a terrific herb for treating any cardiovascular symptom. For intermittent claudication prevention or therapy, eat at least one raw clove a day. There are all kinds of yummy ways to enjoy raw garlic. I suggest chopping a clove and tossing it into a salad or sprinkling it over a pasta dish.

✺✺✺ Ginkgo (*Ginkgo biloba*). Ginkgo is the premier plant medicine for intermittent claudication. It improves blood flow through the legs just as it does through the heart and brain by opening (dilating) the arteries.

Nine excellent studies that I've reviewed show that 40 milligrams of ginkgo extract twice a day provide better relief than pentoxyfilline (Trental), the standard medicine prescribed for intermittent claudication. People suffering from intermittent claudication found that they could go 75 to 110 percent farther without pain if they took the herbal extract. People using Trental, on the other hand, increased their pain-free walking distance by only 65 percent.

Not only that, but ginkgo is cheaper—about $20 a month compared to more than $50 for Trental. And ginkgo side effects are minimal, consisting of occasional abdominal distress, headache or dizziness.

If you're going to use ginkgo, you need to use extracts rather than taking the leaf itself. The active compounds in ginkgo are present in very low concentrations in the leaf, too low to be of any significant benefit. When you get a standard ginkgo extract, it's a 50:1 preparation, meaning that 50 pounds of leaves are processed to get 1 pound of extract. You can purchase standardized extracts at many health food stores and pharmacies.

❧❧ **Ginger (*Zingiber officinale*).** In various studies, ginger has been shown to be almost as effective, or as effective, as aspirin and garlic in preventing the blood clots that trigger heart attack. Similar clotting in the leg can trigger intermittent claudication pain. If I had this condition, I'd eat a lot of ginger.

❧❧ **Hawthorn (*Crataegus*, various species).** In studies, people with intermittent claudication showed better blood flow and walking performance after being injected with hawthorn extract. Personally, I don't think you have to inject it to get the benefit.

Naturopaths recommend taking 120 to 240 milligrams of a standardized extract containing 1.8 percent vitexin-4-rhamnoside or 10 percent oligomeric procyanidins three times a day.

Hawthorn is a powerful heart medicine. If you want to use this herb, please discuss it with your doctor.

❧❧ **Purslane (*Portulaca oleracea*).** Saturated fat is a major culprit in causing any form of cardiovascular disease, including intermittent claudication. The beneficial oils known as omega-3 fatty acids help prevent cardiovascular disease, and purslane is our best leafy source of omega-3's. It's also extremely well endowed with antioxidants, substances that mop up free radicals, highly reactive oxygen molecules that damage the body's cells and contribute to heart disease.

Purslane is a delicious vegetable. I steam the leaves and eat them like spinach or add them raw to salads and soups.

Intestinal Parasites

Friends, relatives and strangers often approach me for advice about healing with herbs. One of my most interesting inquiries a few years ago came from a holistically inclined friend who had amebiasis, often known as amebic dysentery.

She'd initially been misdiagnosed, and by the time her doctor figured out what she really had, she was in a bad way, with diarrhea, flatulence and severe abdominal distress. Her doctor prescribed the standard drug, metronidazole (Flagyl), but like many people, she was concerned about its potential side effects. Her question to me was, What did I think about her trying the Chinese herb *qing hao?*

I replied that qing hao, which we Americans call sweet Annie, was being prescribed for amebiasis by three physicians I knew in New York City, with good results. I knew this because some of their patients had come to me seeking a free source of this herb. One young lady who had a bad case of intestinal parasites (giardia) had apparently achieved relief for the first time in over two years by using qing hao in combination with another Chinese herbal ingredient, gossypol.

Amoebas among Us

Worldwide, an estimated 500 million people are infected with intestinal parasites, and these microorganisms contribute to thousands of deaths each year. Amebiasis and giardiasis, both of which are caused by tiny parasites known as amoebas, are increasingly common in the United States.

Many travelers bring them home from abroad, but you don't have to leave our shores to come down with a case. Giardia has become endemic in North American wildlife. Twenty years ago, it was safe to drink from wilderness streams in the West without boiling the water, but no longer. Giardia-contaminated wildlife wastes have introduced the parasite into just about every once-pristine waterway.

Metronidazole is the medical drug of choice for getting rid of intestinal parasites. While it is effective and generally safe, the woman who didn't want to take it was right to be cautious. It can cause severe side effects, including abdominal distress, nausea and vomiting (especially if you drink alcohol while taking it). More serious side effects are also possible, notably seizures and nerve damage to the extremities, a condition known as peripheral neuropathy.

Green Pharmacy for Intestinal Parasites

I wouldn't criticize anyone for taking metronidazole. After all, if you have intestinal parasites, you want them *gone*. But if you'd rather not take this drug, it's nice to know that there are a number of herbal alternatives.

Some of the herbs mentioned in this chapter can produce side effects such as nausea when taken in doses high enough to dislodge and kill parasites. On the other hand, some of these parasites can be life-threatening if you don't take aggressive action. So, whatever you do, be sure to work with your doctor, even if you're taking the herbal approach. Here are the herbs that might help.

✿✿✿ **Cinchona (*Cinchona*, various species).** Cinchona bark is the herbal source of the antimalarial drug quinine. Amoebas are close kin to the microbes that cause malaria, and the same kinds of compounds seem to work on both.

There are more than 20 active compounds in cinchona besides quinine and quinidine. Many of these will also work against amoebas. Cinchona bark is available from some herbalists and can be made into a tea, which, I should warn you, tastes quite bitter. But if you want to try it, steep about a half-teaspoon of powdered bark in a cup of boiling water for ten minutes. I'd suggest drinking two or three cups a day.

✿✿✿ **Goldenseal (*Hydrastis canadensis*).** The compound berberine, a proven amebicide, occurs in five herbs that have yellow roots, most notably goldenseal but also goldthread, barberry, Oregon grape and yellowroot. But you have to be careful with it. The LD50 (the technical term for the dose that kills half of those who take it) is only about ten times higher than the therapeutic dose for getting rid of intestinal parasites. The lesson? Don't go overboard with goldenseal.

If you'd like to try this herb, please discuss it with your doctor. The recommended dose for killing parasites is $\frac{1}{3}$ to $\frac{1}{2}$

ounce of dried herb divided into three parts and taken over the period of one day, in tea or capsules.

Another word of warning: Because this much goldenseal might cause miscarriage, don't use this treatment if you're pregnant.

Having said all this, I should add that I don't know of anyone who has ever suffered serious side effects from this herb, and the research is clear that many have benefited.

One study compared pure berberine compound with metronidazole. Of 40 children with giardia, 48 percent of those treated with berberine stopped experiencing symptoms, while only 33 percent of those treated with metronidazole felt similar relief.

Some pharmacognosists (natural product pharmacists) come out in favor of taking berberine sulfate but advise against taking goldenseal and other herbs containing this compound. If I had intestinal parasites, I'd still try the herbal approach. I think it works.

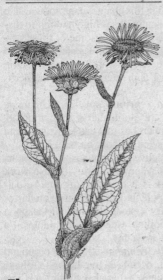

Elecampane

Elecampane, also known as wild sunflower, was used as a veterinary as well as a human medicine in the Middle Ages.

🍂🍂🍂 **Ipecac (*Cephaelis ipecacuanha*).** Here in the United States, we think of ipecac as an emergency treatment to induce vomiting when a child ingests a poison. But this herbal root has another major role in the tropics, where it comes from: It kills amoebas. It contains at least three amebicidal compounds, cephaeline, dehydroemetine and emetine.

Germany's Commission E, the expert panel that judges the safety and effectiveness of herbal medicines for the German government, recommends taking 30 drops of an ipecac tincture (part ipecac and part alcohol). This is a one-time only treatment.

❦❦ **Elecampane (*Inula helenium*).** This common North American herb contains two anti-amebic compounds, alantolactone and isoalantolactone. If I had intestinal amoebas, I'd certainly give elecampane a try, since it appears to be safe. Typically, herbalists recommend bringing a cup of water to a boil, then dropping in one teaspoon of herb and simmering for 20 minutes. You can drink up to three cups a day.

❦❦ **Papaya (*Carica papaya*).** This fruit contains both antiseptic and antiparasitic compounds, including one called carpaine. I have chewed the piquant seeds on occasion, and if I had amebiasis, I would not hesitate to add a few crushed seeds to any fruit juice. The active ingredients give a pungent bite to the seeds.

❦❦ **Sweet Annie (*Artemisia annua*).** As far as I know, neither sweet Annie nor its active ingredient artemisinin has been approved as safe and effective for treating intestinal parasites. Nonetheless, both the herb and the pure active ingredient are being used successfully for just this purpose.

Sweet Annie has been proven by research in China and at the Walter Reed Army Research Institute in Washington, D.C., for fighting the malarial organism that is kin to the amoeba, so there is some rationale for using this herb to treat amebiasis.

It's hard to get a handle on the safe and effective dose of this herb, as the doctors, vendors and consumers I've spoken to all suggest different amounts. For that reason, this would not be among my top choices of herbs for treating amoebas. Because of its reputation, though, I would certainly try this herb judiciously if I had any of the amebic ailments and did not have an effective doctor and/or drug at hand. I suggest making a tea using two to five teaspoons of the herb and drinking one to three cups a day.

❦ **Cubeb (*Piper cubeba*).** Cubeb is a spice that is related to but not as well-known as black pepper. My good friends, pharmacognosist Albert Leung, Ph.D., and Arkansas herbalist Steven Foster, have teamed up on an update of Dr. Leung's *The Encyclopedia of Common Natural Ingredients*. In this update they cite studies showing that ground cubeb is very effective in treating amebic dysentery. Cubeb has long been important in the traditional Ayurvedic medicine of India, and it looks to me as if its popularity in the United States is due to rise. You can use the powder like pepper in cooking.

Laryngitis

It was my 32nd wedding anniversary, and my bluegrass band, Durham Station, was getting together for a cookout dinner and evening picking party. I had promised to tape a couple of herbal songs for radio people who needed something unique to use as background music. (The songs I've written about herbs most definitely qualify as unique.)

At noon I called our banjo picker, who is also our high tenor singer, to remind him to bring his recording equipment. "Don't expect me to sing," he whispered. He'd sung his heart out the night before and awakened that morning with chest congestion and laryngitis.

Talk about dire emergencies! I fixed him my best herbal remedy, something I call Cineolade, a pineapple-ginger juice in which I steep herbs high in the chemical cineole, which is reportedly useful in relieving laryngitis. As I recall, I used rosemary, spearmint, cardamom and lavender and sweetened the drink with licorice.

Well, the banjo picker drank the brew, and he sang reasonably well. No one who heard him talk before he drank the tea could quite believe how good he sounded when he got around to singing. Our recordings turned out okay, too.

Green Pharmacy for Laryngitis

Laryngitis is an inflammation of the vocal cords that causes hoarseness or voice loss and usually a dry, sore throat. More and more these days at pharmacies and health food stores, you can find herbal lozenges for sore throat and laryngitis. They taste pretty good. If you have chronic laryngitis, though, see your doctor: It may be a symptom of a serious condition. But for an occasional bout of laryngitis, you can turn to the Green Pharmacy for help. Here are several good herbs to try.

✿✿✿ Cardamom (*Elettaria cardamomum*) and other herbs containing cineole. The cineole contained in the Cineolade I gave to my banjo-picking buddy is an expectorant that can help bring relief.

Here are several herbs with high cineole content, in descending order of potency: cardamom, eucalyptus, spearmint, rosemary, sweet Annie, ginger, nutmeg, lavender, bee balm, peppermint and tansy. I suggest making a tea using a selection of these herbs, and go heavy on the ginger. Add some pineapple juice before drinking.

❦❦ Ginger (*Zingiber officinale*). After reading New England herbalist Paul Schulick's nice book, *Ginger: Common Spice and Wonder Drug*, I feel pretty confident in recommending this herb. I'm more a tea man than a candy man, but if I had laryngitis, I might try candied ginger.

❦ ❦ Horehound (*Marrubium vulgare*). This herb has been used for centuries to treat coughs and other respiratory problems like laryngitis. Commission E, the body of experts that advises the German government about herbs, endorses horehound for bronchial problems, including laryngitis. The suggested dosage is a tea made with one to two teaspoons of dried herb per cup of boiling water.

But wouldn't you know that the Food and Drug Administration declared horehound ineffective in treating sore throat and laryngitis? The problem is not with horehound but rather with the agency charged with protecting and promoting the public health. Horehound is one of the first herbs I suggest for throat problems. I'd recommend a strong horehound tea with lemon, licorice and stevia, which is available in many health food stores. You

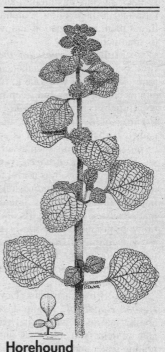

Horehound

Horehound tea, made from dried leaves and flower tops, is a popular folk remedy for coughs and colds.

can open a tea bag and add a pinch of herb in place of artificial sweetener.

❧❧ **Mallows** (*Althaea*, **various species**). The mallows, including marsh mallow, the herbal forerunner of our pillowy candy treat, have been used for thousands of years as throat soothers. They are useful in treating laryngitis, colds, coughs, sore throat and bronchitis.

Mallows contain a special gelatinous fiber, mucilage, that soothes mucous membranes and helps protect them from bacteria and inflammation. Commission E approves mallows for throat pain, inflammation and irritation. Sounds like a laryngitis treatment to me.

❧❧ **Mullein** (*Verbascum thapsus*). Like mallow, mullein flowers have constituents that can help relieve laryngitis symptoms. Make a tea with one to two teaspoons of dried herb per cup of boiling water and steep for ten minutes.

❧ **Couchgrass** (*Agropyron repens* **or** *Elymus repens*). Because of its other name, quackgrass, this is my favorite-named herbal medicine. It is approved by Commission E for respiratory problems such as laryngitis and cough.

❧ **Echinacea** (*Echinacea*, **various species**). Echinacea, also known as coneflower, is useful for relieving or treating laryngitis, according to Commission E. Echinacea also enhances immune function, which should help the body fight any virus that's causing the laryngitis. (While it may make your tongue tingle or go numb temporarily, this effect is harmless.)

❧ **Elecampane** (*Inula helenium*). Elecampane is an antiseptic expectorant that is useful in treating laryngitis. This herb's benefits have been confirmed clinically and experimentally to my satisfaction.

Noted British herbalist David Hoffmann, author of *The Herbal Handbook*, whom I respect, suggests a three-herb combo tea made with equal parts of elecampane, horehound and mullein. You might try one teaspoon of each per cup of boiling water and steep for ten minutes. Other elecampane fans suggest pouring one cup of cold water over one teaspoon of shredded elecampane and steeping it for ten hours. You can drink the tea three times daily.

❧ **Ivy** (*Hedera helix*). Ivy is an old folk remedy for whooping cough. Commission E suggests taking a pinch of dried ivy (0.3 gram) to relieve inflammatory conditions of the respiratory tract, including laryngitis. Ivy has expectorant action, and it helps minimize bronchial secretions that can cause cough and throat irritation.

❧ **Knotgrass (*Polygonum aviculare*).** Commission E approves making a tea with two to three teaspoons of dried knotgrass per cup of boiling water to treat sore throat and laryngitis.

❧ **Plantain (*Plantago*, various species).** Herbalists have used plantain for centuries to treat sore throat, laryngitis, cough and bronchitis. Commission E concurs, noting that English plantain (*P. lanceolata*) in particular is a safe, effective antibacterial, astringent throat soother. The suggested dosage is one teaspoon per cup of boiling water. Steep until cool.

❧ **Primrose (*Primula veris*).** Commission E suggests using one to two teaspoons of dried primrose flowers or one teaspoon of the plant's dried root as a respiratory remedy for laryngitis, bronchitis, colds and coughs. (Note that this recommendation is for primrose, not evening primrose.)

❧ **Soapwort (*Saponaria officinalis*).** Chemicals (saponins) in soapwort reportedly have pain-relieving, anti-inflammatory activity that may help laryngitis. Commission E recommends making a tea with one teaspoon of dried herb per cup of boiling water for treating respiratory complaints, including laryngitis.

❧ **Stinging nettle (*Urtica dioica*).** In recent years, stinging nettle leaves and root juice have received considerable attention because of studies suggesting their usefulness in treating asthma, bronchitis and hay fever. I'd also try stinging nettle tea for laryngitis.

❧ **Sundew (*Drosera*, various species).** If your laryngitis is due to a hacking cough, sundew is worth trying. It contains a cough suppressant compound (carboxy-oxy-napthoquinone), which is comparable to codeine, and other constituents that calm the muscle spasms that can trigger coughing. German studies of sundew as a treatment for laryngitis, sore throat and bronchitis show good results in more than 90 percent of users, with no significant side effects.

One of the compounds in sundew, plumbagin, inhibits several types of bacteria that cause laryngitis.

❧ **Hot, spicy foods.** If you look at the ethnobotanical literature from around the world, you'll find that spicy foods have been used traditionally to treat laryngitis and other respiratory conditions. It makes sense to me. Garlic, ginger, horseradish and mustard all seem useful for relieving laryngitis, especially when it is associated with thick secretions in the airways.

Lice

A while back, after staying at one of the "country hotels" in Madagascar's rain forest, I developed an itchy case of lice.

At least I think I had lice. My 65-year-old eyes were too weak to see any real lice crawling over me. Perhaps it was just my imagination. But even if I just imagined those lice, there could not have been a more appropriate place to do so. The hotel was filthy and very bug-ridden.

Since I didn't have any offhand knowledge of herbal lice remedies, I threaded my way through the tropical foliage to a good doctor. My friend Linnea Smith, M.D., searched but saw no lice. Just in case, however, she gave me a bottle of Kwell shampoo, the classic lice medicine. I dutifully shampooed. Well, I must have had lice or a similar infestation, because after that Kwell treatment, my itch-misery ceased.

Lice are a familiar—and "lousy"—problem for some ten million Americans each year. That adds up to a lot of Kwell and other delousing products. But what else is there? Here goes.

Green Pharmacy for Lice

Few herbal reference books recommend botanical remedies for lice, so I hope herbalists notice this chapter and begin including lice-killing herbs (pediculicides) in their works. Here are a few herbs that can send lice packing.

🌿 **Neem (*Azadiracta indica*) and turmeric (*Curcuma longa*).** In one study done in India, researchers treated 814 people complaining of lice with a combination of these two herbal remedies.

Neem is a large oaklike tree that's native to India and is now planted around the subtropical world, including Florida and Southern California. The leaves and seed oil contain compounds that appear to be active against many insect pests. For this reason, U.S. companies that market nontoxic pesticides now offer several neem products to organic farmers. (Some friends of mine in Hawaii are now growing and harvesting neem.)

Turmeric has a long history in Asian folklore as a vermin killer, and it's especially good at fighting scabies, which are parasitic mites. It makes sense that researchers would try turmeric for lice. In one study, they prepared a neem-turmeric paste by pulverizing fresh neem leaves and turmeric root (four parts neem to one part turmeric). The people in this study rubbed the paste all over their bodies and allowed it to dry. They repeated the treatment until they no longer felt or saw lice. Meanwhile, they also boiled their clothes and bedding, a standard recommendation for delousing.

Researchers reported that 98 percent of the people in the study were completely cured within 3 to 15 days. They also noted that the 2 percent who remained infested had not followed the program.

❧ **Sweetflag (*Acorus calamus*).** The American species of this plant, which grows in temperate regions around the world, has proven lice-killing properties. The aromatic root is pounded into a powder and either made into poultice or rubbed directly onto the afflicted areas.

Liver Problems

I had hepatitis in Panama 25 years ago, and I did what my doctors told me: I stopped drinking alcohol until I recovered, which was a challenge because in Panama, the rum is cheap and tasty. And I rested. That was it. Mainstream medicine just didn't have a whole lot to offer people with hepatitis then—and it still doesn't.

But herbal medicine does. When my son developed hepatitis a few years ago, his doctor gave him the same advice mine gave me in Panama years ago. But this time around, I knew more about medicinal herbs, so I gave my son two bottles of milk thistle capsules.

Milk thistle is my top-choice herb for all kinds of liver ailments, including everything from hepatitis to cirrhosis to *Amanita* mushroom poisoning.

Liver Troubles

The leading cause of liver disease is alcohol, which causes cirrhosis. Alcoholism affects an estimated ten million Americans, causing some 200,000 deaths a year and making it one of our most serious health problems. Alcoholic liver disease is the fourth leading cause of death in 25- to 64-year-old men.

After alcohol, hepatitis is the number two cause of liver disease. Hepatitis, which simply means inflammation of the liver, is not one disease but many. There is acute hepatitis (which eventually heals) or the chronic variety (which can continue for a long time). Hepatitis can be caused by viruses; the types are indicated with letters—A, B, C, D or E—and other letters are sure to be added as new viruses are identified. It can also be caused by alcohol, medications (even acetaminophen products like Tylenol) or overexposure to industrial chemicals, such as fumes from dry-cleaning chemicals like carbon tetrachloride.

There are more than 300,000 cases of the various forms of hepatitis each year in the United States. Hepatitis B is particularly insidious. It is spread like AIDS, sexually and by blood-to-blood contact.

About 5,000 people a year die from hepatitis B, and if you survive it, you're at risk for liver cancer years later. Fortunately, there's now a hepatitis B vaccine. But there are no vaccines for the other forms of hepatitis.

Green Pharmacy for Liver Problems

Since mainstream medicine does not have much to offer in the way of hepatitis treatment beyond rest, I think it's too bad that our high priests of medicine don't read the herbal literature more often. They might learn something about milk thistle and the many other herbs that can help treat liver disease.

✿✿✿ **Carrot (*Daucus carota*).** Scientists in India have discovered that carrots afford significant protection for the liver, at least experimentally in laboratory animals. When liver cell injury was induced experimentally with chemicals, paralleling the liver damage inflicted by chemical pollutants, experiments showed that lab animals could recover with the help of carrot extracts. These extracts increase the activity of several enzymes that speed up detoxification of the liver and other organs.

❧❧❧ **Dandelion (*Taraxacum officinale*).** "Dandelion root heads the list of excellent foods for the liver," writes herbal pharmacologist Daniel Mowrey, Ph.D., author of *The Scientific Validation of Herbal Medicine* and *Herbal Tonic Therapies*. The leaves are a diuretic, meaning that they help flush excess water from the body. And the roots have been used for centuries to treat jaundice, the yellowing of the skin that occurs as a result of a seriously malfunctioning liver.

I recommend using both the leaves and flowers. Dandelion flowers are well-endowed with lecithin, a nutrient that has been proven useful in various liver ailments.

Since dandelion is a food plant, I suggest steaming the leaves and flowers like spinach and eating a lot of this delicious vegetable. If you don't care for the bitter taste, herb shops and health food stores sell capsules and tinctures. Follow the package directions.

❧❧❧ **Indian almond (*Terminalia catappa*).** Extracts of this herb have been shown in studies to prevent chemically induced liver damage in laboratory animals. Unfortunately, Indian almonds are unlike any of the almonds for sale here in America, but I hope they'll be more available here someday. They can be found growing wild on all tropical coasts, including Florida and Hawaii.

❧❧❧ **Milk thistle (*Silybum marianum*).** Milk thistle has been used as a liver remedy for at least 2,000 years. Research shows that compounds from the seeds help protect the liver against damage from alcohol and hepatitis and can even regenerate liver cells that have been damaged. That's why Commission E, the German expert panel that judges the safety and effectiveness of medicinal herbs for the German government, approves

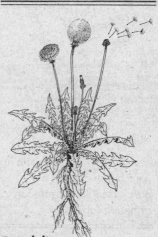

Dandelion

This common weed was prescribed by Chinese physicians for a wide range of problems.

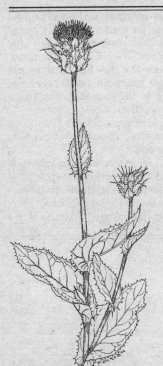

Milk Thistle

You can grow milk thistle in your home garden or purchase it in capsule form at health food stores.

milk thistle seeds or seed extracts as supportive treatment for cirrhosis and chronic inflammatory liver conditions.

Other studies show that the compound silymarin, which is found in milk thistle, helps protect the liver from many industrial toxins, such as carbon tetrachloride.

Even if you don't have liver damage or liver disease, milk thistle helps improve liver function by helping the liver remove toxins from your body.

You can buy milk thistle capsules at health food stores or herb shops. Follow the package directions.

If you're the gardening type, you can grow your own. Very young leaves of this herb can be used in salads, although they contain only traces of silymarin. In addition to their medicinal value, the seeds can be roasted, ground and used as a substitute for coffee. (Milk thistle is a relative of chicory, which is another coffee substitute.)

Given the amount of alcohol abuse in this country, I sometimes have a fantasy about getting rich by selling my Beer Beans, a mixture of 20 parts (by weight) roasted milk thistle seeds, soybeans (which are reputed to curb the desire for alcohol) and ginkgo nuts (proven to speed alcohol metabolism). I'd roast these and offer them to heavy-drinking friends.

❧❧❧ **Schisandra (*Schisandra chinensis*).** Widely used in Chinese medicine as a male tonic, this herb also has strong liver-protecting properties, according to pharmacognosist (natural product pharmacist) Albert Leung, Ph.D. Chinese doctors use its extracts effectively to treat viral hepatitis and other liver ailments. The seeds contain more than a dozen liver-protective compounds.

I really wouldn't be surprised if one day schisandra is right up there with milk thistle as a top herb for liver complaints. You should be able to find the dried berries in some herb shops and health food stores. In China, people take approximately one to seven teaspoons a day for up to a month after the hepatitis has subsided.

<hr>

❧❧❧

Liver-Protecting Salad

Salads are a great place for liver-protective ingredients. When you make a salad, try adding young milk thistle leaves, carrots and dandelion flowers. Use ginger and turmeric in the dressing.

❧❧❧

<hr>

❧❧❧ **Tamarind** (*Tamarindus indica*). In Latin America, tamarind juice is the chaser of choice when you're drinking alcoholic beverages. That's because it has a reputation for preventing hangover. Having tested it on occasion, I think it helps. This strengthens my suspicions that tamarind just might help protect the liver. These suspicions were at least partially confirmed by a study showing that extracts of tamarind prevented liver damage in experimental animals that were given liver-damaging chemicals.

The sugary pulp around the seeds is used to make a sweetened beverage that is consumed more as a food than a medicine. I drink two glasses a day if it is available. So far, however, I have found the dried pulp only in a few Latin American markets. Happy hunting.

❧❧ **Chicory** (*Cichorium intybus*). Acetaminophen in high

doses is toxic to the liver, and if the doses are high enough, it can be fatal. In one study, 70 percent of mice given chicory extracts survived a dose of acetaminophen that killed 100 percent of untreated animals. I'm not surprised, since chicory is related to milk thistle.

For home medication, I dig my own roots, scorch and pulverize them to make a chicory "coffee" and drink two to four cups a day. Chicory makes a wonderful, caffeine-free substitute for coffee. You don't need to go to this much trouble, however. Standardized extracts of the roots are available in herb shops, health food stores and some markets.

❧

A Tea for Your Liver

This is a grab-bag tea recipe made with herbs that reportedly have liver-protective benefits. Mix to taste: licorice, dandelion, chicory, turmeric and ginger. If you like, you can also add anise, caraway, celery seed, dill, clove, fennel, peppermint, rosemary and vanilla bean. You can mix up a jar of dried herbs and keep the mixture handy for whenever you want an herbal tea.

❧

❧❧ **Chinese angelica (*Angelica sinensis*).** Also known as *dang-quai*, this Chinese herb is revered in the Orient as an aid for women's health. It also helps protect the liver, apparently by helping it use more oxygen. Chinese herbal physicians favor it for treating cirrhosis.

The usual recommendation is to take two to six teaspoons a day in teas, tinctures or pills for as much as a month. Here in the United States, you'll find Chinese angelica in Chinese herb shops and some health food stores. (Do not take this herb if you are pregnant, however.)

❧❧ **Javanese turmeric (*Curcuma xanthorrhiza*).** In Asian

folklore, this herb has been highly regarded for conditions related to the liver, particularly gallstones and jaundice. Taiwanese scientists have discovered why: Extracts of this yellow root are significantly protective for the liver. You probably won't find this herb except in Indonesian or other South Asian markets, but you may well have such a market in your area.

If you can find it, I suggest taking up to five teaspoons a day for a month. Have it with food or tea.

❧❧ **Licorice (*Glycyrrhiza glabra*).** The active compound in licorice root, glycyrrhizin, inhibits liver cell injury caused by many chemicals and is used in the treatment of cirrhosis and chronic hepatitis, especially in Japan. Unfortunately, the Japanese inject it, which I would not recommend.

Russian studies suggest that an herbal combination that includes licorice, peppermint, rose, tansy and stinging nettle can help stabilize liver cell membranes in experimental animals, thus protecting the animals from liver damage.

Closer to home, noted naturopaths Joseph Pizzorno, N.D., president of Bastyr College of Naturopathy in Seattle, and Michael Murray, N.D., co-authors of *A Textbook of Natural Medicine*, mention well-designed clinical trials showing glycyrrhizin to be quite effective in treating viral hepatitis.

You can buy standardized extracts at health food stores. Follow the package directions.

❧ **Bottle gourd (*Lagenaria siceraria*).** Scientists at the University of North Carolina School of Medicine in Chapel Hill have found that in experimental animals, a deficiency of the B vitamin choline causes liver damage and is associated with the development of liver cancer. Whether choline can help heal the human liver is uncertain, but it can't hurt to get a little more of this nutrient.

According to my database, the best source of choline is bottle gourd (1.6 percent on a dry-weight basis). Eat bottle gourd as you would squash. If you can't find it at markets near you, you might consider growing your own. Other herbs high in choline include fenugreek leaves, shepherd's purse, horehound, ginseng, cowpeas, English peas, mung beans, sponge gourds, lentils and Chinese angelica.

❧ **Ginger (*Zingiber officinale*).** According to research by yours truly, along with molecular biologist Stephen Beckstrom-Sternberg, Ph.D., ginger contains eight liver-protecting compounds. I won't go so far as to say that it could treat hepatitis, but if you love ginger, as I do, you get a little liver protection every time you use it in cooking or tea.

🌿 **Tea (*Camellia sinensis*).** Tea is clinically effective in treating acute infectious hepatitis, note Dr. Leung and Arkansas herbalist Steven Foster in *The Encyclopedia of Common Natural Ingredients*. If I had hepatitis, I'd drink two to four cups a day.

🌿 **Turmeric (*Curcuma longa*).** This spice, often included in curries, contains several related compounds that protect the liver. If I had hepatitis, I would add more turmeric to my cooking.

Lyme Disease

Pliny the Elder, a Roman naturalist of the first century A.D., made no attempt to hide his loathing: "Ticks are the foulest and nastiest creatures that be," he said. So just imagine how much contempt he'd have today for the deer ticks that are now known to be carriers of Lyme disease.

My Herbal Vineyard in Maryland is a lush six-acre spread filled with upward of 300 species of herbs, shrubs, trees and welcome weeds. It has attracted visitors (and television crews) from around the world. It has also attracted less welcome guests, notably the deer that bring their unwelcome hitchhikers, deer ticks.

Not too long ago, after a three-hour video session out in my ginseng patch with me showing off my Siberian ginseng plants and talking about this herb, I swatted reflexively at something tickling my thigh. It went *splat!* and while there wasn't much left to identify, what remained looked vaguely ticklike.

A day later, a small red spot appeared on my thigh. It grew to look suspiciously like the characteristic bull's-eye rash caused by the tickborne bacteria *Borrelia burgdorferi*, which cause Lyme disease. By the next day, the bull's-eye had become more pronounced, measuring nearly three inches in diameter. So I took some echinacea and garlic.

The day after that, my wife, Peggy, coerced me into visiting our HMO. Without the tick, they couldn't test for *Borrelia*, so they couldn't be certain that I had Lyme disease. But all the physical signs pointed in that direction. The doctor recommended a course of doxycycline (Bio-Tab, Monodox), a bactericidal antibiotic, just in case.

Antibiotics and Herbs to the Rescue

We picked up the prescription, but I wavered about taking it. Doxycycline can make the skin more sun-sensitive, leading to rashes. And I couldn't really stay out of the sun because I had yet another video crew due for yet another tour of the Herbal Vineyard.

I weighed my options. I could take the antibiotic and take my chances in the sun. I could opt for an herbal alternative—echinacea, for example—hoping to boost my immune system for its confrontation with *Borrelia*, plus take antibiotic garlic tablets to fight the bacteria. Or I could combine the conventional and herbal medicines.

After considerable soul-searching, I went with the combination approach: doxycycline plus garlic capsules, equivalent to 1,200 milligrams of fresh garlic a day. I also took six echinacea capsules a day, each containing 450 milligrams of the immune-boosting root, and I juiced up some carrots and tomatoes. These vegetables are rich in vitamin A–family carotenoids, and a good deal of research shows that carotenoids help fight infection. And of course I added plenty of fresh garlic while I had the carrots and tomatoes in the juicer.

I finished my three-week doxycycline regimen in Nashville, and I even sang a song about the antibiotic at Opryland. By then the bull's-eye had disappeared, and I showed no signs of Lyme disease. We'll never know whether I really needed the garlic or the doxycycline. But I surely didn't need the crippling arthritis that often ensues with Lyme disease.

Beware the Bull's-Eye

Lyme disease, named for the town of Old Lyme, Connecticut, where it was first identified about 20 years ago, is a zoonosis, a human infection caused by an animal-borne pathogen or infectious agent. How did this relatively new disease appear? Blame it on real estate development. More and more housing is being built in and near wildlife areas, bringing deer and people into closer contact. Since bobcats and other such predators are rare, the deer populations have increased, and there are more hungry deer than ever munching our gardens.

Lyme disease generally causes the characteristic bull's-eye skin rash, but in about 10 percent of cases, no rash appears. After a few weeks to several months, some 70 percent of those who remain untreated suffer bacterial invasions of the joints and possibly other organs, notably the central nervous system, causing chronic arthritis.

Currently, in areas without major Lyme disease problems, 1 to 2 percent of people show antibodies to *Borrelia*, signifying that they have at some point been exposed to the virus. In some Lyme-endemic areas, however, the figure is 10 percent.

Because of all the publicity about Lyme disease, we not only have an epidemic of this infection, we also have an epidemic of overdiagnosis. Doctors are too willing to diagnose Lyme disease, apparently because the early symptoms—skin rash, headache, fever, nausea and muscle pain—are common to so many other maladies.

In a 1995 survey by the American Medical Association, only about half of those diagnosed with Lyme disease actually had it. If that's true, then there may be only 5,000 infections a year in the United States, not the 10,000 figure you see bandied about. Did I really have Lyme disease? I think so, but these statistics certainly make me wonder.

Green Pharmacy for Lyme Disease

One thing I don't wonder about is my decision to combine my conventional medical treatment with herbs. There are a number of helpful herbs that you and your doctor might consider using in addition to any medical treatment you're receiving for the disease. And two of them, garlic and mountain mint, might prevent the disease, because they act as natural tick repellents.

❧❧❧ **Echinacea (*Echinacea*, various species).** Varro Tyler, Ph.D., dean and professor emeritus of pharmacognosy (natural product pharmacy) at Purdue University in West Lafayette, Indiana, is outspoken in his support of echinacea, noting that the herb has been extensively studied as an immunostimulant and that it increases the body's resistance to bacterial infection.

A century ago, here in the United States, the recommended dose of echinacea rhizome and root was one gram (approximately a half-teaspoon) per day. During my Lyme treatment, I took about four grams (two teaspoons)—that's how afraid of *Borrelia* I was.

Echinacea comes in teas, tinctures and capsules. I often add a dropper or two of tincture to juices or beverage teas. (Although echinacea can cause your tongue to tingle or go numb temporarily, this effect is harmless.) To treat my suspected Lyme infection, though, I took capsules to get a lot down quickly.

❦❦❦ **Garlic (*Allium sativum*).** Louis Pasteur was the first to describe the antibacterial effect of garlic juices. More recently, we've found that garlic even works against many antibiotic-resistant strains of bacteria, and given the speed with which bacteria become resistant, I doubt that it will be long before *Borrelia* develops resistance to doxycycline.

Dutch studies suggest that getting the best antibiotic action from garlic requires ingesting 5 to 15 average-size cloves a day. It's hard to get that much fresh garlic down, but I find that juicing it with carrots works.

If you just can't make yourself consume that much garlic, don't despair. I believe that while lower doses may not eradicate infection by themselves, they can still help when combined with other herbs and antibiotics.

❦❦❦ **Mountain mint (*Pycnanthemum muticum*).** A welcome weed at Herbal Vineyard, this plant provides me with my tick repellent, day after day, in summer. When I spend time outdoors, I crush mountain mint leaves and rub my legs with the juice, which is well-endowed with the bug- and tick-repelling compound pulegone. But on the fateful afternoon of my tick encounter, I didn't anticipate spending so long outside with that camera crew, and I did not use the herb. I won't make that mistake again. (It's probably best not to use this herb on your skin if you're pregnant, however.)

❦❦ **Licorice (*Glycyrrhiza glabra*).** Once I queried my database about which herb contained the most bactericidal compounds. The answer was licorice, which is up to 33 percent antibacterial compounds on a dry-weight basis. Small wonder that the Chinese have used licorice for centuries to treat bacterial infections such as tuberculosis. I often use licorice roots, which are also antiviral, to treat both viral and bacterial infections. Compounds known as saponins, which are found in licorice, also increase the availability of other antibiotic compounds.

Other herbs well-endowed with bactericidal compounds, in descending order of potency, include thyme, hops, oregano and rosemary. Sounds like the makings of a good tea, which can be sweetened with licorice extract.

Macular Degeneration

Being an Alabama-born redneck who was raised on fruits and vegetables, I'm happy to tell all who will listen that the antioxidants and other plant chemicals (phytochemicals) in these foods help prevent heart disease and cancer. Of course, nowadays that's probably not news to you. But maybe here's a new one for you: Did you know that antioxidant nutrients also help save eyesight?

I can't guarantee that if you eat your veggies you'll have good vision when you're as old as Methuselah. But if the studies I've reviewed are correct, you'll certainly have better vision than you would if you ate junk food instead.

Here's why: There is some indication that cell damage caused by highly reactive oxygen molecules (free radicals) plays a role in an eye condition known as macular degeneration. Antioxidants are substances that neutralize these free radicals and prevent them from doing harm. And fruits and vegetables, especially leafy vegetables, are simply your best sources of these beneficial substances.

The macula is the central and most sensitive portion of the retina, the nerve-rich area in the back of the eye that is necessary for sight. For unknown reasons, after around age 60, the macula begins to break down. As it degenerates, central vision and fine detail perception deteriorate. (Peripheral vision remains unaffected.)

Macular degeneration affects more than 25 percent of Americans over 65 years old. It is the leading cause of blindness in the elderly. You're at somewhat greater risk of having macular degeneration if you are farsighted or smoke cigarettes. People with light-colored eyes and a family history of the condition are also at greater risk.

Green Pharmacy for Macular Degeneration

Conventional medical therapies don't help much with macular degeneration, which makes nutritional approaches look all the more appealing. Quite a few foods and herbs might help.

❧❧❧ **Bilberry (*Vaccinium myrtillus*).** This fruit and its relatives, blueberry, cranberry, huckleberry, blackberry, grape, plum and wild cherry, have been used traditionally for problems with visual acuity. And scientific research has validated this folk medicine approach.

All of these fruits contain compounds known as anthocyanosides, which are potent antioxidants. In one study, daily treatment with 400 milligrams of bilberry and 20 milligrams of the famous antioxidant beta-carotene improved many participants' night vision and enlarged their visual fields.

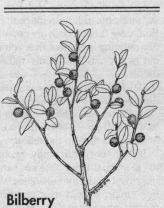

Bilberry anthocyanosides also strengthen the capillaries in the retina, which helps slow macular degeneration. Herbal pharmacologist Daniel Mowrey, Ph.D., author of *The Scientific Validation of Herbal Medicine* and *Herbal Tonic Therapies*, suggests a tea of bilberry, butcher's broom, centella and ginger for the prevention and treatment of several types of macular degeneration. I agree.

I suggest using a lot of bil-

Bilberry

Bilberries contain a powerful antioxidant that was once used by eighteenth-century herbalists as an ingredient in mouthwash.

berries and adding the other herbs based on whatever you have on hand and how you feel about the taste. Steep the herbs in boiling water for 15 minutes; you can drink a cup of this Eye Tea up to four times a day.

❧❧ Collard greens (*Brassica oleracea*), spinach (*Spinacia oleracea*) and other vegetables. One study, done by ophthalmologist Johanna Seddon, M.D., of the Massachusetts Eye and Ear Infirmary in Boston, involved surveying almost 900 people, 326 of whom had macular degeneration. Dr. Seddon found that eating antioxidant-rich fruits and vegetables at least five times a week cut the risk of macular degeneration in half.

Collard greens, the popular soul food, and spinach, Popeye's favorite food, stood out in Dr. Seddon's study. These vegetables contain the beneficial compounds lutein and zeaxanthin. Vegetables that contain similar compounds that may provide eye protection include bok choy, broccoli, brussels sprouts, cabbage, kale, kohlrabi, mustard greens, radishes, turnip greens and watercress.

Dr. Seddon's study also found that taking vitamin C and E supplements didn't do much to help prevent macular degeneration, even though both are potent antioxidants. This strengthens my ongoing argument that you're better off with whole, nutrient-rich foods and herbs rather than single-nutrient supplements.

If I had macular degeneration or any risk factors for it, I'd dine regularly on my Cruci-Fix, a steamed mixture of all the cruciferous vegetables I had on hand.

❧❧ Ginkgo (*Ginkgo biloba*). Ginkgo extracts help maintain good blood flow to the retina.

In one six-month study, people who received 80 milligrams of a standardized ginkgo extract twice daily significantly improved their long-distance vision. Another study suggests that ginkgo extract may even reverse damage in the retina. To me this suggests that you should try mixing ginkgo with antioxidant mint teas.

Ginkgo leaves actually contain very little of the active compounds. The best way to get the full benefits of this herb is to use a standardized extract—a 50:1 preparation, which means that 50 pounds of leaves have been processed to make 1 pound of extract. (I occasionally add a few leaves to my blended fresh fruit juices anyway.) The suggested dose of standardized extract is 150 to 300 milligrams a day. (In amounts higher than 240 milligrams, ginkgo may cause diarrhea, irritability and restlessness, so if you experience any of these symptoms, opt for a lower dose.)

Peanut (*Arachis hypogaea*). A good deal of research shows that soybeans help prevent the retinal breakdown that happens to people with diabetes, a condition known as diabetic retinopathy. It seems that the active constituent in soybeans is genistein. If genistein helps prevent diabetic retinopathy, it also might help prevent macular degeneration.

Many other legumes besides soybeans contain a generous portion of genistein. From a taste standpoint, I go for peanuts, which actually contain more genistein than soybeans. In fact, I munch on peanuts nearly every day. Spanish peanuts are also well-endowed with antioxidant compounds known as procyanidins.

Clove (*Syzygium aromaticum*). Clove oil is a powerful antioxidant. Studies show that it helps prevent the breakdown in the retina of a substance known as docosahexaenoic acid. This action helps preserve vision in old age. I'd suggest adding one or two drops of oil to antioxidant mint teas and enjoying up to four cups a day.

Wolfberry (*Lycium chinese*). This is a traditional Chinese treatment for blurred vision and other problems with sight. In one study, participants consumed about two ounces (50 grams) of wolfberries a day. Their vision improved significantly. Wolfberries are high in antioxidants and beneficial plant pigments known as carotenoids.

Menopause

Here is an excerpt from a letter I received in 1991: "I am a 59-year-old woman who has gone through menopause. As a result, my skin has become extremely thin, and my hair has thinned as well. I would like to inquire if there are any natural alternatives to hormone replacement therapy (HRT). I feel very unsure of HRT and don't want to take it. I fear it has too many risks."

This is just one of the more than 10,000 letters I received that year, which was a bumper-crop year for mail because I did a three-minute spot on food pharmacy on the CBS national morning show. The phones rang off the hook at the U.S. Department of Agriculture (USDA), where I worked at the time. And all of the USDA secretaries, mail staff and operators—as well as the bosses—regretted my three minutes of fame. Of course, I didn't. It was another chance to get people excited about herbs and other natural medicines.

The Big Hormone Question

I, too, have misgivings about HRT. Although the female sex hormone estrogen evidently relieves hot flashes, vaginal dryness and other discomforts of menopause, a good deal of research shows that it may increase a woman's risk of getting breast cancer. (Researchers have found that including progesterone as part of the therapy may reduce the risk of breast cancer.)

I like to quote Andrew Weil, M.D., an herb advocate who teaches at the University of Arizona College of Medicine in Tucson and author of *Natural Health, Natural Medicine*, who warns friends contemplating HRT: "You should avoid estrogen replacement altogether if you are at increased risk of cancer of the breast or reproductive system, including having a personal or family history of these cancers or ovarian cancer. If you do decide to take replacement therapy, use a low dose of estrogen (1.25 milligrams a day, maximum) and never take it without progesterone for at least part of the monthly cycle." This sounds like good advice to me. In fact, it's not unique to Dr. Weil. Many gynecologists also take this approach.

I know a naturopath who is very opposed to HRT and instead recommends eating lots of veggies and legumes high in phytoestrogens, which are estrogen-like compounds. He says, "If you add up all the warnings, cautions, contraindications and side effects, the number comes to over 100." My friend is amazed that any physician would prescribe this therapy. Still, the vast majority of doctors do prescribe HRT.

Why? Mainly because HRT also reduces the risk of heart disease and osteoporosis, which pose a greater risk to many women than breast cancer. But in my humble opinion, there are better ways to reduce these risks than taking HRT.

Many doctors disagree with me, though. This is a decision

that you'll have to make yourself, and I suggest that you get the full picture—pro and con—from your own gynecologist. (For more details on heart disease, see page 295; for more on osteoporosis, see page 411.)

. When there are alternatives to dangerous drugs, those approaches should be given a chance before you resort to more drastic, expensive approaches that have the potential to cause damaging side effects. I fear that for economic reasons the pharmaceutical firms are not interested in proving that natural approaches to menopause, or anything else for that matter, are safer and more effective than synthetics. I personally believe that the natural approaches are better, and I'm not alone in that opinion. Unfortunately, few doctors share it.

Midlife Discomforts

Menopause means the cessation of menstruation. Most women experience menopause during their late forties and early fifties. Sometimes it happens quickly. More frequently, it takes a few years for menstrual periods to cease.

As menopause develops, estrogen production declines, often causing one or more discomforts: anxiety, breast tenderness, depression, dry skin, headache, hot flashes, incontinence, insomnia, irritability, nervousness, night sweats and vaginal dryness.

Of this list, hot flashes are most common, affecting about 85 percent of menopausal women. Hot flashes usually occur without warning, but some women notice that emotional stress, exercise, alcohol and certain foods may trigger them.

The Fabulous Phytos

Let me remind you that as a botanist, I cannot and do not prescribe. However, I believe it within my botanical prerogative to outline the research on herbal and nutritional approaches to menopause that I would not hesitate to suggest to my wife or daughter.

But before I mention specific herbs that can offer help, let me make an important point about diet. Hot flashes and other menopausal symptoms are rare in vegetarian cultures, especially among people who consume a lot of legumes, like black beans, mung beans and soybeans.

Why? Because beans and many other plants have mild estrogenic activity, thanks to phytoestrogens. These compounds include isoflavones, lignans, phytosterols and saponins.

In addition to acting like estrogen in women whose own sex hormone production has declined, phytoestrogens also appear to reduce the risk of estrogen-linked cancers such as breast cancer. Animal experiments show that phytoestrogens are extremely effective in preventing tumors of the breast tissue.

The Soy Factor

We used to think that Asian women had a low rate of breast cancer simply because they eat a low-fat diet. Now it looks as though their substantial intake of legumes like soy and bean sprouts is also a reason. How is it possible for phytoestrogens to help prevent menopausal symptoms and at the same time also help prevent illnesses associated with estrogen?

Phytoestrogens are weaker than the body's own estrogen. In premenopausal women, phytoestrogens compete with women's own, more potent estrogen, reducing the total effects of estrogen. But as women's estrogen production falls, phytoestrogens supplement this hormone.

Put another way, when women have too much biological estrogen, phytoestrogens lower the burden; when they have too little, phytoestrogens pinch-hit.

I know of no evidence that phytoestrogens in moderation cause harm. One cup of soybeans (about 200 grams) provides about 300 milligrams of the most important class of phytoestrogens, isoflavones. That amount could provide about the equivalent of one tablet of Premarin, the commonly prescribed synthetic hormone used in ERT.

Studies show that women who regularly eat soy foods have few hot flashes, and they have more cells in their vaginal linings. These extra cells offset the vaginal dryness and irritation that are so common in postmenopausal women.

Soybeans are not the only beans high in isoflavones. Most beans and many other legumes contain reasonable amounts. I feel that little harm can be done by enjoying a diet rich in a diversity of beans unless you're allergic to them or strenuously object to the flatus they cause. (I don't, but if you'd like some techniques for reducing the gas-producing effects of beans, see page 244.)

Green Pharmacy for Menopause

In addition to a high-phytoestrogen vegetarian diet, a number of specific herbs can help relieve many symptoms associated with menopause. Here's my selection.

Black cohosh (*Cimicifuga racemosa*). Long recommended for "female complaints," this herb contains estrogenic substances that help relieve menopause discomforts, especially hot flashes. In one study of 110 menopausal women, half were given black cohosh root extract, while the other half took an inactive preparation (a placebo). After eight weeks, blood tests showed significant estrogenic activity in the women taking the herb.

In another study, women with vaginal dryness due to menopause experienced similar relief whether taking black cohosh or pharmaceutical estrogen.

Licorice (*Glycyrrhiza glabra*). Licorice contains natural estrogenic compounds. Like the isoflavones in soy, glycyrrhizin, the active ingredient in licorice, appears to reduce estrogen levels in women when they're too high and increase the levels when they're too low.

Could licorice candy help women with menopausal discomforts? Possibly, but read the label. Most American licorice contains extracts of licorice plus anise, which contains a chemical (anethole) that is less estrogenic

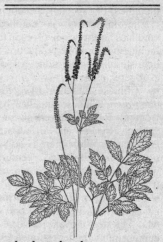

Black Cohosh

This herb grew wild in the Ohio River valley and was used by American Indian women for gynecological complaints and childbirth.

than glycyrrhizin. Many health food stores carry candies made from pure licorice.

Licorice and its extracts are safe for normal use in moderate amounts, but long-term use or ingestion of larger amounts can produce headache, lethargy, sodium and water retention, excessive loss of potassium and high blood pressure. A safe daily dose of a true licorice confection is said to be five grams, or less than a quarter-ounce. It's hard to stop when something tastes that good, but you'll just have to control yourself.

❧ **Alfalfa (*Medicago sativa*).** Alfalfa has demonstrable estrogenic activity. The leaves make a pleasant-tasting tea. If you have lupus or a family history of lupus, however, steer clear of alfalfa sprouts. There's some evidence that they may trigger lupus in sensitive individuals.

❧ **Chasteberry (*Vitex agnus-castus*).** This herb has been endorsed as a normalizing herb for female sex hormones and is thought to be especially beneficial during menopausal changes.

The biochemistry is complicated, but basically chasteberry regulates hormones involved in the menstrual cycle: It increases luteinizing hormone production and inhibits the release of follicle-stimulating hormone. All of this translates into a beneficial estrogenic effect.

❧ **Chinese angelica (*Angelica sinensis*).** Also known as *dang-quai*, Chinese angelica has an age-old reputation as a women's tonic. Believers swear that it relieves hot flashes and vaginal dryness and irritation, thus aiding women during menopause. While there is no scientific backup for this assertion, the herb does have centuries of folk use going for it. I wouldn't hesitate to recommend it to family members and friends.

❧ **Red clover (*Trifolium pratense*).** This herb contains 1 to 2.5 percent isoflavones. In one study, postmenopausal women who ingested clover, flaxseed and soy for two weeks had demonstrably higher estrogen levels, which declined when they went off the special diet. Some clovers are so estrogenic that they cause spontaneous abortion in cattle that overgraze on them. Red clover makes a pleasant-tasting tea.

❧ **Strawberry (*Fragaria*, various species) and other foods containing boron.** There's more to estrogen activity than the hormone itself. USDA research shows that taking as little as three milligrams of boron can double blood levels of circulating estrogen. So I'd recommend that postmenopausal women and those approaching menopause eat foods high in this mineral.

According to my database, the top boron-containing foods, in descending order of potency, include strawberries, peaches, cabbage, tomatoes, dandelion, apples, asparagus, figs, poppy seeds, broccoli, pears, cherries, beets, apricots, currants, parsley, dill and cumin seed.

Working with all the estrogenic and boron-containing plants and herbs, you can concoct some interesting salads and vegetable dishes.

❧ **Assorted herbs.** A number of other herbs contain phytoestrogens that could prove useful in helping with menopause. These include apples, celery stalks, dates, elder, false-unicorn root, fennel, Honduran sarsaparilla, lady's slipper, liferoot, Mexican wild yams, passionflower, pomegranates and sassafras.

Menstrual Cramps

There we were, three investigators, each with American Indian family connections, gazing at a patch of squaw vine. One of my companions was a bona fide Lumbee Indian, whose tribe lives near the border between North and South Carolina. The other was Scandinavian, but she was the mother of an honorary Abenaki (one who had been adopted into the Massachusetts tribe). And I am the Caucasian grandfather of three part-Cherokee grandchildren.

We got to discussing the term *squaw vine* as we considered the plant, a ground-hugging evergreen vinelet with bright red berries. I had been told that there were two possible interpretations of *squaw* in the common names of plants: one, perhaps sexist, that it was used only for women's reproductive ills, and the other, perhaps racist, that it was altogether useless.

The Lumbee discounted the possibility that it was useless, saying that the Indians would not have continued to use such a plant for menstrual difficulties unless it was effective. He agreed with me that the word *squaw* did not sound respectful of Indian women.

We couldn't rename the plant, because every herbalist knows it as squaw vine. But we agreed that from then on, we would take *squaw* to mean useful and beautiful. Still a bit sexist, perhaps, but much more positive.

Green Pharmacy for Menstrual Cramps

There are actually quite a few herbs, including squaw vine, that can help ease monthly cramps.

❦❦❦ **Black haw (*Viburnum prunifolium*).** Under the name crampbark, this herb was recognized as a treatment for menstrual cramps in most pharmacology reference books through the nineteenth century. The bark contains at least four substances that help relax the uterus. Two (aesculetin and scopoletin) also help relieve muscle spasms. With so much folklore and science to recommend it, black haw would be one of the first remedies that I'd suggest to my daughter if she came to me complaining of cramps.

❦❦❦ **Chinese angelica (*Angelica sinensis*).** Also known as *dang-quai*, Chinese angelica is one of the most widely used herbs in Chinese traditional medicine. It is considered a female tonic, especially good for menstrual cramps, and is highly recommended by experts in Oriental medicine.

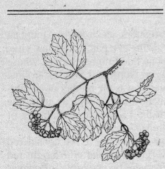

Black Haw

Black haw is a spreading shrub with clusters of white flowers that is related to honeysuckle and elderberry.

❦❦❦ **Raspberry (*Rubus idaeus*).** Many women herbalists I respect recommend raspberry leaf tea for easing menstrual cramps. One study showed that this herb helps relax the uterus. It's also popular for soothing the uterine irritability associated with pregnancy.

Researchers don't know the active compound in raspberry, but they speculate that it might be Pycnogenol (an oligomeric procyanidin, or OPC). That makes sense to me. In one study, taking 200 milligrams of OPC daily over two cycles eliminated or significantly relieved menstrual cramps and/or premenstrual syndrome in 50 to 60 percent of the women who took them. Among women who took OPCs for four cycles, the number who benefited was even higher—66 to 80 percent.

You can buy pure OPC in the form of Pycnogenol, but it's an expensive supplement. I'd suggest trying raspberry leaf tea instead.

❦❦ Bilberry (*Vaccinium myrtillus*). Bilberry contains chemicals called anthocyanidins, which have muscle-relaxant properties, and it also contains OPCs. For menstrual cramps, some herbalists suggest taking 20 to 40 milligrams of concentrated bilberry extract three times a day. If you can't find extracts, try a half-cup of fresh bilberries or blueberries, which have similar properties.

❦❦ Chasteberry (*Vitex agnus-castus*). The small fruits of the chasteberry tree have been used for menstrual disorders since Greco-Roman times. I'm convinced that chasteberry is effective.

❦❦ Ginger (*Zingiber officinale*). Eclectic physicians—turn-of-the-century American doctors who combined natural remedies with mainstream medicine—prescribed ginger to treat painful menstruation.

This herb is also used to induce menstruation in a wide range of cultures from Venezuela to Vietnam. With at least six pain-relieving compounds and another six anti-cramping compounds, ginger tea is a trustworthy remedy for menstrual cramps.

❦❦ Kava kava (*Piper methysticum*). Kava kava contains two pain-relieving chemicals that are as effective as aspirin, according to pharmacognosist (natural product pharmacist) Albert Leung, Ph.D., and Arkansas herbalist Steven Foster in their book *The Encyclopedia of Common Natural Ingredients*. Although kava kava has been described as narcotic and hypnotic, it is neither hallucinogenic nor stupefying. Furthermore, according to Dr. Leung and Foster, it is nonaddictive and does not cause dependency.

Some Europeans use kava kava extracts for its relaxant or anti-anxiety effects. Since the plant also helps relax the uterus, it is used to treat menstrual cramps.

❦❦ Red clover (*Trifolium pratense*). Clover is rich in phytoestrogens, plant chemicals that act on the body in the same

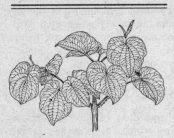

Kava Kava

An ingredient in a traditional Polynesian beverage, kava kava has antispasmodic effects and can help ease menstrual cramps.

way as the female hormone estrogen. Herbalists believe that phytoestrogens help minimize menstrual cramps by bringing the body's hormone levels into better balance.

One phytoestrogen in red clover is the compound formononetin. Although "clover disease" has been known to cause infertility in sheep that graze on it, you won't get enough clover to be even remotely concerned about this effect. Have red clover in tea, and it just might relieve cramping problems.

🌺🌺 **Squaw vine (*Mitchella repens*).** Cherokee women routinely took squaw vine for "period pains," according to Daniel Moerman, Ph.D., professor of anthropology at the University of Michigan and author of some excellent books on American Indian uses of medicinal plants. They also used it to ease childbirth and to treat sore nipples while nursing. The Oklahoma, Delaware, Iroquois and Menominee tribes used squaw vine similarly. Today's herbalists generally recommend it (along with raspberry) for the discomforts of pregnancy. You can try using it as the Cherokees did, to ease menstrual cramps.

🌺 **Strawberry (*Fragaria*, various species).** Like raspberry, strawberry leaf may help relieve cramps, according to Germany's Commission E, the body of scientists that advises that country's government about herbs.

The commission also notes that this action has not been substantiated. But I mention strawberry because there are lots of good reasons to drink it besides its reputed ability to ease menstrual cramps. Its leaves are rich in vitamins and minerals plus ellagic acid, a highly touted cancer preventive. Strawberry leaf tea may be of benefit to almost anyone who might be deficient in any vitamins or minerals. One piece of advice, though: Don't drink strawberry leaf tea if you're allergic to strawberries.

❧ Yarrow (*Achillea millefolium*). Yarrow is useful for relieving women's painful cramps, according to Commission E. I am not surprised at this endorsement, as yarrow contains a number of antispasmodic constituents.

Morning Sickness

A while back, one of my nieces telephoned to ask what I would recommend for morning sickness. She was pregnant and having trouble keeping anything down. I was faced with my usual problem: I'm a botanist, not a clinician. Suppose I'm wrong? I would never want to suggest to my niece that she try anything that might be dangerous to her or her baby.

I'd once told my daughter to try ginger for morning sickness, and now I was prepared to recommend the same for my niece. My only hesitation was the counsel of one pharmacologist, who said that ginger might stimulate miscarriage. But I couldn't imagine a cup or two of ginger tea doing this, so with the one caution I had also given my daughter—to go slowly—I suggested the herb to my niece. She phoned back to say that the ginger helped, with no noticeable side effects.

I'll still counsel ginger until I get more evidence that the pharmacologist's warning has merit. Meanwhile, I've never seen anything safer or better for morning sickness.

Shortly after I talked with my niece, I learned of a study that probably explains the pharmacologist's concern about miscarriage. It turns out that it takes less than 1 gram of ginger to control the nausea of morning sickness, while the Chinese, who use the herb to bring on menstruation (and possibly abortion) use 20 to 28 grams for this purpose.

Very roughly, a strong cup of ginger tea might contain about 250 milligrams of the herb, which is about $\frac{1}{80}$ of the amount necessary to trigger miscarriage. A heavily spiced Chinese dish might contain 500 milligrams—$\frac{1}{40}$ of the miscarriage dose— and an eight-ounce glass of ginger ale could contain 1,000 milligrams—$\frac{1}{20}$ of the menstruation-triggering dose. You'd have to gag down a heck of a lot of ginger before you'd have to be concerned about any kind of problems.

Queasy Times

Morning sickness is the nausea, dizziness and general ill feeling that pregnant women experience on getting up in the morning, or sometimes for much of the day. An estimated 50 percent of pregnant women complain of morning sickness, typically during their first trimester of pregnancy. But some women experience it for much longer.

Scientists are not sure why morning sickness develops. Several folk medical traditions claim it's Nature's way of clearing toxins from the mother's system. I don't know about that, but I do know I'd never suggest that my daughter or any woman take hard-core medications to treat it. So I hope that if you're pregnant, you'll discuss these gentle herbal alternatives with your doctor before resorting to drugs to relieve the problem.

Green Pharmacy for Morning Sickness

If you believe in food as your best medicine, as I do, then just eating might help. Many pregnant women report relief from morning sickness when they snack on dry toast or crackers immediately after rising and eat small, frequent meals during the day. In addition, here are the herbs that can help.

❦❦❦ **Ginger (*Zingiber officinale*).** In a paper I once published called "Foods as Pharmaceuticals," I listed only ginger for morning sickness. Many women have told me since that it helps, and I believe them.

I don't know of any scientific studies showing that ginger helps relieve morning sickness, but there's no shortage of research demonstrating that the herb treats motion sickness, a closely related stomach-upsetting condition. One excellent study showed ginger to be far superior to the commonly prescribed dimenhydrinate (Dramamine) as a treatment for nausea induced by motion.

In several studies, ginger has also been shown to relieve dizziness. This chapter lists other remedies for morning sickness, but in my opinion, ginger still ranks number one. I'd suggest up to two cups of ginger tea a day.

❦❦ **Peppermint (*Mentha piperita*) and other mints.** Peppermint owes its medicinal value to menthol, a cooling, anesthetic stomach soother. The eclectics, nineteenth-century physicians who combined herbs with the mainstream medicine of the time, recommended menthol vapors for morning sickness. The ancient Romans chewed mint sprigs to soothe their stomachs after large meals, hence our after-dinner mints (which don't contain real peppermint, despite their name).

Peppermint certainly works to relieve stomach distress, but according to my database, it is not the best source of menthol. Cornmint tops the menthol list, followed by mountain mint (which you should not use during pregnancy), watermint and Virginia mountain mint.

Just don't drink large amounts of strong peppermint tea, as some herbals warn that large amounts may trigger miscarriage. If my niece wanted to use peppermint tea, I'd suggest she drink no more than a cup or two at a time.

❧ **Black horehound (*Ballota nigra*).** This herb has a good reputation as a treatment for the nausea of motion sickness. I believe it's also useful as a treatment for vomiting due to pregnancy or nervousness.

Try black horehound alone or in this combination: one part black horehound, one part camomile and two parts meadowsweet. Meadowsweet contains an aspirin-like compound, so if a little aspirin upsets your stomach, you might replace this herb with ginger and/or citrus rind. Try a cup or two a day.

❧ **Cabbage (*Brassica oleracea*).** Raw or cooked cabbage, cabbage juice and/or sauerkraut are old-time remedies for stomach distress. Sauerkraut juice in particular is reportedly soothing to the overactive intestines that contribute to morning sickness.

❧ **Peach (*Prunus persica*).** The Chinese use the leaves and Europeans use the bark of the peach tree to make a tea for morning sickness. The leaves contain the compound benzaldehyde, which should be of some help in relieving this condition. If you opt for bark, don't use more than a teaspoon.

❧ **Raspberry (*Rubus idaeus*).** Tea made from raspberry leaves has been widely recommended for curbing the nausea of morning sickness. This use has not been investigated adequately enough. Still, I believe that folklore carries a good deal of weight, and the tea has a persistent reputation as a treatment for women's conditions, from menstrual cramps to morning sickness and labor pains.

Raspberry leaf is said to contain a constituent, readily extracted with hot water, that relaxes the smooth muscles of the uterus. I'd suggest drinking up to three cups a day. Or combine it with ginger, mint and a little lemon for a very pleasant anti-queasiness tea.

🍀 **Citrus fruits.** A little piece of grapefruit, orange or tanger-ine rind added to beverage teas has been reported to help relieve morning sickness.

🍀 **Juices.** Those who have juicing machines might consider a combination of ginger, kiwi, mint and pineapple; apple, carrot and ginger; or apple, fennel, ginger and peppermint or spearmint. The chemical constituents of these herbs lead me to suspect that they would all be useful in easing morning sick-ness. And what better way to banish this problem than with a healthy, tasty juice for breakfast?

Motion Sickness

O ur word *nausea* comes from the Greek word *naus*, mean-ing "ship." *Naus* is also the root of our word *nautical*. What does nausea have to do with nautical? If you've ever had seasickness, you know. Those old Greek sailors battled sea-sickness as well as actual storms at sea and mythical sea mon-sters.

Seasickness is just one form of motion sickness, the nausea, dizziness and I'd-rather-be-dead feeling that many people expe-rience on boats, cars, trains or planes.

Drugstores stock several different motion sickness remedies, most notably the antihistamine dimenhydrinate (Dramamine). Transderm Scōp, a patch that delivers the drug scopolamine through the skin, is a popular treatment, but it can cause side effects that prompt concerns about its safety. It has been known to cause hallucinations and convulsions in some people. And dimenhydrinate can also cause problems, making you drowsy and dopey.

Green Pharmacy for Motion Sickness

Fortunately, there's one herbal alternative that beats motion sickness drugs every time. I'm talking about ginger. It's not the only effective herbal remedy, but it's certainly the best that I'm aware of.

❦❦❦   Ginger (*Zingiber officinale*). Some years ago out in Utah, herbal pharmacologist Daniel Mowrey, Ph.D., author of *The Scientific Validation of Herbal Medicine* and *Herbal Tonic Therapies*, tested ginger head-to-head against dimenhydrinate. He rigged up a motorized chair guaranteed to cause nausea in anyone susceptible to motion sickness. The chair had a handle, allowing those seated in it to turn it off at will.

Dr. Mowrey recruited a bunch of people who got motion sickness. He gave half of them a standard dose of dimenhydrinate; the other half got one gram (about a half-teaspoon) of ginger. They all rode the chair and turned it off when they started feeling nauseated. Those taking the ginger lasted almost twice as long as those in the dimenhydrinate group.

Not long after Dr. Mowrey's study, other researchers recruited 80 naval cadets who were prone to seasickness and gave each of them one gram of powdered ginger. The researchers reported 38 percent less seasickness and 72 percent less vomiting among those cadets. Ever since those studies, every herbalist I know has trumpeted ginger for motion sickness.

Varro Tyler, Ph.D., dean and professor emeritus of pharmacognosy (natural product pharmacy) at Purdue University in West Lafayette, Indiana, endorses ginger: "To prevent motion sickness, swallow two capsules 30 minutes before departure and then one or two more as symptoms begin to occur, probably about every four hours."

I use ginger myself. It works. Sometimes I munch the ginger raw, but chances are that you'd prefer a few teaspoons in tea. You can also buy ginger capsules at health food stores. Or you can simply drink ginger ale, but if you do, make sure the label says that it's made with real ginger. A lot of ginger ale these days is artificially flavored.

Yet another ginger-filled remedy is my Stomach-Settler Tea: Chop up a two-inch section of ginger root and stir it in with dashes of camomile flowers, fennel, orange peel, peppermint and/or spearmint. Steep these with a few cups of water for 15 minutes. (You might also add a dash of cinnamon. Back in King Solomon's time, cinnamon tea was used to prevent nausea. Queen Peggy, Mrs. Duke, still uses it this way.)

If you have a juicer on hand, you might try juiceman Jay

Kordich's Ginger Jolt—two apples, one pear and a one-inch section of ginger root. If all you have is a blender, try this Digestive Delight from naturopath Michael Murray, N.D.: one cup of fresh pineapple chunks, one or two kiwifruits, a one-inch section of ginger root and a few pinches of mint.

☙ **Raspberry (*Rubus idaeus*).** Raspberry leaf tea is widely recommended for the nausea of morning sickness. Some herbalists also suggest it for motion sickness. I have no problem with that: Ginger and raspberry tea mix nicely.

Multiple Sclerosis

My best friend from college, now a dentist and jazz saxophonist who plays with a group imaginatively named Group Sax, was hit with multiple sclerosis (MS) around age 55. He asked my advice about this mysterious and elusive disease. I told him what I knew and about natural healing techniques that might be promising—some herbal oils and a few dietary approaches.

That was ten years ago. Apparently my advice helped. Like most MS patients, he has ups and downs, but when I last talked with him, he had a new girlfriend and was planning to attend the reunion of our Satterfield Big Band Jazz Orchestra. He and I both played with Satterfield during college at the University of North Carolina at Chapel Hill. For nearly 15 years now, we've been having reunions in Chapel Hill each August, playing big band numbers for one fun weekend a year. Despite my friend's MS, he's outlived quite a few other Satterfielders.

The Young People's Disease

Multiple sclerosis is a baffling, heartbreaking chronic illness of the nervous system that afflicts an estimated 350,000 Americans, about 60 percent of them women. Two-thirds of MS cases are diagnosed in people ages 20 to 40.

In MS, the protective myelin sheath that covers the major nerves breaks down, causing minute electrical malfunctions within the nerves. People with MS may experience an enormous array of possible symptoms, from minor weakness to paralysis. In most, however, the symptoms come and go. After each attack, or exacerbation, some people return to normal, while others experience residual disability.

Scientists are not sure what causes MS, but there are two major theories: MS often appears in clusters, leading some experts to theorize that a virus or viruslike microorganism is the culprit. Others believe that MS is an autoimmune disease. In this view, the immune system mistakes the myelin sheath for a threatening invader and attacks it.

A third theory has also been proposed, but it has received scant attention from conventional medicine. It links MS to a high-fat diet. Its originator, Roy L. Swank, M.D., Ph.D., professor emeritus of neurology at Oregon Health Sciences University in Portland and author of *The Multiple Sclerosis Diet Book*, claims impressive results in treating MS with a low-fat elimination diet.

Green Pharmacy for Multiple Sclerosis

Most dietary approaches to MS stress the importance of decreasing the amount of saturated fat in the diet—the kind of fat found in meat and dairy products. In addition, I'd also suggest some herbs.

🌿🌿🌿 **Stinging nettle (*Urtica dioica*).** I'd certainly flail myself with nettle if I had MS. This practice, known as urtication, involves taking the fresh plant, which is covered with tiny, hairlike stingers, and simply slapping it against your exposed skin. (Remember, you need to wear gloves whenever you handle this plant.) It stings and is irritating as all get-out, but it does provide microinjections of a number of potentially beneficial chemicals.

Among these compounds is histamine, the chemical that often induces allergies like hay fever. Several compounds in stinging nettle might have effects similar to bee stings. I know it sounds far-fetched, but some people with MS have benefited from being stung by bees, a form of therapy that is occasionally recommended by proponents of alternative healing methods for people with this condition.

I personally think people are better off using a potted stinging nettle plant rather than bees. Unlike the bees, which die after stinging you, the plant recharges its microinjector needles and can be used again and again. I don't consider nettle curative, but I believe it would help, and as I mentioned, I have heard testimony to this effect.

There are no reports in the United States of serious allergic reactions to stinging nettle, but there have been severe reactions to bee stings, including some fatalities.

❧

Dr. Swank's Low-Fat Diet

In the late 1940s, Roy L. Swank, M.D., Ph.D., professor emeritus of neurology at Oregon Health Sciences University in Portland and author of *The Multiple Sclerosis Diet Book*, who is now almost 90, first became interested in multiple sclerosis (MS). At that time, scientists were puzzled by the observation that the disease becomes more prevalent as one moves away from the equator. Rates in the United States, Canada, England, Scandinavia, Germany and Switzerland were higher than rates in Mexico and southern Europe.

A half-century ago, MS statistics were sketchy in most countries except Norway, which had instituted one of the first comprehensive disease-reporting systems. Dr. Swank looked at MS there, expecting to find more cases in the northern part of the country than in the south. Instead he found a completely different pattern. The MS rate was low along the entire north-south Norwegian coast, but considerably higher inland. What could account for the difference?

Using Norwegian diet surveys, Dr. Swank determined that the farm-based inland population ate a diet that was considerably higher in saturated fat (meats and dairy products) than the fishing-based coastal population. Intrigued, he reinterpreted the strange geographic distribution of MS: All of the northern countries with high

MS rates also consumed more saturated fats than the southern countries with low MS rates.

To test his theory, beginning in 1950—decades before dietary fat was linked to cancer, heart disease and other ills—Dr. Swank recruited 150 people with MS, placed them on a diet low in saturated fats and compared the course of their disease to that of a similar group who ate an unrestricted diet. After 20 years, those on the Swank diet experienced substantially fewer MS flare-ups, fewer deaths and less disability. (Their blood cholesterol levels also fell to an average of less than 150, substantially reducing their risk of heart disease.) The details of Dr. Swank's diet are available in his book.

There are many stories of the neurological deterioration of MS substantially slowing, and sometimes stopping, on the Swank diet, but it remains very controversial. The MS organizations do not endorse it.

I think it's probably worth trying. Even if the Swank diet doesn't help your MS, it would certainly help prevent cancer and heart disease because it is low in fat and high in fiber.

❧❧

Black currant (*Ribes nigrum*). Black currant oil contains a compound known as gamma-linolenic acid (GLA) that is thought to be useful in treating MS. Herb advocate Andrew Weil, M.D., professor at the University of Arizona College of Medicine in Tucson and author of *Natural Health, Natural Medicine*, strongly endorses GLA as an effective anti-inflammatory for treating autoimmune disorders. He recommends taking 500 milligrams of black currant oil twice a day and says improvement can be expected after eight weeks.

GLA can also be found in borage and evening primrose oil (EPO), but black currant oil may be cheaper. (I'm partial to EPO myself.)

Blueberry (*Vaccinium*, various species). These berries contain compounds known as oligomeric procyanidins (OPCs).

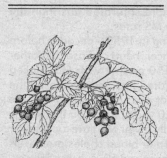

Black Currant

Black currant seeds contain the same anti-inflammatory substance that's found in evening primrose oil.

The biochemistry of OPCs is complicated, but there's good evidence to show that they help prevent the breakdown of certain tissues, such as the myelin sheaths that surround the nerve fibers. OPCs also have anti-inflammatory activity that might help relieve MS symptoms. This sounds like a good reason to eat more blueberries.

🌸🌸 **Evening primrose** (*Oenothera biennis*). Like black currant oil, EPO is rich in GLA. British herbalist David Hoffmann, author of *The Herbal Handbook*, says that EPO is "recommended in all cases" of MS.

🌸🌸 **Pineapple** (*Ananas comosus*). Pineapple contains enzymes, pancreatin and bromelain, that break up protein molecules. Besides being anti-inflammatories, these enzymes have been shown to help reduce the level of circulating immune complexes (CICs). High levels of CICs occur in a number of autoimmune diseases, including MS. These immune complexes activate the immune system to attack the body, ultimately leading to tissue damage.

🌸🌸 **Purslane** (*Portulaca oleracea*) **and other foods containing magnesium.** In a letter to the British medical journal *Lancet* some years ago, a British biochemist with MS said that supplemental magnesium by itself worked better for him than all other supplemental vitamins and minerals. He took 375 milligrams a day. (The Daily Value is 400 milligrams.) This is just one man's story—an anecdote—even though it comes from a biochemist and was printed in a respected journal. Still, from my point of view, it means that purslane and other sources of magnesium are worth trying. I know I would try them if I had MS.

If you'd like your magnesium from an herbal source, purslane is the herb richest in this mineral, at nearly 2 percent on a dry-weight basis, followed by poppy seeds, cowpeas and spinach. I steam purslane like spinach and eat it raw in salads. A heaping serving of steamed greens could provide as much magnesium as the biochemist took. So would eight ounces of fresh greens.

Nausea

One day a co-worker, who was also a friend and a registered nurse, told me that a friend of hers was experiencing a lot of nausea. She casually asked me what I'd recommend for relief. I immediately suggested ginger.

Six months later, she mentioned in passing that the ginger had worked. Only later did I realize that she wasn't asking for help for a friend. She herself had been on chemotherapy to treat cancer, and based on my recommendation, she had used ginger to relieve the nausea it often causes. Ginger's ability to treat nausea is that impressive.

This incident took place several years before I saw the published studies showing that ginger is helpful in relieving chemotherapy-induced nausea. (Chemotherapy patients should not take ginger if their blood-clotting ability is impaired, however.)

Nausea, as I'm sure you know, is that horrible abdominal sensation that makes you feel as if you're going to vomit. And vomiting means losing your lunch, plus a good deal of stomach acid as well, which is why it causes a burning sensation in the chest and throat.

Nausea and vomiting can be caused by many things: infections of the digestive tract (gastroenteritis), inner ear disorders, overindulgence in alcohol or foods, intestinal parasites, morning sickness in pregnancy, motion sickness, emotional stress and toxic overloads on the liver.

Green Pharmacy for Nausea

Frequently, one good upchuck is all it takes to relieve nausea. You just vomit and get it over with. But in other cases, nausea persists even after the stomach has emptied, and you try to vomit without result, a condition known as dry heaves. That's when the herbal remedies in this chapter might help.

❧❧❧ **Ginger** (*Zingiber officinale*). One study showed that ginger appears to be as effective as the prescription drug metoclopramide (Reglan, Clopra) in reducing the nausea and vomiting caused by cancer chemotherapy. This is one use for ginger that you should discuss with your doctor. If he says that your blood-clotting ability is impaired, you should not take this herb while undergoing chemotherapy.

Of course, ginger helps with nausea from less extreme causes as well. I discuss its anti-nausea benefits at some length in the chapters on morning sickness and motion sickness, but suffice it to say that for nausea and vomiting, ginger is many good herbalists' herb of choice.

Powdered ginger makes a pleasant-tasting tea, but when you're experiencing nausea, nothing seems to do the trick quite as well as ginger ale. Just check the label to make sure that it is made with real ginger; many ginger ales are artificially flavored.

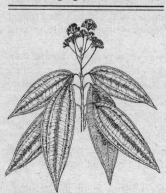

Cinnamon

Originally grown in southern Asia, cinnamon was used as a treatment for fever and diarrhea long before it became known as a kitchen spice.

❧ **Cinnamon** (*Cinnamomum*, **various species**). My wife takes cinnamon tea when she feels nauseated. It helps, and I'm not surprised. Cinnamon contains chemicals called catechins, which help relieve nausea.

Catechins also occur in agrimony, barley, bilberries, chinaberries, dog rose, English oak, hops, hawthorn, motherwort, northern red oak, olives, pears, pecans, sage, strawberries, tea and white willow.

❧ **Peppermint** (*Mentha piperita*). Peppermint tea is a powerful antispasmodic, meaning that it stops muscle spasms in the digestive tract, including those involved in vomiting. (But I wouldn't drink much of it if you're pregnant, since some herbalists have noted that large amounts of peppermint tea may lead to miscarriage.)

🐾 **Assorted essential oils.** Aromatherapy can also help relieve nausea and vomiting. Essential oils of peppermint and rosewood have been suggested for treating nausea. Oils of black pepper, camomile, camphor, fennel, lavender, peppermint and rose are recommended for relieving vomiting.

Place a drop or two of the essential oil or oils that you're trying in a tablespoon of vegetable oil and massage the mixture into your chest so the aroma can be inhaled easily. Remember, though, that essential oils are for external use only.

🐾 **Carminative herbs.** *Carminative* means "stomach-soothing." Carminatives are used mostly to treat indigestion and infant colic, but many respected herbalists also recommend them for nausea.

The carminative herbs I like best include camomile, dill, fennel, lemon balm and any of the mints. I'd suggest trying a tea made with a few teaspoons of one or more of these.

Osteoporosis

Osteoporosis, as you probably know, is a disease caused by loss of the mineral calcium and involves a weakening of bone. It is one of the most common conditions associated with aging, and it affects many more women than men. About 25 percent of women over 65 show signs of osteoporosis, while the figure for elderly men is less than 10 percent. Thin, petite women are at greatest risk. (My wife, Peggy, who is under 65 and formerly thin, has been diagnosed with osteoporosis.)

Osteoporosis causes a variety of possible symptoms: lower back pain, loss of height (up to several inches), stooped posture (dowager's hump) and increased risk of fractures, particularly of the hip. Currently, management of osteoporosis costs the United States some $6 billion a year.

Until quite recently, the Food and Drug Administration and

most physicians told us that supplements, including calcium, were a waste of time and money. Now, very belatedly, they tell us that we're not getting enough calcium. According to the 1995 National Institutes of Health (NIH) Consensus Development Panel on Optimal Calcium Intake, Americans (especially women) should get 1,000 to 1,500 milligrams a day. Unfortunately, most get much less than that, and many don't get even half that amount.

Getting the Full Spectrum of Nutrients

Ironically, the very doctors and federal officials on the NIH panel who would have said "food over supplements" a few years ago now seem to be saying "supplements over food" when it comes to calcium.

The panel did say that, ideally, people should get their calcium from foods such as low-fat dairy products, broccoli, tofu, kale, legumes, canned fish, nuts and seeds. But the panel's report also implied that this is impossible or at least impractical for the vast majority of Americans. The report spent a good deal of space telling people how to take calcium supplements—between meals, to minimize interference with iron absorption.

❧

Bone-Strengthening Broth

Here's a recipe that will appeal to the economy-minded woman who is eager to explore every possible avenue for preventing osteoporosis. Both the fish bones and the veggies provide generous amounts of calcium and other nutrients that prevent this debilitating disease.

In a large pot, place some leftover fish bones in a few quarts of water. (If the bones are really tiny, you might want to tie them in a cheesecloth bag to make it easier to retrieve them later.) Bring to a boil, then cover and simmer for 30 minutes. Add a couple of handfuls each of finely chopped cabbage, dandelion greens, stinging nettle greens, parsley, pigweed and purslane. (You'll need to wear gloves when harvesting stinging nettle greens, but the leaves lose their sting when the plant is cooked.) Simmer until the greens soften slightly.

Season to taste with salt and pepper and any other seasonings that appeal to you. Remove the fish bones before serving. Serve as a vegetable/herb soup topped with avocado slices and black pepper. Or use it as a stock for even heartier bean soups.

Properly prepared, a generous serving of my Bone-Strengthening Broth could easily contain generous amounts of calcium, magnesium, boron, beta-carotene (plus other vitamin A–like carotenoids) and vitamin C, as well as some vitamin D, fluorine and silicon.

❧

I have nothing against calcium supplements, but I firmly believe that everyone should get as much calcium as possible from foods. It's not only possible to do this, it's also better for your bones, because the mineral strength of bone depends on more than calcium. For calcium to actually strengthen bone, it must be consumed along with several other nutrients that few experts seem to talk about. Phosphorus is particularly important, but you also need magnesium, boron, zinc, vitamin D and vitamin A. You can get all of these nutrients from supplements, but I prefer to get them the way Nature intended—packaged all together in food.

The other news about osteoporosis that few people know is that high-protein diets leach calcium from bone. Nutrition experts I rely on suggest that people at risk for osteoporosis limit their protein intake to no more than one gram of protein per kilogram of body weight, which translates into around two to three ounces of protein—on the order of one chicken breast—daily for the average woman. Most Americans eat considerably more protein than this, thus running a risk of calcium loss even if they consume a lot of the mineral.

Green Pharmacy for Osteoporosis

If you're looking to consume less protein and more nutrients that help prevent osteoporosis, here are the plant foods I'd suggest.

🌿🌿🌿 Cabbage (*Brassica oleracea*). Boron helps raise estrogen levels in the blood, and estrogen helps preserve bone. In my database, cabbage ranks highest in boron content among leafy veggies with 145 parts per million (ppm) on a dry-weight basis.

I eat a lot of coleslaw, and it's easy to combine cabbage with high-calcium broccoli, kale, beans and tofu in salads and steamed vegetable dishes. Cabbage is also a key ingredient in my Bone-Strengthening Broth.

🌿🌿🌿 Dandelion (*Taraxacum officinale*). Speaking of boron, dandelion shoots run a close second to cabbage, with 125 ppm. Dandelion also has more than 20,000 ppm of calcium, meaning that just ten grams (just under seven tablespoons) of dried dandelion shoots could provide more than 1 milligram of boron and 200 milligrams of calcium.

Dandelion is also a fair source of silicon, which some studies suggest also helps strengthen bone. I recommend including it in my Bone-Strengthening Broth.

🌿🌿🌿 Pigweed (*Amaranthus*, various species). On a dry-weight basis, pigweed leaves are one of our best vegetable sources of calcium, at 5.3 percent. This means that a small serving of steamed leaves (⅓ ounce or ⅒ cup) provides a hearty 500 milligrams of calcium. Other good plant sources of calcium, in descending order of potency, include lamb's-quarters, broad beans, watercress, licorice, marjoram, savory, red clover shoots, thyme, Chinese cabbage (bok choy), basil, celery seed, dandelion and purslane.

🌿🌿 Avocado (*Persea americana*). As one reputed vegetable source of vitamin D (and the tastiest), avocado can help the body turn calcium into bone. Some people shun avocados because they are fairly high in fat, but if you eat a generally low-fat, vegetarian or semi-vegetarian diet, I don't see much harm in them, especially if you're at risk for osteoporosis. I suggest mashing an avocado into nonfat cottage cheese or yogurt so you get your calcium and some vitamin D at the same time. Avocados are also rich in heart-healthy vitamin E.

🌿🌿 Soybean (*Glycine max*) and other beans. Vegetarian

and Japanese women have a lower incidence of osteoporosis and fractures than Western or meat-eating women. The reason, according to James Anderson, M.D., of the University of Kentucky College of Medicine in Lexington, appears to be that Western-diet meat-eaters excrete more calcium in their urine.

Beans are a good source of protein, but they cause less calcium loss in the urine than meat. In addition, soybeans and other beans contain genistein, a plant estrogen (phytoestrogen) that acts like the female sex hormone in the body.

Pharmaceutical estrogen replacement helps preserve bone and prevent heart disease, but it also increases the risk of breast cancer. Genistein from beans has never been shown to increase cancer risk, and I'd be willing to bet that a diet rich in beans would strengthen bone and prevent heart disease almost as well as, or equally as well as, estrogen pills.

❧ **Black pepper (*Piper nigrum*).** According to my database, black pepper contains four anti-osteoporosis compounds. If you like pepper, you might consider sprinkling it generously on your avocado or bean soup or salad, assuming that every little bit helps.

❧ **Horsetail (*Equisetum arvense*).** French research suggests that silicon helps prevent osteoporosis and can be used to treat bone fractures. Horsetail is among the richest plant sources of this mineral, in the form of the compound monosilicic acid, which the body can readily use.

Aging and low estrogen levels decrease the body's ability to absorb silicon. Some people recommend up to nine 350-milligram capsules a day. You should use this herb only in consultation with a holistic practitioner. If you're advised to use horsetail tea, add a teaspoon of sugar to the water along with the dried herb. (The sugar will pull more silicon out of the plant.) Bring it to a boil, then let it simmer for about three hours. Strain out the leaves, then let the tea cool before drinking.

❧ **Parsley (*Petroselinum crispum*).** That dark green garnish, which is so often thrown away instead of eaten, is generously endowed with boron. It would take about three ounces of dried parsley to provide the three milligrams deemed useful in raising estrogen levels. That's more than most people want to consume, but every sprig helps.

In my database, parsley is also among the highest food sources of fluorine, another bone strengthener. Freshen your breath while you save your bones by routinely eating every sprig of parsley garnish placed on your plate in restaurants.

Overweight

I've always liked this letter:
"Please, please, please!!! I know how busy you must be, Dr. Duke, but I hope I'm not being too presumptuous asking for the recipe for those Lean Mean Bran Muffins that you mentioned in *USA Today*. Oh, do I need to activate my serotonin!!

"I never had a weight problem until ten years ago, when old age caught up with me. Please find it in your generous heart to honor my request, and help me shed those 25 unwanted pounds. Thank you for sharing your expertise (kiss, kiss, kiss!!!)."

That's what happens when you lay a little biochemistry on the national press. A few years back, a *USA Today* reporter interviewed me about natural secrets of weight control. For the most part, there are no secrets: Just eat a low-fat diet heavy on fruits, vegetables, herbs and whole grains and get plenty of exercise.

But you know the media—always looking for something new. So I mentioned to the reporter that serotonin is the brain chemical responsible for the feeling of satiety, and that pumping up one's serotonin might help people shut the refrigerator.

A key ingredient in serotonin is the amino acid tryptophan. Perhaps you've heard that tryptophan is a sedative. A few years back there was a big market for tryptophan supplements. Then some people got sick after taking supplements from a contaminated batch, and the Food and Drug Administration (FDA) overreacted by banning it from health food stores. But the FDA can't ban the tryptophan in food.

That's where my Lean Mean Bran Muffins come in. (The recipe is on page 418.) They provide plenty of tryptophan to support serotonin synthesis in the brain, which helps you get the message that you're full.

Green Pharmacy for Overweight

If muffins don't move you, you might try the herbs that may help people control their weight.

✺✺✺ **Plantain or psyllium (*Plantago*, various species).** Plantain is a leafy plant, and psyllium is the seed of the plant. In one Italian study, scientists gave women who were seriously obese—at least 60 percent over their recommended weight— three grams of plantain in water 30 minutes before meals. The plantain group lost more weight than a similar group of women who simply cut back on their diet.

Russian researchers have found that the weight-loss effect of plantain and psyllium is related to the spongy fiber (mucilage) in the seeds and to specific chemicals (polyphenols) in the leaves.

It may not be practical to make a plantain-in-water mixture, but getting psyllium is no problem at all, since Metamucil and similar products contain psyllium. Just mix a teaspoonful with juice or water and have it before each meal. You should watch how you react to this herb if you have allergies, however. If allergic symptoms develop after you take it once, don't use it again.

✺✺✺ **Red pepper (*Capsicum*, various species) and other hot spices.** In one experiment, researchers at Oxford Polytechnic Institute in England measured the metabolic rates of people on a standardized diet, then added a teaspoon of red-pepper sauce and a teaspoon of mustard to every meal. The study showed that the hot herbs raised metabolic rates by as much as 25 percent.

If you're trying to lose weight, you get another benefit from eating spicy foods. The hot spice stimulates thirst, so you drink more liquids. If you fill up on water instead of food, you'll obviously take in fewer calories and gain less weight.

So hot, spicy foods just might help you keep your weight down. One caveat, though: Many people use hot spices in barbecue sauce on high-fat foods such as spareribs, hot dogs and sausages. If you have a yen for barbecue sauce, skip the fat with my Hot Doggone. To a hot dog bun, add coleslaw, barbecue sauce, mustard and onions. I know it sounds weird, but this concoction is surprisingly satisfying. (It's best to leave out the hot dog, but if you must have one, make it vegetarian.)

✺✺ **Chickweed (*Stellaria media*).** This herb has quite a folk reputation as a slimmer. Try adding some to your diet and see what happens.

❧❧

Lean Mean Bran Muffins

After *USA Today* mentioned my Lean Mean Bran Muffin recipe, I got dozens of letters asking for it. Little did the letter writers know that I never make my concoctions— muffins, teas, soups, salads—the same way twice. I just use a handful of this and a pinch of that, depending on my mood and what I have on hand. But I know that most people prefer specific recipes, so I had my good friend, nutritionist Leigh Broadhurst, Ph.D., put this one together just for this book.

This recipe requires that you have access to evening primrose plants. Before starting the recipe, collect some evening primrose seeds. Store them in the refrigerator and just before making the muffins, grind them in a spice mill or an electric coffee grinder.

2	ounces bran flakes
¼	cup walnut pieces, sunflower seeds, or both
¼	cup raisins or dried cherries
2	tablespoons evening primrose seeds, ground
1	cup (4.5 ounces) unbleached all-purpose flour
⅔	cup (2 ounces) old-fashioned rolled oats
½	cup (2.5 ounces) stone-ground cornmeal
½	cup sugar
1–1½	teaspoons cinnamon, apple pie spice or pumpkin pie spice (optional)
2	teaspoons baking powder
¾	teaspoon baking soda
½	teaspoon sea salt
1	apple or pear, chopped
1	cup low-fat or nonfat buttermilk
1	large egg
3	tablespoons cold-pressed unrefined sesame oil
	Sesame seeds (optional)

Preheat the oven to 475°. Place the rack in the center of the oven.

Line a 12-cup muffin pan with paper muffin cups. (For best results, do not use a nonstick pan without paper liners.)

With your hands, crush the bran flakes into uniform small pieces, but not crumbs. In a small bowl, mix the bran flakes with the walnuts and/or sunflower seeds, raisins or cherries and evening primrose seeds. Set aside.

In a large bowl, stir together the flour, oats, cornmeal, sugar, baking powder, cinnamon or pie spice (if using), baking powder, baking soda and salt. Add the bran flake mixture and stir together.

Place the apples or pears, buttermilk, egg and oil in a food processor or blender and process until the fruit is coarsely pureed. Fold the fruit mixture into the flour mixture, stirring gently to combine.

Fill the muffin cups to the top and sprinkle the tops with the sesame seeds (if using). Place the pan in the center of the oven and immediately reduce the temperature to 375°. Bake for 20 to 25 minutes, or until the muffins are lightly browned and firm to the touch.

Let cool in the pan for a few minutes, then remove the muffins from the pan and place them on a rack to cool completely. Serve within 24 hours or store in an airtight container or a bag in the freezer.

Notes: Since cereals vary, you can use the label information on the bran flakes package to convert from weight to volume. Two ounces can be 1⅓ to 1½ cups, depending on the cereal.

Sesame oil is available in many health food stores and in Indian grocery stores.

Variation: Substitute 1 banana or 1 cup applesauce or other fruit sauce for the apple or pear.

Makes 12 muffins

❧

Some people eat it raw in salads, and some steam it and eat it like a vegetable. Personally, I prefer to disguise it by including it with other greens. If you want to try my Weed Feed mixture of slimming, edible weeds, mix chickweed, dandelion, evening primrose, stinging nettle (cooked and cooled), plantain and purslane. You can eat this mixture of fresh herbs in a salad. You can also cook all of the greens and perhaps spice them up with slimming hot sauce.

🌿🌿 **Evening primrose (*Oenothera biennis*).** If you'd rather not grind evening primrose seeds into flour as I suggest in my Lean Mean Bran Muffin recipe, try taking a half-teaspoon of evening primrose oil three times a day. The oil contains some tryptophan, but not as much as the flour.

🌿🌿 **Pineapple (*Ananas comosus*).** When I was in Costa Rica, staying at the Monte Verde Lodge and enjoying the beauty and comfort of the Monte Verde cloud forest, the owner of the lodge told me that he had lost 100 pounds on a pineapple regimen. He ate one whole fresh pineapple per day.

Although his story might sound apocryphal, there's more to a pineapple diet than you might think. Pineapple contains an enzyme called bromelain, which helps digest both proteins and fats.

🌿🌿 **Walnut (*Juglans*, various species).** You might think that nuts, which are high in fat, should be avoided by anyone who is trying to lose weight. But a study of more than 25,000 Seventh-Day Adventists showed that those who ate the most nuts were the least obese. Walnuts are our richest dietary source of serotonin, which, as mentioned earlier, helps make us feel full. Possibly the nuts produced feelings of satiety.

It is important to understand, however, that Seventh-Day Adventists are vegetarians who live a much healthier lifestyle than the typical American. It's not clear that nuts would help you control your weight if you're an omnivore eating both meat and vegetables. But you might experiment to see if eating a handful of walnuts helps you control food cravings.

Pain

The worst pain I ever had was caused by a slipped disk. It was just like the pain I'd experienced from time to time with gout—unbearable. My doctor did what doctors do: He gave me potentially addictive pain pills and nonsteroidal anti-inflammatory drugs. I took more drugs for that slipped disk than I'd ever taken in my life. I also took more herbs than I'd ever previously taken, trying to minimize the side effects of the pharmaceuticals.

Doctors recognize two kinds of pain, acute and chronic. Acute pain comes on suddenly, typically subsides with time and usually is alleviated with common pain relievers. Examples would be a headache or the pain of an injury. Chronic pain may begin as acute pain, but it lasts much longer—months or even years—and often cannot be relieved using standard therapies. Those with chronic pain often wind up in a personal hell. Their pain can make them depressed, and with depression the pain may become worse and be more difficult to treat.

If you have persistent pain, see a doctor for a diagnosis. Once the cause has been figured out, rational treatment becomes possible. But if, like many people who have chronic pain, you don't get a clear diagnosis and your pain goes on and on, I'd suggest consulting a pain clinic. These medical clinics, which are relative newcomers to the health-care scene, use a variety of drugs and alternative approaches to help you control your pain even if you can't completely eliminate it. Among the alternative approaches used in some pain clinics are exercise, meditation and biofeedback.

Green Pharmacy for Pain

There are also a number of herbs that can help.

✺✺✺ **Clove (*Syzygium aromaticum*).** Dentists around the country recommend clove oil as first aid for toothache, and in fact, it's what my mother used to give me for toothache. It works, and its use is endorsed by Commission E, the group that advises the German government on herbal medicine. You apply this oil directly to the painful tooth.

❧❧❧ **Red pepper (*Capsicum*, various species).** Red pepper contains pain-relieving salicylates, chemicals that are similar to salicin, the herbal equivalent of aspirin. In fact, red pepper once ranked as the best food-grade source of salicylates, although a new study has downgraded it considerably. This herb also contains capsaicin, a compound that stimulates the release of the body's natural painkillers, called endorphins.

Some folks like the spicy taste of red pepper. I know I do. I suggest using more of this wonderful spice in your cooking.

Capsaicin also works when used externally by interfering with substance P, a pain transmitter in the skin. So many studies have shown benefits from applying capsaicin externally that the Food and Drug Administration approved pain-relieving skin creams containing 0.025 percent capsaicin (Zostrix, Capzasin-P) for the treatment of arthritis and rheumatism. (If you use a capsaicin cream, be sure to wash your hands thoroughly afterward: You don't want to get it in your eyes. Also, since some people are quite sensitive to this compound, you should test it on a small area of skin to make sure that it's okay for you to use before using it on a larger area. If it seems to irritate your skin, discontinue use.)

❧❧❧ **Willow (*Salix*, various species).** Willow bark contains salicin. In fact, most plants contain some salicin or related salicylates. Just 100 years ago, aspirin was derived from several plants that contain more of these compounds than most: willow, meadowsweet and wintergreen. When medicines have been in short supply during wartime, doctors in some countries have successfully gone back to using willow bark for pain relief.

Commission E recognizes willow bark as an effective pain reliever for everything from headache to arthritis.

For many kinds of pain relief, I'd start with about a half-teaspoon of salicin-rich willow bark or up to as much as five teaspoons of white willow (*S. alba*), which has a lower salicin concentration. Of course, not everyone knows which species they have, and salicin content varies from species to species. So I'd suggest starting with a low-dose tea and working your way up to a dose that provides effective pain relief.

If you're allergic to aspirin, you probably shouldn't take aspirin-like herbs, either. Also, you should not give either aspirin or its natural herbal alternatives to children who have pain with viral infections such as colds or flu. There's a chance that they might develop Reye's syndrome, a potentially fatal condition that damages the liver and brain.

❧❧ **Evening primrose** (*Oenothera biennis*). This herb is one of our best sources of the amino acid tryptophan. In studies, tryptophan supplements have reduced pain caused by acute and chronic illness and also increased people's ability to tolerate pain. Naturopaths often recommend taking one gram of evening primrose oil four times a day to relieve the pain and nerve damage of diabetic neuropathy, a particularly painful condition that sometimes develops in people with diabetes. I'd suggest taking powdered seeds instead, because evening primrose loses much of its tryptophan in the oil-extraction process.

❧❧ **Ginger** (*Zingiber officinale*). Few people think of ginger as a pain reliever, but it is. In one study, researchers recruited 56 people—28 with rheumatoid arthritis, 18 with osteoarthritis and 10 with the painful muscle condition fibromyalgia—and gave them two to four teaspoons of powdered ginger a day. After three months, more than 75 percent reported significant pain relief with no side effects.

You can also use ginger externally. Hot ginger compresses seem to help relieve abdominal cramps, headache and joint stiffness. I'd suggest adding hot pepper to these compresses.

❧❧ **Kava kava** (*Piper methysticum*). This tropical herb contains two pain-relieving chemicals, dihydrokavain and dihydromethysticin, which have analgesic effectiveness comparable to that of aspirin. Although kava kava has been described as a narcotic, it is nonaddictive. When you chew the leaf, your mouth goes numb. As a result, this plant might be used to relieve the painful symptoms of sore throat, sore gums, canker sores or even toothache.

❧❧ **Lavender** (*Lavandula*, **various species**). Lavender oil is aromatherapy's top treatment for pain, and in fact, this oil was in on the ground floor of aromatherapy's beginnings. In the 1920s, aromatherapy's founder, French perfume chemist René-Maurice Gattefossé, happened to burn his hand in a laboratory accident. Plunging his hand into the nearest cool liquid, lavender oil, Gattefossé experienced rapid relief. Since then, researchers have discovered that some essential oils reduce the flow of nerve impulses, including those that transmit pain. In lavender oil, the key constituents appear to be linalool and linalyl aldehyde.

You can mix a few drops of lavender oil in a tablespoon of vegetable oil and massage it into the painful area.

❀❀ Mountain mint (*Pycnanthemum muticum*). This herb is high in pulegone, a chemical similar to capsaicin that also has pain-relieving effects. I suggest making a tasty tea, then using the spent leaves (or fresh ones) as a poultice on painful areas. (Don't use this treatment if you are pregnant, however.)

❀❀

Analgetea

Here's a pain-relieving herbal blend to keep on hand: willow bark, red pepper, cloves, ginger, peppermint and mountain mint. Just mix whichever of these herbs are available in proportions that appeal to your taste. You can use this mixture to make a tea whenever you feel the need, or you can make a poultice to apply directly to painful areas.

❀❀

❀❀ Peppermint (*Mentha piperita*). Menthol, the active constituent in peppermint, has anesthetic effects. In one study, scientists asked 32 people who had headaches to massage tincture of peppermint oil on their temples. This had significant pain-relieving effects. But if you try peppermint oil, be sure to dilute it by adding a few drops to a couple of tablespoons of any vegetable oil. Pure peppermint oil can be irritating to the skin. And never ingest the oil; a very small amount can be toxic.

❀❀ Sunflower (*Helianthus annuus*). Sunflower seeds are among the best sources of phenylalanine, a chemical involved in pain control. Studies suggest that phenylalanine helps reduce pain by inhibiting the breakdown of enkephalins, chemicals involved in pain perception. In studies with both humans and animals, phenylalanine makes acupuncture more effective at reducing pain. In laboratory rats, the chemical enhanced the effect of morphine and made it last longer.

If I were in pain, I'd eat a handful of sunflower seeds—I'm a habitual seed muncher anyhow—and use ground seeds in a poultice on painful areas.

✒✒ Turmeric (*Curcuma longa*). Many clinical studies agree that the curcumin in turmeric has anti-inflammatory effects, including a significant beneficial effect in relieving rheumatoid arthritis. But it takes more than a shake of the spice jar to gain this benefit. The dose naturopaths recommend is 400 milligrams three times a day. To get that much, you'd have to consume at least one-third of an ounce of this herb. So if you'd like to try turmeric for pain, I'd suggest taking capsules, even if you have to make your own. (Empty gelatin capsules can be purchased at health food stores.)

✒ Eucalyptus (*Eucalyptus globulus*). Aromatherapists often suggest adding eucalyptus oil to the pain-relieving essential oils of lavender and peppermint. The compound cineole, which is found in eucalyptus, speeds absorption of the other aromatic pain relievers through the skin. Remember, though, that these oils are best reserved for external use only.

✒ Rosemary (*Rosmarinus officinalis*). Commission E recommends using two to three teaspoons of dried rosemary to make a cup of pain-relieving tea. For a bath that will certainly relax you and may provide pain relief, fill a cloth bag with two ounces of rosemary and toss it into your bathwater.

Parkinson's Disease

B ack in 1991, I spent three minutes on the *CBS Morning Show* with Paula Zahn. The show, which was called "Meals That Heal," was about one of my favorite topics, using food as medicine. I happened to mention that fava beans have the potential to treat a variety of conditions, including Parkinson's disease. Shortly afterward, I received the following letter from a young woman: "Please send me . . . any research pertaining to Parkinson's. I coordinate a national group called Younger Parkinson People. An increasing number of people are now diagnosed in their early thirties. I am 43, diagnosed at 36. Please send any new information that might help us."

I sent the woman information on my top choice herb for treating Parkinson's disease—fava beans. But before I discuss these tasty and versatile beans in detail, I'd better say a word about Parkinson's disease.

It's actually a group of neurological disorders characterized by trembling and shaking, slowing of movement, loss of muscle control and muscle rigidity. An estimated 450,000 Americans have Parkinson's; most are over 60. Among the elderly, about 1 in 200 people has Parkinson's. There are approximately 50,000 new diagnoses each year. Men are more susceptible than women.

Parkinson's is a serious condition. Anyone who has it should be under a physician's care.

Green Pharmacy for Parkinson's Disease

In addition to following your physician's advice, there are several herbs that you might want to investigate. But if you're under a doctor's care for Parkinson's, you'll certainly want to confer before trying any natural therapies. Here are some options.

🌿🌿🌿 **Fava bean (*Vicia faba*).** These beans are one of Nature's best plant sources of a compound called L-dopa, the natural precursor of dopamine in the brain. In Parkinson's, an imbalance develops in the brain between two chemicals, dopamine and acetylcholine, usually due to degeneration of the cells that produce dopamine. If your brain makes less dopamine, taking L-dopa can help things along. L-dopa is a standard therapy for Parkinson's.

The trouble with L-dopa is that as a pharmaceutical it's very expensive, and lots of people with Parkinson's can't afford it. But fava beans are cheap. According to my calculations, it takes about a 16-ounce can of fava beans to get enough L-dopa to have a physiological effect on Parkinson's. At my supermarket, a 16-ounce can costs $1.15. Try buying pharmaceutical L-dopa for anywhere near that.

Even more intriguing, the latest news is that fava bean sprouts contain ten times more L-dopa than the unsprouted beans. That reduces the cost of a physiological dose to just over 10 cents—the cost of a handul of sprouts. Even though I've discussed the potential of fava beans with dozens of people over the last five years, I know of no one with Parkinson's disease who has taken the food approach seriously.

If you'd like to add fava beans to your diet, it's vitally important that you let your doctor know that you are doing so, and why. (It might help to take along a copy of this book.) Most cases of Parkinson's get off to a slow, mild start, and doctors don't usually prescribe L-dopa until the disease is more advanced. I suspect that eating more fava beans at this early stage would be really helpful. If you are already taking L-dopa, however, do not start eating these beans unless you discuss it with your doctor.

In addition to L-dopa, fava beans (and other legumes) also contain choline and lecithin. Some research suggests that these compounds might have positive effects in preventing Parkinson's or might help relieve some of its symptoms.

Fava beans are also high in fiber, which helps prevent constipation, a common problem in Parkinson's. But as I mentioned, to get a physiologically meaningful dose of L-dopa from fava beans, you have to eat a pound of them (or about two ounces of sprouts).

If you do decide to go with the beans, you have to deal with their notorious problem—gas.

For some people, beans get easier to handle intestinally as you eat more of them. In preparation for the CBS morning show, I ate a 16-ounce can of fava beans one day at lunch. Within two hours, the expected side effect ensued. The next day, I ate a second can. Again I became gassy, but not until four hours later. By the third can, on day three, my gut seemed to have adjusted, and gas wasn't much of a problem.

So, bean eaters, there is hope. And if your gut doesn't adjust, you can try Beano, an over-the-counter product that helps reduce flatulence from beans. It's available at most drugstores; just follow the directions on the label.

🦋🦋🦋 **Velvet bean (*Mucuna*, various species).** Like fava beans, velvet beans contain a generous amount of L-dopa, around 50,000 parts per million. But unlike fava beans, velvet beans have actually been used in clinical trials to treat Parkinson's.

The study with velvet beans was done by researchers at Southern Illinois University School of Medicine in Springfield under the leadership of B. V. Manyam, M.D. The researchers used a velvet bean preparation called HP-0, which is derived from the inner part of the bean. The HP-0 was standardized so that each gram of the preparation contained 33.33 milligrams of L-dopa.

From the trials, researchers concluded that their bean preparation was effective. Unfortunately, as far as I know, this preparation is still proprietary and experimental, so it's not available. But plain old velvet beans are. Like fava beans, they are high in fiber.

❧ ❧ Evening primrose (*Oenothera biennis*). Evening primrose oil (EPO) improved Parkinson's-induced tremors in 55 percent of those who took the equivalent of two teaspoons a day for several months. The oil contains traces of the amino acid tryptophan, which boosts the effectiveness of L-dopa. (Ground evening primrose seeds contain even more.)

Melvyn Werbach, M.D., assistant clinical professor of psychiatry at the University of California, Los Angeles, School of Medicine and author of *Nutritional Influences on Illness*, suggests taking two grams of tryptophan three times a day in combination with L-dopa for treating Parkinson's. Unfortunately, you can't get a tryptophan supplement because the Food and Drug Administraion banned it some years ago after a batch turned out to be contaminated. While you can still get tryptophan in evening primrose seeds, it would take nearly a quarter-pound of seeds to provide two grams of tryptophan.

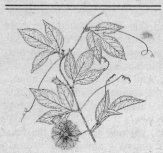

Passionflower

Passionflower, which is more widely used in Europe than in its homeland, America, may help combat Parkinson's disease.

As far as I'm concerned, every little bit helps. I think taking a couple of teaspoons of EPO a day or including ground seeds in your baked goods might be helpful.

❧ Ginkgo (*Ginkgo biloba*). Ginkgo is more widely used in stroke recovery and to treat Alzheimer's disease, but I believe it may also help with Parkinson's, because it improves blood circulation through the brain, delivering more L-dopa where it's needed. I suggest trying three capsules a day, each containing 300 to 500 milligrams of a standardized 50:1 ginkgo extract with 25 percent flavonoids. (This information will be on the label.) Just be aware that more than 240 milligrams a day may cause diarrhea, irritability and restlessness. If you experience any of these symptoms, try a lower dose.

🌹 **Passionflower (*Passiflora incarnata*).** Two herbalists whom I particularly respect, David Hoffmann, author of *The Herbal Handbook*, and Michael Tierra, recommend passionflower for treating Parkinson's disease. Many other herbalists do, too. Passionflower contains two reportedly effective anti-Parkinson's compounds—harmine and harmaline alkaloids. If I had Parkinson's, I would take 10 to 30 drops three times a day of a standardized tincture containing 0.7 percent flavonoids. (Again, you'll find this information on the label.)

🌹 **St.-John's-wort (*Hypericum perforatum*).** It's a curious thing: Smokers have an unusually low risk of Parkinson's.

Why? Apparently it's because nicotine increases the release of dopamine in the brain. Meanwhile, the enzyme monoamine oxidase (MAO) depresses dopamine, so it would make sense that medications that inhibit MAO (MAO inhibitors) would boost dopamine and decrease Parkinson's risk, just as nicotine does.

MAO inhibitors are a major class of antidepressant medications, and St.-John's-wort is one reported herbal MAO inhibitor. If I had Parkinson's, I'd try a St.-John's-wort tincture standardized to 0.1 percent hypericin and take 20 to 30 drops three times a day. Remember, though, that if you take an MAO inhibitor, whether pharmaceutical or herbal, on a regular basis, there is the possibility of interaction with some foods and medications. You should avoid alcoholic beverages and smoked or pickled foods, as well as cold and hay fever remedies, amphetamines, narcotics, tryptophan and tyrosine. You should not take St.-John's-wort if you're pregnant, and you should avoid intense sun exposure while using it, since this herb can make the skin more sensitive to sunlight.

Pneumonia

There we were in October of 1995, three musicians from different musical traditions trading tunes at the Napo Camp in Amazonian Peru. My shaman friend Antonio Montero Pisco was chanting his personal songs to the spirits of medicinal plants. While Antonio chanted, Joe Moreno, a music therapist from Maryville University in St. Louis, deftly scribbled away, transcribing the chants into musical notation.

Meanwhile, yours truly, a bad but enthusiastic bluegrass guitarist and bass fiddle player, sat there in awe of both of them. The year before, we had asked Antonio to tape record his chants to some 30 medicinal plants, including one called mucurita (*Petiveria alliacea*), an herb that smells like onion.

Later, Joe amazed Antonio by singing his chant back to him. Then Antonio and Joe sang it together, with Antonio accompanying them on his *shacapa*, a grassy fan that when shaken, sounds like brushes on a drum. It was one of those moments that only happen in the Amazon and keep me going back for more.

I tell this story because the plant my friends sang about is one of Antonio's mainstay treatments for respiratory infections. If I developed pneumonia, an American doctor would probably prescribe an antibiotic on the chance that I had a bacterial lung infection and not a viral one. But Antonio would prescribe mucurita, probably with some onions and garlic.

The sulfide compounds responsible for the aromas of these three plants have antiseptic, antibiotic and antiviral properties, and the bad breath they cause is a sign that the sulfides go right to the lungs, where they're needed.

Deep-Down Trouble

Pneumonia is a general term meaning any infection deep in the lungs. (Bronchitis, by contrast, is an infection in the gateway to the lungs, the bronchial tubes.)

Among infectious diseases in the United States, pneumonia is currently the leading killer and the nation's fifth leading cause of death overall, claiming more lives each year than

AIDS. Most of those deaths come from two sources: influenza, which may progress to pneumonia, especially in the elderly, and hospital-acquired infections in those who are ill from other causes but develop pneumonia because their weakened immune systems can't fight it off. Bacteria that cause pneumonia are so abundant in hospitals that according to *Consumer's Report on Health*, an estimated 4 percent of all patients develop the infection, probably as a direct result of their hospital stay.

Some 40,000 older Americans die of pneumonia every year, so it's nothing to fool around with. Others at risk include those with alcoholism, cancer, cirrhosis, heart or kidney failure, sickle-cell disease, spleen disorders or recent organ transplants.

Pneumonia may be caused by bacteria, fungi, protozoa or viruses, hence it is inappropriate to self-diagnose, much less self-medicate. Symptoms include shortness of breath, chest pain, coughing, difficulty breathing, fever and chills with shaking. If you develop pneumonia symptoms, you must see your doctor promptly.

Green Pharmacy for Pneumonia

In addition to taking whatever your doctor prescribes, you might try some herbal and nutritional alternatives, with your doctor's permission.

✿✿ **Astragalus (*Astragalus*, various species).** Also known as *huang qi*, astragalus is an immune booster and the Asian answer to our own echinacea. There's no reason not to use both.

✿✿ **Baikal skullcap (*Scutellaria baicalensis*).** Experimental data from China show that the root of this plant, which is close kin to our own skullcap, has broad-spectrum antimicrobial action. It inhibits flu viruses and several pneumonia-causing fungi. Chinese physicians sometimes inject a mixture of Baikal skullcap, goldthread and amur cork tree extracts to treat pneumonia, flu and other respiratory infections.

I'm not recommending injections. But if I had pneumonia, I would take mixtures of Baikal skullcap and our own golden antibiotic herbs: barberry, goldthread, goldenseal, Oregon grape and/or yellowroot. While baikal, the Asian form of skullcap, is hard to find in many herb shops and health food stores, it's not difficult to obtain in Chinese herb stores.

✿✿ **Dandelion (*Taraxacum officinale*).** Numerous clinical trials have demonstrated dandelion's effectiveness against pneumonia, bronchitis and upper respiratory infections, according to pharmacognosist (natural product pharmacist) Albert Leung, Ph.D.

I suggest cooking the greens and roots. Remember to drink the potlikker, the juice that remains after the greens are cooked. Although I can find dandelion 12 months of the year in Maryland, you may not have access to the fresh herb all year long where you live. You can also drink tea made from the dried herb, or you can take capsules.

✒✒ Echinacea (*Echinacea*, various species). Antibiotics may be indicated in bacterial pneumonia, but in any type of infectious pneumonia—bacterial, viral or fungal—I'd recommend herbs that enhance the immune system. Echinacea is one of the best. A wealth of scientific studies shows that it helps the body fight off all sorts of bacteria, viruses and fungi.

Echinacea preparations—teas and tinctures—have become very popular health food store products for treating colds, flu and bronchitis. If I had pneumonia, I'd take a teaspoon or two of tincture in juice or tea several times a day. (Although echinacea can cause your tongue to tingle or go numb temporarily, this effect is harmless.)

✒✒ Garlic (*Allium sativum*). Mary Bove, N.D., chair of the botanical medicine department at Bastyr University in Seattle and one of the nation's most highly trained herbalists, developed pneumonia when she was eight months pregnant. Her physician, predictably, prescribed antibiotics, but she rejected them in favor of six to ten cloves of chopped garlic a day, along with echinacea. She began feeling better after two days and was cured in two weeks.

Not surprisingly, Dr. Bove prescribes this treatment for pneumonia in her own naturopathic practice. Other naturopaths do, too. Jill Stansbury, N.D., a faculty member at the National College of Naturopathic Medicine in Portland, Oregon, urges her students to use garlic to treat respiratory and digestive tract infections. In fact, garlic is about the closest thing we have to an herbal wonder drug for treating infections.

✒✒ Goldenseal (*Hydrastis canadensis*). American Indians used goldenseal to treat all manner of infections, and white settlers adopted it because it works. It turns out that goldenseal has two broad-spectrum antimicrobial constituents, hydrastine and berberine.

To use this herb, buy a tincture at a health food store and follow the package directions. Other herbs with similar action include barberry, goldthread, Oregon grape and yellowroot. They are all fine used on their own, but I'd also suggest trying a mixture. And I would also encourage use of goldenseal as part of a comprehensive plan for treating pneumonia.

✺✺ **Honeysuckle (*Lonicera japonica*).** Chinese herbalists suggest honeysuckle for treating pneumonia, bronchitis, flu and colds, but they use the flowers in a preparation taken by injection. I don't recommend injecting this herb, but you can take it orally. Flower extracts are strongly active against many kinds of bacteria and viruses, and I wouldn't hesitate to use it myself.

In summer, you can boil a cup of flowers in a cup of water, then strain the tea before drinking it. In winter, you can strip off the old, dried leaves from a vine and use them to make a tea. Even better, you can take your honeysuckle in combination with forsythia. Forsythia also contains several potent antiseptic and some antiviral compounds. In winter, I sometimes make a tea with bare twigs of honeysuckle and forsythia and sweeten it with lemonade powder.

✺✺ **Onion (*Allium cepa*).** Onions are closely related to garlic, with many similar sulfur-containing compounds. Most herbalists consider garlic more effective, but onions are certainly beneficial. I recommend onion soup for respiratory complaints, including pneumonia. And if you prefer chicken soup for treating colds, flu, bronchitis and pneumonia, be sure to add some onions and garlic to the recipe.

✺ **Osha (*Lomatium dissectum*).** American Indians used this herb, rather suggestive of a parsley or dill plant, to treat all manner of respiratory ailments: pneumonia, influenza, colds, bronchitis, tuberculosis, hay fever and asthma. Some naturopaths have been calling for clinical trials to see if it might help treat pneumonia, which sounds like a good idea to me. In the meantime, you could try chewing on the root as American Indians do.

✺ **Sundew (*Drosera*, various species).** A major constituent of sundew, plumbagin, inhibits several of the bacteria that can cause pneumonia. The herb also contains a cough suppressant.

Commission E, the body of experts that advises the German government about herbs, recommends taking about two teaspoons of tincture a day to treat respiratory problems, including pneumonia.

Poison Ivy, Poison Oak and Poison Sumac

I'm about to confess to one of the reasons that I went into botany. One time, long ago when I was a kid, I was playing in a vacant lot on Mordecai Drive in Raleigh, North Carolina, and unknowingly used poison ivy as toilet paper. I got a bad rash in a bad spot, and it tormented me for more than a week. To avoid a repeat of that experience, I figured it would serve me well to learn how to recognize poisonous plants. Well, one thing led to another, and I wound up as a botanist.

Although I never repeated that particular mistake, I still have a fairly close, although mostly rash-free, relationship with poison ivy. A big patch of it has practically surrounded the mailbox at my Herbal Vineyard. If I don't thin it periodically, it becomes a problem for my neighbor, whose mailbox is next to mine and who is extremely sensitive to the plant.

So when the poison ivy grows into a sizable clump, I go out and grab a bunch of jewelweed, a succulent, orange-flowered annual that grows in moist meadows on my land. I crush a ball of it in my hands and rub myself down with its juice. Then I spend 15 or 20 minutes pulling up the poison ivy, rubbing myself with jewelweed juice periodically. The result? My neighbor is happy, and I never get a poison ivy rash.

Most but not all Americans are sensitive to the irritating oil, urushiol, that's found in plants like poison ivy, poison oak and poison sumac. Those who are sensitive develop a nasty, persistent, blistering rash after contact. It's not clear why some people are relatively or even completely immune to these oils. While it's estimated that some 350,000 Americans experience an episode of poison-plant rash each year, I suspect that figure is low. Many people never call their doctors, so it's hard to get a decent estimate.

Green Pharmacy for Poison Ivy, Poison Oak and Poison Sumac

The traditional drugstore remedy for reactions to poisonous plants is calamine lotion. It cools the hot rash and relieves some of the itching. But personally, I think several herbal approaches work even better.

⚘⚘⚘   Jewelweed (*Impatiens capensis*). I'm not the only fan of jewelweed for preventing the unpleasant symptoms that develop following exposure to poisonous plants. Increasingly, at workshops where I mention it, participants chime in with their own jewelweed stories. I'm well aware that these stories, and my own, are what scientists call anecdotes and therefore are open to scientific skepticism. But seeing is believing. Pile up all the anecdotes, and they make a pretty convincing case.

Of course, experimental evidence is even better. That's why, whenever I teach a three-day class on medicinal herbs, I treat my students to a dramatic little demonstration. I find a poisonous plant, usually poison ivy. I apply its juice to the sensitive undersides of both of my wrists. A minute or two later, I wipe one wrist with a ball of crushed jewelweed leaves and stems. Three days later, the wrist that I didn't treat with jewelweed shows the typical itchy, blistery poison-plant rash. The wrist rubbed with jewelweed invariably shows much less of a rash, and sometimes none at all.

My friend Robert Rosen, Ph.D., a chemist at Rutgers University in New Brunswick, New Jersey, is a whiz at isolating chemical substances from plants. He may have come up with an explanation for jewelweed's effectiveness. Urushiol does its dirty work by binding to skin cells and triggering the rash-producing irritation. A mere one-billionth of a gram of urushiol is enough to affect those who are highly sensitive.

Dr. Rosen has identified the active ingredient in jewelweed as a chemical called lawsone. This substance binds to the same molecular sites on the skin as urushiol. If applied quickly after contact with a poison plant, lawsone beats the urushiol to those sites, in effect locking it out. The simple result is that you don't get the rash.

The greatest concentrations of lawsone are not necessarily found in jewelweed leaves. Although the leaves have some lawsone, there may be more in the reddish protuberances that resemble little prop-roots extending out from the lower stem near ground level. Apply the juice from the crushed red knobs, and you'll probably get better protection.

∾∾ Aloe (*Aloe vera*). The gel inside leathery aloe leaves has been shown again and again to help heal burns and other skin problems. Herbalists also recommend using it to help soothe and heal the rash that follows contact with poisonous plants. If I got a rash that I suspected came from a poisonous plant, I'd slit open a fresh aloe leaf and wipe the gel on the affected area.

∾∾ Plantain (*Plantago*, various species). The prestigious *New England Journal of Medicine* reported that poultices made from plantain leaves can help control the itching of poison ivy.

∾∾ Soapwort (*Saponaria officinalis*). Doctors used to recommend that as soon as you realize you've been exposed to a poisonous plant, you should vigorously wash the area with soap and water to get rid of the urushiol. If you're outdoors without ready access to soap, you can try the juice of the soapwort plant to wash yourself.

I'm singling out soapwort here, but I believe that any of the "soapy" plants that contain compounds known as saponins might work better than soap and water in minimizing the irritating effects of urushiol. Other plants high in saponins include horse chestnut, licorice, seneca snakeroot, soapbark, rose leaves and gotu kola. (Remember, I'm calling for external use of these plants. Horse chestnut and seneca snakeroot are inedible.)

Pregnancy and Delivery

I'm very pleased with my part-Cherokee, part-redneck grandson, John James Duke, born August 13, 1993. I have enjoyed introducing him to the pleasures and perils of my raspberry patch, a tangle of vines where the sweet berries beckon and the thorns threaten.

The way we work it, I pull out a fruit-bearing branch with gloved hands, and he picks off the ripe, sweet berries.

Whenever we do this, I can't help but consider the raspberry's popularity among herbalists for calming the uterus during pregnancy and facilitating delivery.

Green Pharmacy for Pregnancy and Delivery

Raspberry is probably the best-known herb for pregnancy, but it's just one of many that are useful.

Before I discuss the individual herbs, I should mention that these days obstetricians insist that their patients let them know about any over-the-counter medications, vitamins, supplements or herbs that they take. This is a good rule to follow. The herbs I'm listing here have centuries of safe use behind them, but every woman—and every pregnancy—is different. Please let your doctor know about any herbs that you want to try.

And do pay careful attention to the properties that these herbs have. Some help settle an irritable uterus and help make pregnancy more comfortable. Others can hasten delivery.

❀-❀-❀ Partridge berry (*Mitchella repens*). Around 1860, in an old, long-gone medical journal called *Botanic Physician*, a Dr. Smith heaped praise on partridge berry: "This is an invaluable plant for child-bearing women. I first obtained knowledge of its use from a tribe of Indians in the west part of New York. The squaws drank it in decoction for two or three weeks previous to and during delivery, and it was the use of it that rendered that generally dreaded event so remarkably safe and easy with them."

Partridge berry remains popular today, particularly with women herbalists. Jeannine Parvati, author of a fascinating book, *Hygieia: A Woman's Herbal*, calls partridge berry her favorite pregnancy herb. She often combines it with raspberry, black haw, blessed thistle, licorice or sarsaparilla. Parvati suggests using the herb just before delivery.

❀-❀-❀ Raspberry (*Rubus idaeus*). I'm sold on raspberry for complaints of pregnancy. One study identified a chemical in raspberry that relaxes the uterus. For centuries, women prone to miscarriage have been urged to drink raspberry leaf tea throughout their pregnancy to help them carry the baby to term. The herb is also reportedly useful in preventing many of the discomforts of pregnancy, including morning sickness.

Chances are that this herb's close botanical relatives, blackberries, dewberries and wineberries, would offer similar benefits.

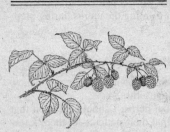

Raspberry

Raspberry, a member of the rose family, was recommended by seventeenth-century herbalists for pregnancy complaints.

❧❧ **Black haw (*Viburnum prunifolium*).** Also called crampbark, this herb was recognized in most nineteenth-century pharmacy reference books as a treatment for painful menstrual cramps and threatened miscarriage. Today herbalists continue to recommend it for those conditions as well as to treat the discomforts of pregnancy. It seems to soothe the uterus.

❧❧ **Blue cohosh (*Caulophyllum thalictroides*).** Several years ago, a chemist friend came out to Herbal Vineyard with his wife, a nurse, who was close to full term and obviously ready to bear fruit. She said that she wanted to get it over with and asked what I recommended. I said that as a botanist I could not recommend, but if I were in her shoes and trying to speed up delivery, I might try blue cohosh.

American Indians used blue cohosh to induce labor, and with good reason. This plant contains the compound caulosaponin, a powerful stimulator of uterine contractions.

I need to let you know that there are a few anecdotes suggesting that getting an overdose of blue cohosh might be harmful before term, possibly even causing loss of the baby. So I would strongly advise against using this herb unless you discuss it with your doctor.

But remember my oft-repeated lament. If there's an anecdote about some harm caused by an herb, the medical establishment latches onto it as a fact. But if there are 100 anecdotal accounts of benefits from an herb, those anecdotes remain "just anecdotes."

The bottom line here is that if my own daughter were blue about a slow delivery and wanted to get on with it, I would suggest using blue cohosh tincture.

Maine herbalist Deb Soule, founder of Avena Botanicals and author of an interesting and well-reasoned feminist herbal, *The*

Roots of Healing, suggests using 20 to 30 drops of blue cohosh tincture to induce labor. Having spent some time with her in the North Woods, I have great respect for Soule and her women's health herbal formulas.

❦❦ **Jute (*Corchorus olitorius*).** Jute is one of the best natural sources of folate (32 parts per million on a dry-weight basis). Folate (the naturally occurring form of folic acid) is the B vitamin that helps prevent the often-fatal spinal malformation known as spina bifida. (For just this reason, an obstetrician will usually recommend a folic acid supplement to pregnant women.) Lentils also contain fairly high levels of folate.

❦❦ **Parsley (*Petroselinum crispum*).** Parsley contains the compound apiole, a uterine stimulant that was once used to induce abortions. In Russia, a product called Supetin that contains mostly parsley juice is used to stimulate uterine contractions during labor.

The herb contains such a small amount of apiole that there's little need for concern if you use culinary amounts. I even encourage eating parsley for its folate. You might want to avoid eating large amounts of parsley, such as you might find in tabbouleh salad, while you're pregnant, however. And do avoid using parsley for medicinal purposes unless you're about to deliver and are not concerned about hastening things along. There's an unconfirmed rumor from Germany that parsley contains progesterone.

❦❦ **St.-John's-wort (*Hypericum perforatum*).** Soule suggests that this herb's blood-red oil is "a must to have at all births." The oil is very soothing when rubbed on the perineum, the tear-prone area between the vagina and anus, during labor. Following delivery, it's even more valuable. Its soothing, anti-inflammatory action eases burning and swelling and speeds the healing of perineal tears.

❦❦ **Shepherd's purse (*Capsella bursa-pastoris*).** Soule suggests taking 40 to 60 drops of tincture soon after giving birth to help stop bleeding. This advice makes good sense, as the herb's ability to constrict blood vessels has been documented scientifically.

❦❦ **Spinach (*Spinacia oleracea*).** Because it's so rich in folate, spinach ranks second highest in my database among plants that might help prevent spina bifida and other related defects. Spinach is also relatively high in zinc. When women are deficient in zinc, they experience birthing difficulties and slower wound healing. Nonvegetarians get most of their zinc from meat, so if you're a vegetarian, be sure to eat spinach, especially if you're pregnant.

You could also make a soup that includes some or all of the following ingredients: spinach, endive, asparagus, parsley, okra, pigweed and cabbage. And make sure that you have whole-wheat bread with your soup, since you can get twice as much folate from whole-wheat as from white bread.

❧ **Herbal formulas.** The following are some of Soule's sensible formulas for pregnancy, based on her 12 years of experience with backwoods medicine in Maine.

To prevent miscarriage, she recommends two parts black haw, one part false-unicorn root and one part wild yam. Mix their tinctures using 20 drops of black haw and 10 drops each of false-unicorn root and wild yam, she suggests. Drink this mixture two to four times a day as a general preventive. If there's a problem with spotting, take the formula every two hours until spotting stops.

For a tea to prevent miscarriage, Soule suggests two tablespoons of lemon balm (also known as melissa) and partridge berry leaves and one tablespoon each of stinging nettle leaves, oatstraw and raspberry leaves steeped in a quart of boiling water. Drink up to three cups a day.

For delivery, she recommends a tea made with two parts each of holy basil, lavender and lemon balm and one part each of borage and pansy flowers. Alternate this with raspberry leaf tea.

For postpartum support, especially after cesarean sections, Soule recommends a tincture of three parts bupleurum, two parts dandelion root and one part each of astragalus, blessed thistle and wild yam.

To help repair perineal tears, she suggests herbal sitz baths with calendula, yarrow flowers and comfrey leaves added to the water.

Because I know Soule and have a great deal of respect for her herbal wisdom, I would not hesitate to suggest her books and these formulas to my daughter, were she in a birthing mode. They all seem like safe and sound formulas to me.

Premenstrual Syndrome

I recently read about a bumper sticker that said: "Warning: I have PMS and I have a gun." Maybe the woman driving the car should take a bead on the Food and Drug Administration (FDA), which has tried mighty hard over the years to discourage the use of evening primrose oil (EPO) for treating the irritability and other symptoms of premenstrual syndrome (PMS).

I'm a botanist, not a doctor, so I'm leery of prescribing medicine, especially in the realm of women's health. But from everything I know about primrose oil, I would encourage my daughter, or any other woman, to try EPO. I have also taught many women who have PMS to gather this American Indian food plant and make a cereal containing EPO out of the seeds.

PMS describes a variety of possible symptoms that can occur as a woman approaches menstruation: anxiety, bloating, breast tenderness, irritability, moodiness and weight gain. Most authorities believe that all of these symptoms are caused by changes in the levels of female sex hormones, estrogen and progesterone, that precede menstruation.

The higher the estrogen level, scientists say, the greater the risk of PMS. Estimates vary, but some 25 to 50 percent of menstruating women suffer some degree of PMS, with 8 to 15 percent experiencing severe symptoms.

Green Pharmacy for Premenstrual Syndrome

Fortunately, there are any number of herbs, including evening primrose, that can help relieve the symptoms.

🌿🌿🌿 **Chasteberry (Vitex agnus-castus).** The small fruits of the chaste tree have been used for menstrual disorders since Greco-Roman times.

Researchers have found that chasteberry helps relieve PMS because of its effects on female sex hormones. It helps balance hormones produced during women's monthly cycles, increasing production of luteinizing hormone and inhibiting the release of follicle-stimulating hormone. This leads to a shift in the estrogen-progesterone ratio, resulting in less estrogen to cause or aggravate PMS.

The only caveat is that women who have PMS with significant depression should probably steer clear of chasteberry. Some research suggests that PMS with depression is caused by excess progesterone, and chasteberry is said to raise progesterone levels.

For most women, though, chasteberry works. In one year-long study, women with PMS took either 175 milligrams a day of chasteberry extract or 200 milligrams a day of vitamin B_6, a frequently touted supplement that is said to quell PMS. Chasteberry proved clearly superior to the B_6.

At least one chasteberry product is approved in Germany for use as a treatment for PMS, menstrual complaints and breast tenderness. You can buy both the herb itself and herbal tinctures in many stores that carry herbal products.

꒰꒰꒰ Chinese angelica (*Angelica sinensis*). One of the most respected herbs in Chinese traditional medicine, Chinese angelica, or *dang-quai*, is used primarily as a women's tonic to treat PMS and menstrual cramps. Many women take two capsules twice a day to prevent PMS. (You should not use Chinese angelica if you are pregnant.)

꒰꒰꒰ Evening primrose (*Oenothera biennis*). For centuries, American Indian woman have been chewing the seeds of the evening primrose for premenstrual and menstrual complaints. And EPO is an approved PMS treatment in Great Britain.

I'm not the only herb lover who touts EPO for PMS. The word is getting out. On my last pharmacy ecotour to Costa Rica, I overheard a conversation between two women pharmacists who did not know that I was within earshot. One said she took one EPO capsule a day all month until she felt her PMS coming on, then upped her intake to four capsules a day until her period was over. She said she'd been doing this for several years and had persuaded all of her co-workers, five other women, to adopt the same regimen.

"The six of us," she said, "have been working together so long that our periods have almost become synchronized. I'd hate to think what would have happened without EPO—all of us with PMS at the same time each month."

I give a lot of speeches about herbal medicine around the

world, and I like to tell my audiences about EPO. After one speech, a woman proudly told me that she'd been taking EPO for her PMS for years, and she had experienced substantial relief. Then, in a whisper, she confided that she worked for the FDA, the very agency whose regulations have sometimes denied this valuable natural treatment to the millions of American women who suffer premenstrual discomfort.

I should make it clear here that EPO is now available commercially for women to use. What I'm complaining about is that the FDA forbids labeling this product as helpful in treating PMS.

The FDA should know that EPO is not harmful. And in addition to the woman I met, many people within the FDA know that it alleviates PMS symptoms. But the agency won't approve it because it does not accept the British safety and effectiveness studies.

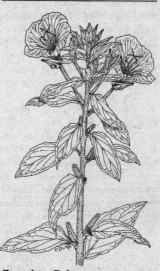

Evening Primrose

The leaves and flowers of evening primrose, an American Indian food plant, produce a valuable seed oil that helps relieve premenstrual complaints.

The FDA needs American studies submitted by a U.S. pharmaceutical company intent on marketing EPO. But a drug company would have to register EPO as a new drug and spend up to $500 million to prove it safe and effective. What pharmaceutical firm in its right mind would invest half a billion dollars to prove that EPO relieves PMS when anyone can simply go out and forage the seeds and use them?

Around Maryland, where I live, evening primrose seeds can be harvested free all winter long. I have gathered as much as a pound during a two-hour outing. And whether you gather the seeds yourself or purchase EPO at a natural food store or pharmacy, there's nothing to stop you from using EPO to treat PMS.

❦❦ Stinging nettle (*Urtica dioica*). This is a traditional liver tonic often recommended for ridding the body of all kinds of toxins. When the liver is sluggish, it processes estrogen slowly, contributing to the high levels that may cause or aggravate PMS. This herb can also reduce bloating and breast tenderness. I suggest trying a tea made with equal parts of stinging nettle and burdock.

❦ Burdock (*Arctium lappa*). Burdock is also a traditional liver tonic, and I believe that its mild stimulating effects on that organ make it useful for treating the irritability of PMS. Burdock is also mildly diuretic, which means it may help relieve PMS-related bloating and breast tenderness, both of which are associated with too much fluid in the system.

❦ Raspberry (*Rubus idaeus*). Raspberry is best known as a pregnancy tonic that quiets an irritable uterus. But I've heard many good herbalists praise it for helping to treat PMS as well. As a safe and tasty beverage, it's probably worth a try.

❦ Skullcap (*Scutellaria lateriflora*) and valerian (*Valeriana officinalis*). Both of these herbs are sedative/tranquilizers that might help relieve the nervous tension and irritability of PMS.

❦ Soy products, peanuts and other legumes. Tofu and other soy products contain natural but weak plant estrogens (phytoestrogens) that limit the uptake of the estrogen produced by the body. This anti-estrogen effect has been credited with helping to prevent breast cancer, and I don't see why it wouldn't also help ease the symptoms of PMS. Although soybeans have gotten a good deal of attention because they contain the estrogenic compound genistein, peanuts, black beans and lima beans often contain even more of this compound. And the scurfy pea (*Psoralea corylifolia*) has some 50 times more genistein than soybeans.

Prostate Enlargement

The prostate is a small gland that only men have. It sits just above the rectum and provides a good deal of the fluid in semen. Unlike most body parts, the prostate gland grows larger as men age, a condition known as benign prostatic hypertrophy (BPH). By age 40, 10 percent of men have some degree of prostate enlargement. But at age 50, the figure is 50 percent, and it keeps increasing as the years pass. Why is this cause for concern?

The male urethra, the tube through which urine passes, is encircled by the prostate gland. As the prostate grows larger, it pinches the urethra, causing BPH symptoms. It becomes harder to urinate forcefully, and men with BPH have difficulty emptying the bladder completely. The hallmark symptom is having to get up at night to urinate.

Throwing Down the Gauntlet

I'm betting my own prostate gland that herbal treatments work better than the most commonly prescribed drugs or surgery for controlling BPH, also called noncancerous prostate enlargement.

The prescription drugs finasteride (Proscar) and terazosin (Hytrin) have become big moneymakers because they are the only pharmaceuticals that are approved to prevent prostatic proliferation, the growth of new prostate cells that causes BPH in men over 50.

I announced my intentions to challenge Proscar with the herbal alternatives, saw palmetto, licorice and pumpkin seeds, in the early 1990s, shortly after the Food and Drug Administration (FDA) approved the drug. I did it publicly at a conference in front of dozens of officials from the FDA and the National Institutes of Health (NIH). I wanted all of the "magic bullet" proponents to see that not everyone thought that a prescription drug was the best answer for BPH.

I publicly bet my prostate gland that my mixture of saw palmetto, licorice and pumpkin seeds, which I blend into something I call Prosnut Butter (see page 449), would do the same thing that Proscar does. I also declared that it was cheaper and probably safer.

The other reason that I bet my prostate in public was that I wanted to make some progress toward fulfilling my life's ambition, which is getting the FDA to make the drug companies test their new synthetic drugs not only against an inactive substance (a placebo) but also against any known or suspected herbal alternative.

If the synthetic proves to be better than the placebo and the herbs, then, fine, approve the drug. But if the herbs prove to be better, or even reasonably close in effectiveness, then both should be approved. To recoup its investment in the research, the pharmaceutical firm could get some marketing privileges for the processed herb extract as well as its new synthetic. This way, people could have a choice between the pharmaceutical, which is always much more expensive, and the herbal alternative, which is always cheaper.

A year's supply of Proscar costs about $800. A year's supply of saw palmetto and licorice would be only a small fraction of that, and if you stocked up on pumpkin seeds around Halloween, you could get them dirt cheap, possibly even for free.

Until Proscar and Hytrin came along, the only medically recognized treatment for BPH was surgery. One procedure is known as transurethral resection of the prostate (TURP). TURP is the most common operation performed on men over 65. During a TURP, the urologist threads an instrument up the urethra and cuts away part of the prostate gland to enlarge the opening for the urethra, thus easing urine flow. TURP generally works well, but it is expensive and carries the usual risks of surgery, and recovery takes a week or two.

Proscar and Hytrin have been widely hailed as alternatives because they're cheaper and less traumatic than surgery. But herbs are cheaper still.

Herbs on Trial

The drugs keep prostate cells from proliferating by preventing the gland from converting the male sex hormone testosterone into a related compound, dihydrotestosterone, that stimulates prostate cell proliferation.

While the drugs do indeed prevent this process from occurring, the natural alternatives that I mentioned work at least as well. In fact, in my opinion, and in the opinions of many naturopathic physicians, the herbs work a whole lot better.

Proscar, especially, has definite drawbacks. Most men must take it for at least six months before any significant improvement becomes apparent. And it doesn't work for everyone. Fewer than half of men taking Proscar experience significant clinical improvement even after one year.

Proscar also has some disturbing side effects, among them decreased libido, ejaculatory problems and erection loss. In contrast, herbs like saw palmetto, licorice and pumpkin seeds are not reported to cause any of these problems.

Green Pharmacy for Prostate Enlargement

Here are the details about the herbs that I can say without reservation provide the best results.

❧❧❧ **Licorice (*Glycyrrhiza glabra*).** Licorice contains a compound that prevents the conversion of testosterone to dihydrotestosterone. Taking very large doses of licorice for a long period of time can produce headache, lethargy, sodium and water retention, excessive loss of potassium and high blood pressure. Some 25 cases have been documented in the world medical literature, and the people who developed problems ate two to four ounces of real licorice candy a day for years.

I doubt that the licorice extract in my Prosnut Butter would cause any problems. I've personally experienced no symptoms. But if you try the herbal approach to BPH, be alert to any symptoms and cut down drastically on your licorice intake if you experience them.

❧❧❧ **Pumpkin (*Cucurbita pepo*).** Pumpkin seeds were the traditional treatment for BPH in Bulgaria, Turkey and the Ukraine. The recommendation was a handful of seeds a day throughout adulthood.

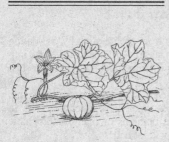

Pumpkin

This orange fruit is more than a Halloween prop: Its seeds contain a substance that can help relieve prostate problems.

The fatty oil in pumpkin seeds is a powerful diuretic, a fact that has caused some nay-sayers to assert that any increased urine flow has nothing to do with relief from BPH. Pumpkin seeds, however, also contain chemicals called cucurbitacins that appear to prevent some transformation of testosterone into dihydrotestosterone.

In addition, pumpkin seeds can contain as much as eight milligrams of zinc per half-cup serving. Naturopaths Joseph Pizzorno, N.D., president of Bastyr University in Seattle, and Michael Murray, N.D., co-authors of *A Textbook of Natural Medicine*, suggest taking 60 milligrams of zinc per day for treating BPH. (This is much more than the Daily Value, so be sure to check with a doctor before you begin taking this much zinc.)

Zinc has been shown to reduce the size of the prostate, presumably by inhibiting the conversion process mentioned earlier. Pumpkin seeds are also high in certain amino acids—alanine, glycine and glutamic acid. Dr. Murray and Dr. Pizzorno report that in a study of 45 men who were given supplements of these amino acids (200 milligrams of each) every day, the regimen significantly relieved BPH symptoms.

A half-cup serving of pumpkin seeds can have 1,150 to 1,245 milligrams of alanine, 1,800 to 1,930 milligrams of glycine and 4,315 to 4,635 milligrams of glutamic acid. That's anywhere from 5 to 20 times the doctors' daily recommendation.

For all of these reasons, plus good flavor, I stress a good quantity of pumpkin seeds in Prosnut Butter.

There are some other seeds that contain these beneficial amino acids. Buffalo gourd seeds contain generous amounts of all three, peanuts and sesame seeds are high in glycine, and almonds, butternuts and peanuts are high in glutamic acid.

🌺🌺🌺 **Saw palmetto** (*Serenoa repens*). Shortly after

Proscar was approved by the FDA, the agency banned all non-prescription drugs for BPH. The ban was imposed for two reasons, according to Varro Tyler, Ph.D., dean and professor emeritus of pharmacognosy (natural product pharmacy) at Purdue University in West Lafayette, Indiana. First, the FDA said that no credible evidence was presented to show that any over-the-counter (OTC) products were effective. Second, the agency expressed the view that people who used the OTCs might delay getting proper medical treatment as their condition worsened.

❧

Prosnut Butter

Do you like peanut butter and crackers? Do you think maybe you could munch a few every day as a snack? If your answer is yes, then you might even enjoy this "medicine" for benign prostate enlargement (BPH).

The three ingredients in this nutty spread, pumpkin seeds, saw palmetto and licorice, have all been shown to help prevent and relieve BPH:

To make the spread, place a half-cup or so of fresh pumpkin seeds in a blender or food processor. Open one saw palmetto capsule and pour in the contents, then add a few drops of licorice extract and blend until smooth. (You can add a few drops of Brazil nut oil if you need to make the mixture a little more spreadable.) All of these ingredients are available in most health food stores.

Use Prosnut Butter like peanut butter, eating a couple of tablespoonfuls every day. You can eat it on crackers or on bread, if you prefer, or try it with a little jelly. Since you want the ingredients to be fresh, don't mix up a big batch at once. Make just enough to last a couple of days.

❧

"What the FDA overlooked," says Dr. Tyler, "was the considerable evidence in Western Europe that certain phytomedicinals (plant-based medicines) are effective in treating BPH and that people using them experience an appreciable increase in their comfort level. Perhaps the most popular of these is saw palmetto. . . . The beneficial effects include increased urinary flow, reduced residual urine and decreased frequency of urination."

Saw palmetto is a small palm tree that grows in the southeastern United States, particularly in Florida around the Everglades. Seminole Indians ate the saw palmetto seed as food; perhaps they noticed that it helped urinary problems. Whites adopted it as a diuretic to help flush excess water from the body, and over time it came to be used for BPH.

It works because it contains a compound that inhibits the action of the enzyme (testosterone-5-alpha-reductase) that turns testosterone into dihydrotestosterone. Preventing this transformation of testosterone is also the way Proscar works, but saw palmetto does the job in a different and apparently more effective way.

To date, a half-dozen well-designed studies have shown the effectiveness of saw palmetto. In one study, a clinical trial involving more than 2,000 Germans with BPH, a daily dose of one to two grams of saw palmetto seeds (or 320 milligrams of its hexane extract) produced substantial easing of BPH symptoms.

❧❧ **Pygeum (*Pygeum africanum*).** In one study, German researchers gave either pygeum or a placebo to 250 men with BPH. In the placebo group, 31 percent reported improvement, a typical response rate for a placebo. In the pygeum group, the figure was 66 percent.

The recommended dose is 50 milligrams of bark extract twice a day. Depending on the method and concentration of the extract, this could represent a gram or a kilogram of bark. Although the extracts are still available in health food stores, they are made from a species that could be endangered by overharvesting. So you might want to try the other alternatives listed in this chapter before resorting to this one.

❧❧ **Stinging nettle (*Urtica dioica*).** According to the results of another study, extracts of stinging nettle roots have successfully treated BPH. Researchers gave a few teaspoons of the extract daily to 67 men over age 60 with BPH and found that the herb significantly reduced their need to get up at night to urinate. The herb apparently has some inhibitory effect on the conversion of testosterone. German medical herbalists recommend two to three teaspoons of extract a day to treat BPH.

Psoriasis

I first developed something a dermatologist diagnosed as lichen planus, a type of psoriasis, about 20 years ago. Rather symmetrical patches of itchy scales began appearing on both of my legs. Then similar small patches appeared on both arms.

Although my doctor was quick to come up with a diagnosis, he had no idea what had caused what he said was psoriasis or how to cure it. He gave me salves, steroids and vitamins, but nothing seemed to work. I would have tried sunlight, a standard treatment for psoriasis, and a natural one, but it was winter, and there just wasn't much sun. I nearly scratched my skin to the bone.

Then a funny thing happened. When I left the intemperate climate of Maryland for the tropical climate of Ecuador, my "psoriasis" cleared up. Now I'm convinced that the doctor was wrong. I don't think I had psoriasis, just dry skin. We heat our house with oil-fired, hot-water radiators. They produce a dry heat that apparently parched my skin to the point where my symptoms appeared. Every year, a week or two after the first frost, when we start heating the house, my skin acts up by getting dry, itchy and flaky. For me, the best treatment is a trip to the humid tropics, one of many reasons that I love the Amazon. But my skin condition has certainly piqued my interest in psoriasis.

It also leads to the first lesson here: Doctors don't know all that much about treating psoriasis, and sometimes they're wrong when they diagnose it. It makes good sense to investigate gentle herbal approaches before submitting yourself to harsher medical treatments that don't always do the trick anyway.

Skin That Misbehaves

Psoriasis causes red, scaly patches of varying sizes, usually on the scalp and lower back and over the elbows, knees and knuckles. On the toenails and fingernails, it causes pitting and brownish discoloration, and sometimes it causes the nail to lift and crack.

Typically, the rash first appears in teenagers and young adults. It may continue throughout the person's life, increasing and decreasing in severity, often for no apparent reason. Psoriasis leaves no scars and usually itches only when it appears in body creases. In severe cases, it may cause scales, cracks and blisters on the palms of the hands and the soles of the feet. Psoriasis may also cause a rash on the genitals, profuse shedding of dead skin flakes and even (although rarely) arthritis involving the spine and large joints.

Psoriasis afflicts an estimated 2 to 4 percent of Americans, with whites accounting for the overwhelming majority of cases. The condition is a medical mystery. It's not caused by an infection or allergic reaction, nor does it appear to be caused by stress, foods or vitamin or mineral deficiencies. It may be an autoimmune condition, meaning that the immune system attacks the body. It's not contagious.

We also know that psoriasis isn't hereditary, yet for some unknown reason it sometimes shows up in several family members. Illnesses, scrapes and bruises and emotional upsets can make it worse.

Psoriasis somehow interferes with the normal growth and replacement cycle of skin cells. Normally, the body replaces skin cells every 28 days or so. Psoriasis speeds up this process to five to ten times the normal rate, which causes the buildup of scaly patches.

As I've mentioned, sunlight often helps get rid of the patches. Many of us now avoid sunbathing because we know that sun exposure contributes to rising rates of malignant melanoma skin cancer. For people with psoriasis, however, the benefits of sunlight could outweigh the risks. When the weather or the season doesn't allow sunbathing, sunlamps are an alternative.

For mild cases, doctors may recommend over-the-counter 0.5 percent hydrocortisone creams, and stronger prescriptions are also available. The newest treatment for psoriasis, PUVA, involves a combination of exposure to UVA, one type of ultra-violet light, and taking compounds known as psoralens. Psoralens are found in plants and also show up in certain phar-maceuticals. Because PUVA has potentially serious side effects, it should be administered only by a psoriasis specialist.

Green Pharmacy for Psoriasis

Fortunately, there are also a number of herbs that can some-times provide significant relief.

🌿🌿🌿 **Bishop's weed (*Ammi visnaga*).** The "new" PUVA treatment is actually thousands of years old. The ancient Egyptians and Indians rubbed red, scaly skin patches (presum-ably psoriasis) with plants containing psoralens and then had people sit in the sun.

Bishop's weed contains a good deal of one of these psoralens (methoxypsoralen), so its reputation as a psoriasis treatment makes sense. The latest studies have shed light on why psoralen treatment works. These compounds inhibit cell division, slowing down the fast-dividing skin cells that cause psoriasis patches. If you have access to the fresh herb, you might want to give this ancient treatment a try. Do be cautious, however; if this treatment seems to irritate your skin, discontinue use. (High doses of pso-ralens can be carcinogenic.)

🌿🌿🌿 **Red pepper (*Capsicum*, various species).** Thanks to an article in *Prevention* magazine, I have also found one herbal treatment that seems to help both dry skin and psoriasis—hot pepper, specifically one of the many creams containing 0.025 per-cent capsaicin. Capsaicin is the compound that makes hot peppers hot. Capsaicin creams such as Zostrix and Capzasin-P are sold as pain relievers, and they work.

In one study, 98 people with psoriasis used a capsaicin cream, while 99 others treated their skin patches with an inac-tive cream (a placebo). The capsaicin group successfully reduced both scaling and redness, although the hot-pepper cream caused some burning, stinging and itching.

If you use a capsaicin cream, be sure to wash your hands thoroughly afterward so that you won't get it in your eyes. And, of course, if you ultimately get further irritation rather than relief from the cream, don't use it again.

🌿🌿 **Angelica (*Angelica archangelica*) and other herbs**

containing psoralens. Many plants contain psoralens. To get a natural version of a commonly prescribed natural treatment for psoriasis, take any herb or herbs containing psoralens, then spend a little time in the sunlight, which of course supplies ultraviolet light. Food plants that contain psoralens include some of my favorites, such as angelica, carrots, celery, citrus fruits, figs, fennel and parsnips.

Here's a pleasant treatment to try: Pick a sunny afternoon and mix up some of my Psoriaphobic Citrus Juice: Simply toss a mixture of citrus fruits (with a bit of peel), a carrot and a celery stalk into your juicer. Or perhaps you'd rather cook up my Psoralen Soup by adding carrots, celery, parsnips and fennel to your favorite vegetable soup recipe. Remember to go out into the sunlight or get under a sunlamp immediately after eating it. But be very careful if you decide to try herbs that contain psoralens, as large doses of these compounds can be carcinogenic. And if you notice any irritation, stop using the therapy.

✿✿ **Avocado (*Persea americana*).** Folk healers have long recommended rubbing mashed avocado on psoriasis patches. It's certainly cool and soothing. If I had psoriasis, I'd take a piece of the inner peel with a little green pulp adhering to it and rub it on my scaly patches.

✿✿ **Brazil nut (*Bertholettia excelsa*).** These nuts contain an oil rich in vitamin E and selenium. In the Amazon, people use this oil to treat skin conditions, and some skin creams available in the United States contain vitamin E.

Curious about its effects, for a couple of weeks I applied the oil religiously every night before retiring. Like any emollient oil, it soothed and curbed the itching. Brazil nut oil can be purchased at health food stores and seems to be worth trying.

✿✿ **Camomile (*Matricaria recutita*).** Camomile preparations are widely used in Europe to treat psoriasis, eczema and dry, flaky skin. Naturopathic physicians in this country maintain that applying this herb externally works better than commonly prescribed medications for treating psoriasis. Compounds known as flavonoids, which are found in camomile, have significant anti-inflammatory activity. You can buy commercial creams containing camomile at health food stores.

If you have hay fever, however, you should use camomile products cautiously. Camomile is a member of the ragweed family, and in some people, it might trigger allergic reactions. The first time you use it, watch your reaction. If it seems to

help, you can continue to use it. But if it seems to make the itching worse, simply discontinue use.

✌✌ **Flax** (*Linum usitatissimum*). Several plant oils are
chemically similar to fish oils, which have a reputation for helping to relieve psoriasis. Flaxseed oil, for one, contains the beneficial compounds eicosapentaenoic acid and alpha-linolenic
acid. I've reviewed studies showing that 10 to 12 grams (five to
six teaspoons) of these acids can help treat psoriasis. You won't
want to sip this much flaxseed oil, but believing as I do that
every little bit helps, I think that you might want to add some
flaxseed oil to your salad dressings. (Flaxseed oil is very high
in calories, however, so if you use this therapy, be sure to adjust
the rest of your diet accordingly.)

✌✌ **Licorice** (*Glycyrrhiza glabra*). Naturopaths consider
external applications of licorice to be equal or superior to hydrocortisone cream for treating psoriasis. They note that the compound glycyrrhetenic acid (GA), which is found in licorice,
works rather like hydrocortisone in treating psoriasis, eczema
and allergic dermatitis. Other scientists have shown that hydrocortisone works considerably better when used in combination
with GA.

If you'd like to give this herb a try, buy a licorice extract and
apply it directly to the affected areas using a cotton ball or clean
cloth.

✌✌ **Oat** (*Avena sativa*). Oatmeal is a hallowed folk remedy
for relief of itching. Some herbalists recommend using oat-
meal-paste packs or oatmeal baths to treat psoriasis.

You can either scoop a few handfuls of oatmeal into a warm
bath or put the oatmeal in a piece of cheesecloth and tie it up to
prevent the sticky oatmeal from clogging the drain. This treatment relieved my granddaughter's itchy chicken pox, so I've
seen first-hand how well it relieves itching.

✌✌ **Oregon grape** (*Mahonia aquifolium*). All of the anti-
psoriasis chemicals in Oregon grape, and there are several, are
potent antioxidants. This means that they neutralize the highly
reactive molecules known as free radicals that damage cells and
play a role in inflammatory diseases like psoriasis. The same
chemicals are also found in barberry, goldenseal, goldthread
and yellowroot.

In one study, researchers showed that compounds in these
herbs—Mahonia alkaloids—slowed the proliferation of certain
skin cells. If I had a psoriasis flare-up, I'd plan to try the yellow

barks of any of these plants. They can be taken as teas or tinctures or in capsules.

❧❧ Purslane (*Portulaca oleracea*). Herb advocate Andrew Weil, M.D., professor at the University of Arizona College of Medicine in Tucson and author of *Natural Health, Natural Medicine*, recommends several nutrients for treating psoriasis, including vitamins A, C and E, plus the mineral selenium and alpha-linolenic acid. In my database, purslane is the best plant source of vitamins A, C and E. If you have access to fresh purslane, you can enjoy it steamed like spinach or use the young shoots in salads.

❧ Fumitory (*Fumaria*, various species). This herb contains fumaric acid, a compound that seems to be useful for treating psoriasis. Brew a strong fumitory tea and apply it directly to the affected area with a cotton ball or clean cloth.

❧ Lavender (*Lavandula*, various species). Aromatherapists suggest external application of lavender essential oil, followed by an almond oil cream. I'm not surprised, since aromatherapists use lavender for treating all manner of skin problems, including psoriasis. It's worth a try. But do not ingest the oil, as even a small amount can be toxic.

❧ Milk thistle (*Silybum marianum*). Milk thistle has an active ingredient, silymarin, that's reportedly useful in relieving psoriasis. In fact, milk thistle seed contains at least eight anti-inflammatory compounds that may act on the skin. This herb is taken as a tea or tincture or in capsules.

Raynaud's Disease

Have you ever heard the expression, "cold hands, warm heart"? I don't know if one has anything to do with the other, but if you suffer the painfully cold, bluish-white fingers of Raynaud's disease, let me suggest warm soup. I recommend a vegetarian minestrone liberally spiced with cayenne, garlic, ginger and mustard, plus oils of borage, currant and evening primrose.

Make a lot. Eat until you're satisfied. Then strain out some broth and rub it on your frigid fingers. Finally, I would heartily suggest following up your anti-Raynaud's soup by taking the herb ginkgo.

If a doctor heard me suggest this approach, she might think I was off my rocker. I beg to differ. There's reasonably good science behind every one of my suggestions, and this is more than I can say for mainstream medicine's approach to Raynaud's disease.

The Mainstream Approach

Raynaud's disease seems to be caused by constriction and spasms of the small arteries (arterioles) that bring blood to the fingers. As blood flow diminishes, the fingers become painful and turn white or bluish. Raynaud's also occasionally occurs in the nose and toes. It is much more common among women.

While Raynaud's may occur independently of other conditions, sometimes it's a symptom of scleroderma, a rare and serious disease that involves hardening of the skin and damage to the internal organs. Doctors often prescribe corticosteroids such as prednisone (Deltasone, Orasone) to treat both Raynaud's and scleroderma. But corticosteroids have many potentially troubling side effects, such as weight gain, acne and irregular heartbeat. And they sometimes make Raynaud's disease worse.

Green Pharmacy for Raynaud's Disease

Because of the problems sometimes caused by corticosteroids, I think it makes a lot more sense to treat Raynaud's with selections from the Green Pharmacy.

🌿🌿🌿 **Evening primrose (*Oenothera biennis*).** The oil made from evening primrose (EPO) contains a good deal of gamma-linolenic acid (GLA). Some studies suggest that GLA helps relieve symptoms of Raynaud's disease.

In one study, EPO was massaged into the fingers of people with Raynaud's disease. About half improved, more than you would expect if this were simply a placebo response. I suspect that both the massage and the EPO helped.

🌿🌿🌿 **Garlic (*Allium sativum*).** In one excellent study that lasted 12 weeks, researchers gave a daily dose of 800 milligrams of garlic to people with intermittent claudication, a condition caused by a narrowing of the arteries in the legs. People with severe claudication have difficulty walking. By the end of the study, those who took an inactive substance (a placebo) showed no improvement in walking, but the group taking garlic walked significantly better, strongly suggesting that the blood flow to their legs had improved.

Garlic works to improve circulation. In fact, more than one alternative medicine advocate suggests using garlic and ginkgo, which is also known to help circulation, in combination to treat Raynaud's disease. I suggest simply adding more garlic to your diet. You can also take capsules, if you prefer.

🌿🌿🌿 **Ginkgo (*Ginkgo biloba*).** Literally dozens of studies show that ginkgo improves blood circulation. Most of the research has focused on this herb's ability to promote blood flow through the brain, which is why ginkgo extract is widely prescribed in Europe for recovery from stroke and the mental slowing of old age.

But several studies have explored ginkgo's effects on intermittent claudication. When people who have severe claudication take ginkgo, over time the herb improves their ability to walk. While the reasons for the impaired circulation are different, Raynaud's is somewhat similar to claudication, except that it affects the fingers instead of the legs.

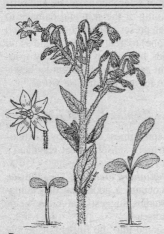

Borage

Borage, an annual that grows about two feet tall, was used by the ancient Greeks to flavor wine.

European physicians frequently recommend ginkgo for Raynaud's, and there are many European case reports of people with Raynaud's experiencing improvement after taking it. It makes sense to me. If I had this condition, I would try ginkgo.

The medicinal part of the plant is the leaf, but the active constituents (ginkgolides) occur in such low concentration that there's little point in using the leaves to make tea.

If you want to try this herb, buy ginkgo pills or capsules made from standardized extract. It's usually a 50:1 ratio, meaning that 50 pounds of ginkgo leaves are processed to yield 1 pound of extract. Look for these extracts in health food stores and herb shops. You can try 60 to 240 milligrams a day, but don't go any higher than that. In large amounts, ginkgo may cause diarrhea, irritability and restlessness.

Borage (*Borago officinalis*). Like evening primrose, borage contains GLA, which helps treat Raynaud's when massaged into the fingers.

Ginger (*Zingiber officinale*). Chinese herbalists often recommend this "hot" herb to treat conditions involving cold, including the cold fingers caused by Raynaud's. Ginger lowers blood pressure and cholesterol levels, and both effects help normalize blood flow all over the body, including the fingers.

Mustard (*Brassica nigra*, *Sinapis alba* and others). I'm sure you've heard of mustard plasters. When applied to the skin, they cause mild irritation that increases the local blood supply, resulting in a warm, tingling sensation. Medically known as rubefacients, mustard and other herbs with this effect have long been used to treat Raynaud's disease.

You can make a mustard plaster by mixing four ounces of fresh ground mustard seed with warm water to make a thick paste. Try applying this to your fingers when symptoms are acting up. Other rubefacients, according to British herbalist David Hoffmann, author of *The Herbal Handbook*, include cloves, garlic, ginger, horseradish, stinging nettle, peppermint oil, rosemary oil and rue. Any of these can be applied to the fingers.

Red pepper (*Capsicum*, various species). This is the classic rubefacient. Back in the old days, people used to sprinkle it in their shoes to keep their feet warm in winter. If I had Raynaud's, I'd try mixing some with vegetable oil and rubbing it on my fingers. (Just be sure not to touch your eyes if you have any on your fingertips.) I might even add some to EPO, borage oil or currant oil. You can use it externally, but of course red pepper is a spicy addition to any food, especially salad dressing.

Indian snakeroot (*Rauwolfia serpentina*). This herb contains the chemical reserpine, which opens (dilates) the blood vessels. It has often been used to treat Raynaud's disease, according to medicinal herb expert Walter Lewis, Ph.D., professor at Washington University in St. Louis, and Memory Elvin-Lewis, Ph.D., authors of *Medical Botany*.

Scabies

More than 30 years ago, Hurricane Hazel forced me to spend a night in a barn in South Carolina. I was hitchhiking along rural roads, innocent of the fact that a serious storm was brewing until I was forced to take refuge. I got shelter from the storm. I also got scabies, probably because the tiny mites that cause it infest animals as well as humans.

Scabies is a highly contagious parasitic skin infestation caused by mites of the genus *Sarcoptes*. Especially common in children, infestations cause small, itchy bumps, sometimes all over the body and sometimes localized between the fingers, on the wrists, on the waist, in the groin or on the genitals.

Green Pharmacy for Scabies

Drug companies have come up with all sorts of over-the-counter and prescription mite killers. But I'd recommend starting with the natural alternatives and moving on to the synthetics only if you find yourself with a really bad case that herbs don't cure. There are a number of herbs that might prove helpful. But whatever you use, other measures are necessary: In addition to treating your body, you have to boil all of your clothes and bedding to kill any mites on them so you aren't reinfected.

🌺🌺🌺 **Evening primrose (*Oenothera biennis*) and St.-John's-wort (*Hypericum perforatum*).** Evening primrose oil (EPO) is approved in the United Kingdom for treating eczema because it soothes the skin. But it's not approved in the United States because the Food and Drug Administration turns a blind eye to European research, and no U.S. drug companies want to invest hundreds of millions to prove the safety and effectiveness of something that they can't patent.

As for St.-John's-wort, I've seen persuasive anecdotal reports that applying this herb to the skin can provide immediate relief from the itching of insect bites.

If I had scabies, I would steep flowering shoots of St.-John's-wort for a few days in enough EPO to cover them, then dab the oil on the affected areas. If you don't have access to the fresh herb, you can use a tincture of St.-John's-wort.

✺✺✺ **Neem (*Azadiracta indica*) and turmeric (*Curcuma longa*).** Neem is an Indian tree with an extract that is powerfully active against many insect pests. Several natural neem-based pesticides are marketed in this country and used by organic farmers and gardeners. Turmeric has a long folk history for treating itchy skin problems.

A few years ago, Indian researcher S. X. Charles, Ph.D., used these two herbs to treat 814 people with scabies. He made a paste with four parts fresh neem leaves and one part turmeric root. The people in his study rubbed it all over themselves daily. Almost 800 of them (98 percent) showed substantial improvement within three to five days and were completely cured within two weeks. You can buy skin-care products containing neem at some health food stores. Just mix in several teaspoons of turmeric and apply it to the affected areas.

✺✺✺ **Onion (*Allium cepa*).** When I was a kid, I boiled onion skins to make a yellow dye. Now in my second childhood, I boil onion skins to extract quercetin, one of Nature's best skin-soothing compounds. Some onion skins are 3 percent quercetin, which translates to considerable soothing power against scabies and other skin problems.

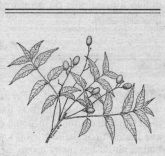

For scabies, I suggest boiling the skins of a half-dozen onions for 15 to 30 minutes in a quart of water. Let the liquid cool; then apply it liberally all over your body. (Save the peeled onions to use in cooking.)

Neem

Originally from India, neem is working its way into the United States as a natural cosmetic, dentifrice and insect repellent.

✺✺ **American pennyroyal (*Hedeoma pulegioides*).** Almost 2,000 years ago, the Roman naturalist Pliny noted that European pennyroyal (*Mentha pulegium*) repels fleas. In fact, this herb's scientific name, *pulegioides*, is derived from the Latin for "flea," and the plant has been popularly known as fleabane for centuries. Pennyroyal oil is the active ingredient in just about every herbal flea collar for pets.

I suggest applying a strong tea or preferably a tincture directly to the affected area to alleviate the itch.

❧❧

Pregnancy Alert

Among the herbs mentioned in this chapter are a few that pregnant women should avoid completely—pennyroyal, peppermint, mountain mint and tansy. If you're pregnant, you shouldn't take these herbs orally or apply them to your skin. When you apply an herb to your skin by adding it to bathwater or in the form of an essential oil, some of the active ingredients do penetrate the skin and get into the bloodstream.

❧❧

❧❧ **Mountain mint (*Pycnanthemum muticum*).** This weedy, three-foot-tall herb is loaded with pulegone, the same insect repellent found in pennyroyal. It's not a popular herb, and I don't understand why. It's a fine weed to grow around the house, and it has many uses.

I often ball up a wad of fresh mountain mint and rub the bruised leaves on my legs to keep the ticks off. I suspect that this herb would be equally effective against mites and lice.

❧❧ **Oat (*Avena sativa*).** While waiting for your herbal mite killers to get the job done, you might want to stop the itching. Oatmeal works quite well. Just scoop a few handfuls into a hot bath and settle in.

❧❧ **Star anise (*Illicium verum*).** The oil of star anise is best known as an antiseptic, but it is also reportedly useful against scabies, lice and bedbugs. Just dab it on the affected areas.

Teatree (*Melaleuca*, various species). Like star anise, teatree oil is best known as an antiseptic, but it's also useful against parasites, including those that cause scabies. Before putting the oil on your skin, you should dilute it by adding several drops to a couple of tablespoons of any vegetable oil.

Remember, though, that you shouldn't take teatree oil, or any essential oils, internally. They are extremely concentrated, and even small quantities of many of them can be poisonous.

Walnut (*Juglans*, various species). Walnuts contain a chemical called juglone that is useful for dealing with mite infestations, according to pharmacognosist (natural product pharmacist) Albert Leung, Ph.D. Dr. Leung recommends making a wash by boiling a few cracked walnut shell pieces in a cup of water until about half of the water has evaporated. To create a concentrated solution, cover several whole walnuts with water and simmer until half of the water is gone. Apply the water liberally to the skin.

Aloe (*Aloe vera*). The soothing gel of aloe contains the compound bradykininase, which should help to relieve the annoying itch and irritation of a scabies rash.

Five-leaved chastetree (*Vitex negundo*). The leaves of this Chinese shrub have a long history of folk use as a poultice for treating scabies, eczema and ringworm. Five-leaved chastetree is available in the United States as an ornamental plant. You can mash the leaves and apply them directly to the affected areas of skin.

Peppermint (*Mentha piperita*). The active ingredient in peppermint is menthol, which has cooling, anesthetic and antiseptic properties. Some respected herbalists frequently recommend menthol and related compounds for treating scabies, so let me propose an herb tea that you can use in your bath to kill scabies mites while alleviating the itch. Mix peppermint, pennyroyal, rosemary, sage, spearmint and thyme in any proportions you like. Make enough tea so that you can toss several cups into your warm bathwater and also enjoy a cup or two as a tasty, stress-reducing beverage.

Tansy (*Tanacetum vulgare*). Practitioners of alternative medicine often recommend washing with strong tansy tea as a treatment for scabies or lice.

Sciatica

I had never used visualization approaches to healing until a story told by one of the few doctors I really admire made me reconsider. This tale comes from Andrew Weil, M.D., professor at the University of Arizona College of Medicine in Tucson and author of *Natural Health, Natural Medicine*, who has become one of the top national experts on natural, alternative medicine.

Dr. Weil tells of a woman who had excruciating sciatic pain for two years, during which time she sought help from some 20 doctors. Her pain continued undiminished.

Sciatica is a condition that involves pain that runs from the lower back to the buttocks and/or the outer back of the leg. It radiates along the sciatic nerve, hence the name. Sometimes the sciatic nerve fibers also become inflamed.

Perhaps you can imagine how this woman felt. I know I can: I suffered through some of the worst pain of my life after slipping a disk in my back, a condition related to sciatica.

After enduring two years of pain, this woman experienced a major breakthrough when her granddaughter paid her a visit. She forced herself to get out of bed to tend to the child. To her astonishment, she found that when she acted as if she felt all right, she actually felt better.

She abandoned her physicians, who apparently weren't able to help her much anyway, and started doing what *she* wanted to do instead of what they prescribed. She sought out acupuncture treatment to relieve her pain. She started taking vitamins, and she began listening to tapes containing visualization exercises aimed at healing back pain.

All of these treatments seemed to help: She felt better and kept improving. And she decided that the most important element of her self-devised program was her visualizations. Her basic technique was to imagine more blood going into her back.

Her pain finally disappeared completely. Dr. Weil checked up on her seven years later, and she was still fine, with no sciatic pain.

Green Pharmacy for Sciatica

Along with the several natural approaches that the woman in Dr. Weil's story tried, there are a number of herbs that might prove helpful in relieving this kind of pain.

❧❧❧ **Hayseed (a mixture of grass seeds, especially** *Anthoxanthon odoratum*). Many years ago, the European naturopath Parson Kneipp learned what people in the Alps did with the seed heads of the various grasses that they stored as hay to feed their animals through the winter. They swept up the hayseed and added it to baths, because they had discovered that this seed has the ability to soothe painful backs, joints and muscles. Kneipp popularized the use of hayseed for this purpose, and today many Europeans subscribe to Kneipp therapy, using hayseed that has been packaged in bath bags or prepared in the form of hot poultices.

The hot hayseed poultices used in Kneipp therapy have been approved by Commission E, the group of herbal medicine experts appointed by the German counterpart of the Food and Drug Administration to judge the safety and effectiveness of herbal therapies. According to Commission E, the poultices are effective for treating a range of rheumatic conditions as well as sciatica.

But how does hayseed work? It contains a good deal of a compound called coumarin, a camphorlike substance that boosts local blood flow when applied externally, according to Rudolph Fritz Weiss, M.D., Germany's leading herbal physician. (Dr. Weiss's book, *Herbal Medicine*, is used in German medical schools.)

I've heard pretty amazing testimonials endorsing hayseed baths and poultices for relieving sciatic pain. If I had sciatica, I would probably give this approach a try. Ask for Kneipp therapy at specialty bath or herb shops.

❧❧❧ **Stinging nettle (*Urtica dioica*).** People have been flailing their bad backs with the stinging nettle plant since Roman times. This is a practice that involves taking sprigs of the fresh plant and slapping it against the painful area.

Be warned, though: This practice stings like crazy. But that is part of the treatment. The sting is a counterirritant, something that causes minor pain and in effect fools the nervous system into disregarding deeper pain. That's not all that stinging nettle does, however. Chemicals in the stingers that cause inflammation seem to trigger the release of the body's natural anti-inflammatory chemicals. So the body's own medicine helps get rid of the sciatic inflammation.

Poultices made from stinging nettle are also good for sciatica, according to Dr. Weiss. (Remember that you need to wear gloves whenever you handle this plant to protect your palms from the stingers.)

❧ ❧ ❧ **Willow (*Salix*, various species).** Willow bark contains salicin, the herbal equivalent of aspirin. It can help relieve sciatic pain, and Commission E recognizes it as an effective pain reliever for everything from headache to arthritis.

The salicin content of willow varies from species to species. I suggest starting with a low-dose tea made with a half-teaspoon of dried herb and working your way up to a dose that provides effective pain relief.

As with aspirin, long-term use of willow bark may cause stomach distress and even ulcers, so I suggest sweetening willow bark tea with a little licorice, which has ulcer-preventing benefits. And if you're allergic to aspirin, you probably shouldn't take herbal aspirin, either.

❧ ❧ ❧ **Wintergreen (*Gaultheria procumbens*).** Wintergreen contains methyl salicylate, a close relative of the salicin in willow bark, and it's about equal in its ability to relieve pain. It has a long history of use both internally in tea and externally in baths and ointments for relieving painful conditions, among them sciatica and gout. I use it both internally and externally myself.

Absorption through the skin may actually be more rapid than through the stomach. In the United States there are more than 40 products on drugstore shelves that contain

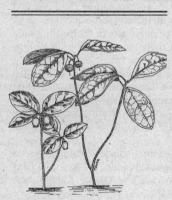

Wintergreen

Wintergreen is a low-growing evergreen shrub with edible red berries; it's also known as spiceberry or teaberry.

methyl salicylate as the active ingredient. All are for external use, and most are used to treat various kinds of pain, most frequently arthritic, rheumatic and sciatic pain.

Warning: You must keep products containing wintergreen oil or any product containing methyl salicylate out of the reach of children. The minty smell can be very tempting, but ingesting even small amounts can prove fatal to young children. In the United States, liquid preparations containing significant amounts of methyl salicylate (more than five milliliters) must have child-resistant packaging. You don't have to worry about wintergreen tea, but do take precautions with commercial pain-relief products intended for external use.

❧❧ **Chinese angelica (*Angelica sinensis*).** Also known as *dang-quai*, Chinese angelica is revered in traditional Chinese medicine as the leading treatment for gynecological complaints. It's often called the female ginseng. But Chinese angelica also has mild sedative, pain-relieving, anti-inflammatory and antispasmodic properties that make it a good herb to try for sciatica.

In China, physicians inject their patients with Chinese angelica extract to treat sciatic pain. I've reviewed data from Chinese clinical trials showing that when this extract is injected into the acupuncture points used to treat sciatica, about 90 percent of people receiving treatment report significant improvement.

I wouldn't recommend injecting it, but it might be useful taken in a tea or tincture. I suggest adding it to wintergreen tea. (Do not take this herb if you are pregnant, however.)

❧❧ **Country mallow (*Sida cordifolia*).** India's traditional Ayurvedic physicians have long used this herb to treat sciatica and other painful muscular and nervous system complaints. The reason appears to be its high concentration of ephedrine: It contains some 850 parts per million. The compound ephedrine is best known as a bronchial decongestant and stimulant, but it also is something of a muscle tonic, which is presumably why it helps relieve sciatica.

❧❧ **Mustard (*Brassica nigra*, *Sinapis alba* and others).** Ever hear of a mustard plaster? This home treatment has a long folk history of use as a treatment for both respiratory complaints and rheumatic problems like sciatica.

Mustard is aromatic, which accounts for some of its use as a bronchial decongestant. But there's a different reason that it's used for sciatica, arthritis, lumbago, neuralgia and rheumatism.

Mustard is a rubefacient counterirritant, which means it causes a soothing feeling of warmth on the skin while its counterirritant properties cause mild irritation, distracting the body from the deeper pain of sciatica. The combination of heat and counterirritation has a pain-relieving effect.

✖.✖. Sciatica cress (*Lepidium*, various species). Down South, this plant is also called peppergrass. Herbalists recommend applying fresh sciatica cress externally as a pain reliever. Like mustard, this herb is both a rubefacient and a counterirritant, and it contains the same hot compounds (isothiocyanates) as mustard.

✖ Ginger (*Zingiber officinale*) and sesame (*Sesamum indicum*). Medical anthropologist John Heinerman, Ph.D., author of *Heinerman's Encyclopedia of Fruits, Vegetables and Herbs*, recommends this Egyptian treatment for sciatica: Mix two tablespoons of grated ginger with three tablespoons of sesame oil and one teaspoon of lemon juice. Rub this mixture into the affected area. My guess is that this helps because ginger, too, is a rubefacient.

Shingles

Shingles is chicken pox returned to haunt you. Like that most common of childhood illnesses, shingles is caused by the herpesvirus. After chicken pox clears up, the virus remains in the body, lying dormant in nerve cells. For reasons that remain a mystery, it can reemerge decades later as shingles.

Symptoms include a painful rash that usually appears on the torso or face. After a few days, chicken pox–like blisters form, then they crust over and eventually heal after two or three weeks. So far it sounds a lot like the childhood disease. In about half of those who develop shingles, however, the pain persists for months and sometimes years. This is called postherpetic neuralgia. Frequently, the pain is quite severe.

Shingles is especially common in people over 60 or those with poor immune function, such as people who are undergoing cancer chemotherapy. If you develop shingles, you should see your doctor immediately for treatment.

Green Pharmacy for Shingles

Nature has given us several herbs that can help treat viral illnesses. If I developed shingles, I would try any of these approaches.

❦❦❦ **Lemon balm** (*Melissa officinalis*). Herbalists recommend many herbs that are members of the mint family, especially lemon balm, or melissa, to treat herpes. There's good reason for this. Lemon balm has been proven to have some effect on viruses of the herpes family. Varro Tyler, Ph.D., dean and professor emeritus of pharmacognosy (natural product pharmacy) at Purdue University in West Lafayette, Indiana, suggests using lemon balm to treat viral infections.

Herpes cold sores are caused by a virus that behaves much like the virus that causes shingles; in fact, both viruses belong to the same genus. In one well-designed study of 116 people with herpes sores, a lemon balm cream healed the sores substantially better than an inactive cream (a placebo).

One European anti-herpes product contains 700 milligrams of lemon balm leaf extract per gram of cream-based ointment. It has been shown to shorten the healing time of herpes sores by several days. You can achieve a similar effect, according to Dr. Tyler, from a tea made with two teaspoons of dried leaf per cup of boiling water. Apply the tea directly to the rash with a cotton pad several times daily.

For shingles, I'd suggest trying a mixed mint tea made with lots of lemon balm plus any other mints that you have on hand: hyssop, oregano, peppermint, rosemary, sage, self-heal, spearmint or thyme. Put a little licorice in the tea as well. Such a beverage would contain quite a few antiviral, anti-herpetic compounds. I suggest drinking the tea as well as applying it directly to the rash.

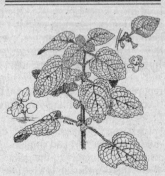

Lemon Balm

This herb, a member of the mint family, helps combat herpes viruses.

❧❧❧ **Red pepper (*Capsicum*, various species).** The fiery ingredient in red pepper, capsaicin, is the hottest thing going for postherpetic neuralgia. Capsaicin brings relief by blocking pain signals from nerves just under the skin. Studies of an ointment containing capsaicin showed such good results that a few years ago, the Food and Drug Administration approved commercial creams such as Zostrix and Capzasin-P, which contain this substance.

You can buy the commercial products if you want. But if you'd like to save money, simply mix powdered red pepper into any white skin lotion until it turns pinkish, then dab it on. Be sure to wash your hands thoroughly afterward so that you don't get pepper in your eyes or on other sensitive areas. And test it on a small area of skin first; if it causes irritation, discontinue use.

❧❧ **Baikal skullcap (*Scutellaria baicalensis*).** The root of this plant, powdered and mixed with water, was used as a folk treatment for shingles in China. It has known antiviral activity, so I think this is worth a try.

❧❧ **Chinese angelica (*Angelica sinensis*).** Also known as *dang-quai*, this herb is revered in Asia as the best herb for menstrual problems and other women's health concerns. In addition, the Chinese have used the powdered root successfully to treat shingles. It can be used in tea or tincture. (Do not take this herb if you are pregnant, however.)

❧❧ **Licorice (*Glycyrrhiza glabra*).** Leading naturopath Joseph Pizzorno, N.D., president of Bastyr University in Seattle and co-author of *The Encyclopedia of Natural Medicine*, reports seeing people with shingles whose pain and inflammation cleared up within three days following application of a licorice ointment on painful areas. Licorice contains several antiviral and immune-boosting compounds and seems to be a rational choice. If I had shingles, I'd drink a weak tea and apply a strong tea directly to the rash.

❧❧ **Passionflower (*Passiflora incarnata*).** Passionflower is a mild tranquilizer, which is not a bad idea if you are being driven to distraction by the pain of shingles. But it also has reputed activity against postherpetic neuralgia. I suggest adding some to a lemon balm–licorice tea.

❧ **Bergamot (*Citrus bergamotia*) and other essential oils.** If you enjoy aromatherapy, you might apply a few drops of essential oils that have been recommended for treating shingles.

They include bergamot, camomile, eucalyptus, geranium, lavender, lemon and teatree oil. Since some full-strength essential oils can be irritating to the skin, dilute them by adding several drops to a couple of tablespoons of vegetable oil and apply them directly to painful areas. (Never ingest essential oils, as even a small amount can be toxic.)

❧ **Pear (*Pyrus*, various species).** Pear juice is rich in antiviral caffeic acid. I'd drink it and eat lots of pears if I had shingles.

❧ **Purslane (*Portulaca oleracea*).** This herb has a folk reputation in China for treating herpes. It's a delicious vegetable that's great when steamed like spinach. It's worth a try.

❧ **Soybean (*Glycine max*) and watercress (*Nasturtium officinale*).** Research by Jean Carper, author of *Food: Your Best Medicine*, suggests that taking two 500-milligram tablets of the amino acid lysine three or four times a day might help relieve shingles symptoms.

If that's true, I'd suggest simply eating more watercress and soybeans. In my database, these are the foods highest in lysine—2.7 percent on a dry-weight basis. Other foods containing lysine, in descending order of potency, include black bean sprouts, carob, lentil sprouts, lentils, spinach, velvet beans, peas, pumpkin seeds, asparagus, butter beans, Chinese cabbage, fava beans, fenugreek and parsley.

You might even want to cook up some of my Lysine Soup. Use several of the high-lysine beans and asparagus and flavor it with fenugreek, parsley and lots of watercress.

Sinusitis

You're probably familiar with Tiger Balm, that strong-smelling oriental ointment that comes in a red tin decorated with a tiger. I have used it for colds and headaches, and I like it. Tiger Balm is filled with potent aromatic herbal extracts—menthol from peppermint, eugenol from cloves, cineole from cajuput (a close relative of teatree), cinnamaldehyde from cinnamon, and camphor. It clears the sinuses faster than a tiger can pounce.

Someone once told me that Tiger Balm was being abused as a hallucinogen. It sounded silly, but just to be sure, I called a friend of mine at the Food and Drug Administration (FDA) to inquire. He laughed and said no, he had not heard of its being abused. I asked why he laughed. He said that every time he had sinusitis, a Chinese colleague pushed Tiger Balm on him. Finally he tried it, and he confided, "It worked."

When I reminded him that it was basically a concoction of herbal aromatics, he replied, "No wonder it works." I wish everyone at the FDA felt as he did. Then maybe we'd see herbs approved for all of the medicinal uses that they're good for.

Sinusitis is inflammation, and almost always infection, of the air-filled bony cavities surrounding the nasal passages. It typically develops following a cold or a bout of hay fever. It may also be associated with a dental infection. Mucus fills the sinuses and then becomes infected, typically with bacteria: haemophilus, pneumococcus, staphylococcus or streptococcus.

Sinusitis causes nasal congestion, sometimes severe pain across the nose and cheeks and often a headache as well. Only a small fraction of colds progress to sinusitis. But in susceptible people, almost anything that starts as a cold can turn into a sinus infection.

Green Pharmacy for Sinusitis

There are a number of herbs that can help treat this condition.

✧✧✧ Garlic (*Allium sativum*) and onion (*A. cepa*). These related herbs are broad-spectrum antibiotics. Garlic is the more potent, but onion still rates in my book. Many studies have confirmed garlic's antibiotic activity, most recently a study of people with AIDS who took the herb to ward off all sorts of opportunistic infections, including sinusitis.

Take capsules if you like, but I prefer to peel and chop whole garlic cloves and use them as food. Naturopath Jane Guiltinan, N.D., chief medical officer at Bastyr University in Seattle, feels the same way.

With my perverse affinity for alliteration, may I suggest my Sinusoup. Begin with your vegetarian minestrone and add heaping helpings of garlic and onions, plus horseradish, hot pepper and ginger. On a cold winter day, it warms the soul as it opens the sinuses.

✧✧✧ Goldenseal (*Hydrastis canadensis*). This is another powerful broad-spectrum herbal antibiotic, with at least two active constituents, berberine and hydrastine. Naturopaths Michael Murray, N.D., and Joseph Pizzorno, N.D., president of Bastyr University, call goldenseal the most effective botanical treatment for acute bacterial infection. I'd have to agree. Lately I've combined goldenseal with echinacea and used it to treat all sorts of minor infections. In fact, I carry it in my travel first-aid kit.

✺✺ Echinacea (*Echinacea*, various species). Native to the American Plains, this herb was a favorite American Indian remedy for all sorts of infections. German researchers have shown beyond any doubt that echinacea is an immune stimulant that speeds the healing of bacterial, fungal and viral infections. Studies in other countries support these findings.

✺✺ Eucalyptus (*Eucalyptus globulus*) and peppermint (*Mentha piperita*). Aromatherapists suggest rubbing diluted essential oils of eucalyptus or peppermint on the forehead and temples to relieve sinusitis. Mix a few drops of either or both oils into a couple of tablespoons of vegetable oil before applying it to your skin. You can also add a few drops of the essential oils to your bathwater. But use these oils sparingly, as too much can be overwhelmingly caustic. And never ingest them; even a small amount can be toxic.

If you don't have these herbal oils on hand, the bruised leaves work well. You can mash some leaves, moisten them with water and make them into a poultice. Either place it on your chest or stuff it into your nostrils (be careful not to push it in too deeply).

In Lesotho, Africa, people push crushed mint leaves up their nostrils to deliver the antiseptic oil to infected sinuses. I have tried this myself and think it helps. If you don't have peppermint on hand, any mint will do, including spearmint, mountain mint (except if you are pregnant) and oregano, all of which contain antiseptic essential oils. I'd also suggest drinking tea made with eucalyptus and any of the mints.

✺✺ Oregano (*Origanum vulgare*). Here's a member of the mint family that's simply loaded with antiseptic compounds. Oregano is useful as a hot tea (inhale the vapors as you drink) or in a massage lotion. You can add a few drops of the essential oil to any skin lotion or to vegetable oil.

✺ Ginkgo (*Ginkgo biloba*). Ginkgo is best known as a treatment for the infirmities of old age, particularly stroke, because it increases blood flow in and around the brain. But this herb also has respiratory benefits. Several herbalists I respect recommend it for sinusitis.

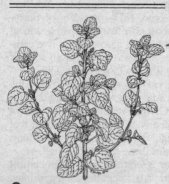

Oregano

Oregano, once prescribed by Chinese physicians to treat fever and other conditions, has proved to be well-endowed with antiseptic compounds.

The active constituents in ginkgo (ginkgolides) occur naturally in a concentration too low to be beneficial. The standard commercial extraction process boils down 50 pounds of leaves to get 1 pound of medicinal extract. When you buy ginkgo, look for a 50:1 extract and follow the package directions. You can try 60 to 240 milligrams a day, but don't go any higher than that. In large amounts, ginkgo may cause diarrhea, irritability and restlessness.

🌿 **Horseradish (*Armoracia rusticana*).** I'm a big believer in horseradish (and Japanese wasabi) for clearing the sinuses. You might try a straight spoonful of ground horseradish if you're extremely brave, or you can add this hot herb to my Sinusoup.

🌿 **Pineapple (*Ananas comosus*).** Bromelain, a compound found in pineapple, is useful for treating sinusitis, according to pharmacognosist (natural product pharmacist) Albert Leung, Ph.D., co-author of *The Encyclopedia of Common Natural Ingredients*.

Naturopaths say that combining 250 to 500 milligrams of pure bromelain with goldenseal enhances the herb's already potent effectiveness. I enjoy pineapple and its juice, so I'd probably chase my goldenseal capsule with the juice rather than taking a bromelain pill.

Skin Problems

Every winter, the baseboard hot-water radiators in our home make the air very dry. And every year, I develop a skin irritation that I call dry winter dermatitis. Over the years, I've found a skin lotion that helps. Its ingredients are water, glycerin and aloe vera, the traditional and very effective herbal treatment for many skin problems. That's my personal Green Pharmacy success story.

I'd also like to mention a case report published in the British medical journal *Lancet*. It seems that there was a physician who moved from a humid subtropical climate to a very dry desert area. He developed a severe dry-skin rash on his hands. He tried steroids, medications that are sometimes prescribed to heal severe rashes. They didn't help, so he decided that he'd just have to live with it.

Four years later, several studies appeared in the medical literature showing that vitamin E reduces heart attack risk by some 35 percent in men. Because he was at risk, the doctor began taking 400 international units of vitamin E a day for his heart. It also helped his skin. In less than two weeks, his four-year-old skin rash cleared up.

Vitamin E is widely touted for skin problems, and it's an ingredient in many skin creams and cosmetics. But like many physicians, this doctor was skeptical of such supplement claims and was not convinced that he actually had vitamin E to thank for resolving his dermatitis. The following year, however, while on a winter vacation, the doctor discontinued his vitamin E, and his dermatitis returned. On returning home, after two weeks without the supplements, he began taking them again, and his rash cleared up again. That made a believer of him.

Allow me to tell you one more story before we get to the herbs. A videographer who worked with me in the Amazon developed a strange and very itchy eczema while in the rain forest. A shamanistic healer I knew suggested that she apply a poultice of crushed petals of Peruvian red hibiscus. The treatment worked.

Oddly, when the videographer returned home to Chapel Hill, North Carolina, her eczema returned, and nothing her physician offered gave her any relief. She continues to import hibiscus from Peru, since it's the only thing that is effective. In a pinch, though, she could splash Red Zinger tea on her rash. The red color of this commercial, mixed-herb tea comes from hibiscus flowers.

Green Pharmacy for Skin Problems

Fortunately, as the stories above demonstrate, herbal approaches have a great deal to offer those with skin problems. In some cases, the herbs help even when pharmaceuticals do not. Here are several of the most helpful herbs.

❦❦❦ **Aloe (Aloe vera).** Aloe has been used since the days of Egypt's ancient pharaohs to treat all manner of skin problems. But aloe is more than an age-old folk remedy. Since the 1930s, when the gel inside aloe's leathery leaves was shown to speed the healing of radiation burns, many studies have shown this herb to be effective in treating a variety of skin problems. In one study of people undergoing dermabrasion, a medical procedure involving removal of the top layer of skin, aloe speeded healing by 72 hours.

Even if you have a brown thumb, aloe is easy to maintain as a potted plant. It requires little water and almost no care. For minor burns, cuts and other skin problems, simply snip off a lower leaf, slit it open lengthwise, scoop out the gelatinous pulp and apply it to the affected area. Or try one of the many commercial skin products that contain this herb.

❦❦❦ **Evening primrose (Oenothera biennis).** Evening primrose oil (EPO) is rich in a compound called gamma-linolenic acid (GLA), which is approved in Great Britain for treating eczema. Research I've reviewed supports this use and suggests that this herbal oil is also helpful in treating other forms of skin irritation (dermatitis).

Although evening primrose is a weed at my place, I buy EPO in capsules at a health food store, and I suggest that this is the easiest way to take this herb. Take the capsules orally, following the package directions. You can also take oils of borage, currant and hops, which are also well-endowed with GLA. As with evening primrose, you can get these other oils in capsule form; follow the package directions when you take them.

❦❦ **Avocado (Persea americana).** There's more to avocado than guacamole. Its oil is actually patented as a treatment for some forms of dermatitis and arthritis. According to Aubrey Hampton, author of *Natural Organic Hair and Skin Care*, long-term treatment with avocado oil helps relieve eczema. I'm not surprised, as avocado oil is rich in vitamins A, D and E, all of which help maintain healthy skin. I suggest applying it directly to any itchy, red or irritated areas. It might also be helpful to ingest the oil and use it in salad dressings.

❧❧ **Calendula (*Calendula officinalis*).** Small wonder that this pretty flower has a folk reputation for treating all kinds of skin problems. Research shows that this herb is antibacterial, antifungal, anti-inflammatory and antiviral. Calendula also stimulates white blood cells to gobble up harmful microbes and helps speed wound healing. I usually buy commercial calendula flower ointments and apply them as needed. That's a good way to use this herb as a skin treatment.

❧❧ **Camomile (*Matricaria recutita*).** Don't just drink your camomile tea—brew it strong and use it in a compress for treating skin problems. This tasty herb is approved in Europe for treatment of inflammatory skin conditions, notably yeast infections. Compounds in camomile (bisabolol, chamazulene and cyclic ethers) are anti-inflammatory, bactericidal and fungicidal.

If you have hay fever, however, you should use camomile products cautiously. Camomile is a member of the ragweed family, and in some people, it might trigger allergic reactions. The first time you try it, watch your reaction. If it seems to help, go ahead and use it. But if it seems to cause or aggravate itching or irritation, discontinue use.

❧❧ **Cucumber (*Cucumis sativus*).** Cool as a cucumber? That's not just a figure of speech. Pharmacognosist (natural product pharmacist) Albert Leung, Ph.D., reminds us that cucumber has a long folk history of use for soothing dermatitis and burns and for treating wrinkles. If I had a skin problem, I'd peel and blend some cucumbers in my blender, with or without avocado, and apply the puree directly to the affected area, leaving it on for 15 to 60 minutes.

❧❧ **Gotu kola (*Centella asiatica*).** This herb, native to India, stimulates the regeneration of skin cells and underlying connective tissue. In clinical trials, gotu kola has proven useful in treating eczema, wounds and other skin conditions. The latest research suggests that one compound (asiaticoside) in gotu kola is among the most promising treatments for one of history's most devastating skin diseases, leprosy. If I developed a skin problem in the tropics, I'd use crushed leaves to make a poultice and apply it to the affected areas. Here in the United States, the leaves are generally unavailable, so I'd buy a commercial tincture and follow the package directions.

❧❧ **Wild pansy (*Viola tricolor*).** This is a traditional herbal treatment for acne, eczema, impetigo, itching and other skin problems. And modern research supports using this herb as a treatment for skin problems. Germany's Commission E, the expert panel that judges the safety and effectiveness of herbal medicines, approves of using pansy tea as a skin treatment. You can make a tea with about one teaspoon of dried herb per cup of boiling water; steep it for ten minutes.

❧❧ **Witch hazel (*Hamamelis virginiana*).** Witch hazel contains generous amounts of tannins, potent astringents that are useful in treating skin problems. According to studies with laboratory animals, witch hazel also increases the tone of the blood vessels in the skin, which enhances blood supply to damaged areas. One sunburn study compared three preparations: a combination of astringent witch hazel and lecithin, a camomile cream and a 1 percent hydrocortisone cream (a standard pharmaceutical anti-inflammatory). The hydrocortisone worked best, but the witch hazel–lecithin combo ran a close second.

Commission E endorses using witch hazel water externally for treating dermatitis and other conditions that damage the skin.

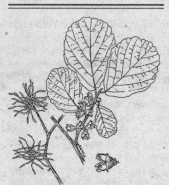

Witch Hazel

Witch hazel, which flowers bewitchingly around Halloween, is an ingredient in astringent lotions.

❧ **Carrot (*Daucus carota*).** Carrots are a rich source of vitamin A–like carotenoids that have been shown to enhance the health of the skin and repair skin damage. Retin-A, the prescription drug used to treat severe acne, is a carotenoid preparation.

Some herbalists recommend applying liquefied carrots (and/or tomatoes and sweet potatoes) to the skin to treat sunburn and other minor skin conditions. I can't see doing that myself, but there's no reason why you shouldn't try it if you want. I eat a lot of carrots and other red and orange fruits and vegetables because I know that ingesting carotenoids not only helps prevent skin damage but can help ward off cancer and heart disease as well.

❧ **English plantain (*Plantago lanceolata*).** External application of cooling, soothing plantain leaves is a time-honored herbal remedy for treating minor skin problems. Modern research has shown that two compounds (aucubin and catapol) in plantain have anti-inflammatory and bactericidal properties.

❧ **Ivy (*Hedera helix*).** Compounds known as saponins, which are found in ivy leaves, are active against several bacteria and fungi that cause skin problems. Commission E endorses using ivy to treat bronchitis, which is an indication of the herb's safety.

Ivy has an extensive folkloric reputation for treating dermatitis. If I had a skin problem, I would chop some leaves in a blender and apply the paste directly to the affected area.

❧ **Marsh mallow (*Althaea officinalis*).** This herb contains a soothing water-soluble fiber called mucilage that has a long history of use for relieving skin problems. In Europe, marsh mallow mucilage is used in ointments for treating chapped skin. If I had a skin problem, I'd put the fresh root through my juicing machine, then apply the liquid directly to the affected areas.

❧ **Pineapple (*Ananas comosus*).** One of the latest buzzwords in skin care is alpha-hydroxy acids (AHAs). AHAs peel off dead skin cells by dissolving the substances that hold the dead skin together.

Dermatologists use AHA preparations clinically to treat acne, chapped skin, fine lines, wrinkles and other skin conditions. They use strong concentrations for face peels, and lower concentrations appear in dozens of over-the-counter skin cleansers, lotions and toners.

What few people know is that AHAs are often herbal products called fruit acids. As the name suggests, AHAs occur in many fruits, notably pineapple, tamarind, gardenia, apples and grapes. They also occur in sour milk. Cleopatra reportedly bathed in sour milk because it brought out the luster in her skin. I can't imagine taking a sour milk bath, but I love pineapple and eat a lot of it, and I could see rubbing the inner peel on damaged skin.

❧ **Purslane (*Portulaca oleracea*).** Like carrots, purslane is generously endowed with carotenoids. I'm not the facial mask type, but if I were, I might try putting a handful of this useful weed into a blender with a carrot and maybe even some pineapple. This would create an invigorating face mask with healing properties. I'd suggest leaving it on for 20 minutes or so.

❧ **Walnut (*Juglans*, various species).** Commission E endorses using walnut leaves for treating mild superficial skin inflammations. Steep two teaspoons of crushed leaves in a cup of boiling water, then apply the tea when cool. Some herbalists suggest adding a handful of crushed walnut leaves to baths for treating eczema.

Smoking

My son and daughter complained about my smoking so bitterly 25 years agò that I quit cold turkey. One day I was smoking some three packs a day of unfiltered, king-size cigarettes, and the next day, none. I occasionally still have dreams in which I give in to the temptation to light up again, but that will never happen.

Quitting for Good Reasons

Smoking is estimated to cause one-third of all cancer deaths and one-fourth of the fatal heart attacks in the United States. The American Lung Association` estimates that 350,000 Americans die every year from smoking. (My own estimate is 500,000.) Forty percent of smokers die before they reach retirement age.

But all the talk about premature death goes over the heads of the teenagers who start smoking and the young adults who won't quit. The hazards of smoking just seem too far off to them.

That's why I like to remind young smokers I know that the

habit hits men in the penis and women in the face. That's right. Smoking damages the blood vessels that supply the penis, so men who smoke have an increased risk of impotence. Smoking also damages the capillaries in women's faces, which is why women smokers develop wrinkles years before nonsmokers. (Smoking develops early wrinkles in men's faces, too, but somehow this particular anti-smoking argument seems to score more points with women than with men.)

Green Pharmacy for Smoking

Years ago, when I kicked the cigarette habit, I didn't know much about herbal medicine. If I were quitting today, I'd use some herbs to help.

❦❦❦ **Licorice (*Glycyrrhiza glabra*).** I don't have much science here, just a gut belief to back licorice as an anti-smoking aid. I've also heard a lot of positive stories about people kicking the habit with the help of licorice.

How does this work? Licorice root happens to look just like an old cheroot cigar. You can keep a stick of licorice root handy and suck on it in place of a cigarette. I believe it works by helping to satisfy the oral cravings that people who are addicted to cigarettes seem to have. If I were still a smoker, I'd give this one a try.

It's interesting that most licorice coming to the United States goes into tobacco products—chewing tobacco and pipe tobacco.

You should be aware that while licorice and its extracts are safe for normal use in moderate amounts—up to about three cups of tea a day—long-term use (more than six weeks) or ingestion of excessive amounts can produce headache, lethargy, sodium and water retention, excessive loss of potassium and high blood pressure.

❦❦❦ **Red clover (*Trifolium pratense*).** A few years back, I got a call from an entrepreneur looking for a source of 50 tons of red clover. He wanted it as a major ingredient in a tobacco-free chewing tobacco product he wanted to market, all tinned up just like the real thing.

I got this call right around the time that I learned about why red clover has an age-old reputation as a cancer preventer. For tumors to grow, they need a blood supply, and they send out biochemical signals that coax the body into growing blood vessels right into them, a process called angiogenesis.

Several leading cancer researchers have been working on ways to stop these new blood vessels from forming, thereby starving tumors. It turns out that one compound with an anti-angiogenic effect is genistein, a constituent of red clover.

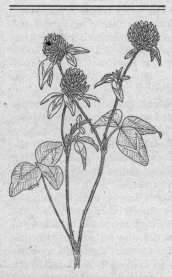

So I welcomed the call from the man seeking red clover. By replacing chewing tobacco with a nontobacco substitute, he was working to prevent the mouth and tongue cancer that chewing tobacco causes. And by replacing tobacco with red clover, he was unwittingly providing anti-angiogenic benefits as well.

I don't know whatever became of the man's tobacco-free red clover chaw, but I have a tin of red clover–based snuff. Aspiring ex-smokers can chew on fresh clover flowers (you can add them to salads) or anything else that contains genistein, such as groundnuts, peanuts or soybeans. These munchies would help satisfy some of the oral needs that smokers and ex-smokers seem to have. At the same time, the genistein in these snacks would be attacking any tumors that might be trying to get a start.

Red Clover

The flowers of red clover, which were widely used for decades in folk remedies for cancer, have been shown to contain the anti-cancer compound genistein.

If you're having a hard time kicking the smoking habit, you might want to develop another habit—drinking red clover tea daily. It seems as if it would offer a measure of protection.

🥕🥕 **Carrot (*Daucus carota*).** Back when I quit smoking, carrots helped me quite a bit. I used to drive to the office munching on a raw carrot or two instead of puffing on a cigarette.

At the time, I chose carrots because I like them, but now we know that carotenoids, the chemical relatives of vitamin A that give carrots their orange color, also help prevent cancer, especially if the carotenoids come from carrots or other whole foods rather than from capsules. (Generally, if you isolate one beneficial chemical—take it out of context—you're missing out on a whole lot of other chemistry that can also help.)

If cigarettes are cancer sticks, carrots are *anti*-cancer sticks. In fact, all fruits and vegetables are. The research is consistent and compelling: The more fruits and vegetables people eat, the less likely they are to develop every major cancer, including lung cancer. So even if you don't quit smoking, you should still be munching on carrots.

❧

Tommie Bass and his "Yallerroot" Cure

I had the pleasure of meeting with the late A. L. "Tommie" Bass in the late fall of 1994, when he was 87, at his Cherokee County farmette just outside Leesburg, Alabama. Bass was the only herbalist I knew who had a permanent official highway sign honoring his calling. As you approached his home, you encountered a sign that read: Arthur Lee "Tommie" Bass, Herbalist, 0.5 mile.

On the day I visited, Tommie also had a sign set up in front of his shack. It announced yellowroot at $1.25 a bunch and prickly ash bark at $5 a bunch.

It was a genuine pleasure for me to visit Cherokee County, because I was born about a hundred miles away, in Jefferson County, back in 1929. By the time I was born, Tommie was already 21 and had been collecting and selling herbs for 11 years.

I was with some friends from Samford University in Birmingham on this visit to this genuine old-time Alabama folk herbalist. We tried calling him ahead of time, but our phone calls went unanswered. So we just jumped in the car and drove up, about a hundred miles from Birmingham, hoping he'd be around. It was a dank, dark, drizzly day, and we found him in his little shack, a disorganized collection of uneven boards tacked together. Although we arrived unannounced, Tommie came out and greeted us warmly.

I was pleased to see Tommie's bundles of yellowroot (*Xanthorrhiza simplicissima*), which resembled yellowish switches, as we walked toward his house. He was enthusiastic about it, saying that it was the best tonic herb he knew. He pronounced it "yallerroot."

Tommie claimed that with this herb he'd helped a lot of people with ulcers abandon their Tagamet. He considered it tops for what he called upstairs hernia, by which he probably meant either hiatal hernia or the heartburn associated with it.

Finally, Tommie said, tucking one of the bitter roots in his mouth, yellowroot is a real help in quitting smoking.

At this point, there's no scientific backing whatsoever for using Tommie's "yallerroot" to help kick the smoking habit. But when I hear an old-time herbalist like Tommie endorse it, I sit up and take notice. I have a lot of respect for Tommie's recommendations. After all, he had nothing whatsoever to gain by promoting yellowroot. When he said that he helped many people quit smoking with it, I believed him. And anyway, it probably can't hurt to give it a try. You can brew up yellowroot as a tea or chew on the bitter twig like a licorice root. It might prevent cavities, too.

❧

Sores

I want to open this chapter with a couple of remarkable stories of just what herbs can do when it comes to healing sores.

I have a friend whose father has diabetes. Like many people with diabetes, he developed foot problems to the point where his doctor advised amputating one of his toes, which had become seriously ulcerated. My friend came to me and asked if I knew of any herbal alternatives to help her father avoid such a drastic measure.

In my usual cautious way, I told her that as a botanist I do not prescribe. But I added that before I had a toe amputated, I'd try comfrey, either as a poultice or a strong wash, to treat the diabetic ulcer. After my friend's father used the comfrey wash for just a week, she reported, his toe improved remarkably. His doctor canceled plans for the amputation.

Here's another true story: A television crew out of Baltimore was doing a feature on medicinal herbs in my herb garden one Friday afternoon. The interviewer spotted some comfrey and asked what it was good for. I answered, "Sores and other wounds, especially indolent ulcers—that is, slow-healing sores."

I started to move on, but then I remembered that I had an indolent ulcer on my right shin. It was a sore, scabbed over, with raised edges, that wasn't getting any worse but certainly wasn't showing any signs of healing, either. It had remained basically the same for weeks.

With the cameras whirring, I raised the leg of my blue jeans and revealed the sore. Then I rubbed it with some fresh comfrey leaves that I had crushed and balled up in my hand. The abraded sore started bleeding. With the cameras still whirring, I grabbed some astringent geranium and rubbed it on to stop the bleeding. It worked. We moved on to other herbs, but just three days later, the following Monday, the sore had healed over.

I wouldn't have believed that story if it had not happened to me. As a scientist, I can't be certain whether the healing came from the comfrey, its abrasive application, the sunshine, the geranium, the comfrey-geranium combination or just good luck. But you can bet your bottom dollar that the next time I am faced with a stubborn sore of any kind, I'll venture back to my herb garden for comfrey and geranium.

Green Pharmacy for Sores

Okay. I've said my piece and I've made my point. I need add only that there are a number of herbs in addition to comfrey that can be used to treat sores.

❧❧❧ **Calendula (*Calendula officinalis*).** Commission E, the group of experts that advises the German government about herbs, endorses calendula as effective for reducing inflammation and speeding the healing of sores. The flowers are used externally in infusions, ointments and tinctures. Calendula also helps prevent staphylococcus infection.

A while back, West Virginia herbalist Jim Foltz gave me some calendula salve. Like Commission E, Foltz firmly believes that this herb is good for treating sores. I found out how good while on a trip to the Amazon. To show some workshop participants how the Peruvian burn-tree got its name, I tied a piece of the tree's inner bark around my right ankle. Soon I had a circular burn where the bark had contacted my skin. Later on, the burn blistered and became somewhat infected. That was when I applied some calendula salve and discovered how well it worked. The burned area healed quite nicely.

You can buy a number of commercial creams and ointments containing calendula. Follow the package directions.

❧❧❧ **Comfrey (*Symphytum officinale*).** Comfrey has a long history of use for treating sores and other wounds. It works because it contains allantoin, a compound that promotes new cell growth. In addition, allantoin is an anti-inflammatory that stimulates the immune system. The astringent tannins in the plant may also help.

I'm not sure if comfrey is a scoundrel or a superstar. It has been vilified by experts who point out that it contains carcinogenic compounds called pyrrolizidine alkaloids that can cause severe liver damage if the herb is ingested. But other experts praise its powers, when it's used externally, for speeding the healing of sores and cuts, including surgical incisions.

I think that there is good reason to use comfrey externally, and little hazard in doing so. I also think that there is much more risk of hazard if you ingest it. But warnings about internal consumption shouldn't stop us from getting it. We would lose a fine medicinal herb if we allowed ourselves to be bullied out of using comfrey externally simply because ingesting it may be hazardous.

You can use fresh comfrey as a poultice or make a strong tea to use as a wash. For treating more serious leg ulcers, Rudolf Fritz Weiss, M.D., the dean of German medical herbalists and author of *Herbal Medicine*, recommends using a leaf or root poultice for the first few days. After that, you can switch to comfrey ointment or make a comfrey paste and cover it with a firm compression bandage.

🌿🌿🌿 **Dragon's blood** (*Croton lechleri*). This is one of the rising herbal superstars from Amazonia. Widely available in Latin America, it's still pretty hard to find in the United States, although I suspect that it will become more available here soon.

Dragon's blood is the source of two drugs now in clinical trials sponsored by Shaman Pharmaceuticals, the South San Francisco pharmaceutical firm that has been working with native healers in the Third World. Unfortunately, like most drug companies, Shaman Pharmaceuticals is going for isolated chemical extracts—the "magic bullet" approach—rather than using the whole herbal product.

My Peruvian shaman friend Antonio Montero Pisco recommends using whole dragon's blood rather than any of its isolated compounds. I agree. When I'm in tropical Peru, I use the whole herb immediately whenever I get a cut or abrasion.

🌿🌿 **Camomile** (*Matricaria recutita*). Most Americans think of this herb as a pleasant beverage tea, which it can be. But camomile is also anti-inflammatory, immune-stimulating and antiseptic. It's widely used in Europe to treat leg ulcers.

The preferred preparation is a camomile extract, but using compresses soaked in a strong tea would be a close approximation. To make the tea, put a large handful of fresh camomile flowers or several teaspoons of dried herb in a cup and cover with boiling water. Let the tea cool, then strain it and apply with a sterile cloth (a cloth bandage works nicely).

If you have hay fever, however, you should use camomile products cautiously. Camomile is a member of the ragweed family, and in some people, it might trigger allergic reactions. The first time you use it, watch your reaction. If it seems to help, go ahead and use it. But if it seems to cause or aggravate itching or irritation, simply discontinue use.

🌿🌿 **Country mallow** (*Sida cordifolia*). The leaves of this wiry perennial weed contain a water-soluble fiber called mucilage, which helps soothe sores when applied in a poultice. In addition, according to unpublished research that I'm familiar with, the plant also seems to possess broad-spectrum antiseptic powers, which would be helpful in treating sores.

❧❧ **Ginkgo (*Ginkgo biloba*).** The Germans use large oral doses of ginkgo to treat leg ulcers, reportedly with good results and no toxicity. I would try it. To use this herb, you'll need to buy a 50:1 extract at a health food store. (Active constituents are not present in high enough concentrations in the fresh leaves to warrant using them.) You can try 60 to 240 milligrams a day, but don't go any higher than that. In large amounts, ginkgo may cause diarrhea, irritability and restlessness.

❧❧ **Teatree (*Melaleuca*, various species).** I'm just one of a growing number of herbalists who now carry teatree oil in my first-aid kit, ready for use as a handy antiseptic. I'm convinced that it's a good one. Teatree oil has been shown effective against a broad range of bacteria.

Since some people find teatree oil irritating to the skin, I suggest diluting it by adding several drops to a couple of tablespoons of any vegetable oil. If this irritates your skin, discontinue use. Just don't take teatree oil, or any essential oils, internally. They are extremely concentrated, and even small quantities of many of them can be poisonous.

❧ **Gotu kola (*Centella asiatica*).** In clinical trials in Brazil and elsewhere, gotu kola has proven useful in treating skin ulcers, surgical wounds, gangrene, skin grafts and traumatic skin injuries. The herb works by stimulating regrowth of normal connective tissue that underlies the skin. The active constituent appears to be asiatic acid. I'd suggest using one of the standardized extracts of gotu kola that are sold here.

To use the extract externally, soak a cotton ball in the liquid and wipe it over the affected area. You can also drink gotu kola: Make a tea following the instructions on the package or bottle.

❧ **Tea (*Camellia sinensis*).** Tea contains many of the same compounds that are found in dragon's blood. It's antiseptic and astringent and helps promote skin healing. You can have a cup of tea and then lay the moist, spent tea bag on your sore.

Sore Throat

I'm not necessarily fond of lawyers, but I hold my lawyer son-in-law in high regard. On one visit, he arrived with a raging sore throat. The over-the-counter throat lozenges that he was using were not helping, so I gave him some slippery elm capsules. They did the trick. (If they hadn't, I would have urged him to take some licorice as well, because it's what I add to my own tea whenever I'm treating myself for sore throat.)

Although slippery elm grows nearby, I rarely collect the bark. It's easier to buy the prepared material.

Sore throat is a typical first symptom of colds. (Many of the herbal suggestions in the chapter on colds and flu on page 164 apply here as well.) But sore throat may also be caused by exposure to chemical irritants or by streptococcus bacteria (strep throat). If you develop a sore throat with a fever and no other symptoms, it might be strep, and a visit to the doctor is strongly advised.

Green Pharmacy for Sore Throat

Most commercial sore throat treatments involve sucking on anesthetic lozenges that deaden the nerve cells in the throat so that you don't feel the pain. I prefer the herbal alternatives, which actually soothe inflamed tissue. Here are the herbs that can help.

✿✿✿ **Eucalyptus (*Eucalyptus globulus*).** Commission E, the body of experts that advises the German government about herbs, approves using eucalyptus to treat sore throat.

Eucalyptus helps in two ways. The aromatic oil has a cooling effect on inflamed tissue, and the tannins in eucalyptus exert soothing astringent action as well. I suggest using a few teaspoons of crushed leaf per cup of boiling water to make a soothing tea.

✿✿✿ **Honeysuckle (*Lonicera japonica*).** The Chinese use honeysuckle flowers extensively to treat sore throat, colds, flu, tonsillitis, bronchitis and pneumonia. In one study of 425 Chinese students with strep throats, positive results were obtained with a treatment that involved blowing powdered

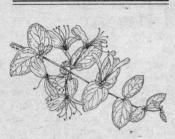

Honeysuckle

The flowers of this plant contain some two dozen antiseptic compounds and are widely used for respiratory problems.

dried honeysuckle flowers, blackberry lily roots and a small amount of borneol into the backs of their throats. (Borneol is just one of more than 20 antiseptic compounds found in honeysuckle flowers.)

I don't think that you need to use powdered honeysuckle to get the benefit of this herb. Honeysuckle flower extracts are strongly active against many microorganisms that cause sore throat and respiratory conditions.

I personally like using honeysuckle in combination with forsythia flowers for my own sore throats, and I often take them in hot lemonade sweetened with licorice, especially in winter.

❧ ❧ ❧ **Licorice (*Glycyrrhiza glabra*).** Licorice has been revered as a sore throat treatment for centuries in both Europe and China.

Commission E approves licorice for treating sore throat, and its effectiveness has been scientifically documented, according to pharmacognosist (natural product pharmacist) Albert Leung, Ph.D.

Dr. Leung recommends starting with three cups of water and five to seven teaspoons of root pieces. Put the herb in the water and bring it to a boil, then simmer until about half of the water has boiled away.

Licorice not only soothes a sore throat, it also has an expectorant effect that can help treat colds and other respiratory conditions. (Like most non-nutritive sweeteners, licorice has an "off" taste that some people find less than appealing.)

❧ ❧ ❧ **Slippery elm (*Ulmus rubra*).** This is an all-around soother, helping the throat, the respiratory tract and the digestive tract. And like most if not all woody plants, slippery elm contains compounds called oligomeric procyanidins, which have antiseptic and anti-allergic action.

❧❧ **Balloonflower (*Platycodon grandiflorum*).** The Chinese have great respect for this plant's root as a remedy for sore throat and cough. There's even a Chinese stamp commemorating it. Several Japanese patent medicines for treating bronchitis employ the root extract, and pharmacological studies confirm its anti-cough and expectorant activities. (Balloonflower is also an attractive ornamental. I have one from China that has fared well in my garden at the Herbal Vineyard.) You can take it as either a tea or a tincture.

❧❧ **Burnet-saxifrage (*Pimpinella major*).** Commission E endorses burnet-saxifrage root for treating sore throat and upper respiratory infections. Try simmering three to six teaspoons per cup of boiling water for about 20 minutes, then let it cool before drinking. I'd suggest adding a little licorice.

❧❧ **Garlic (*Allium sativum*).** Garlic is a favorite naturopathic remedy for upper respiratory problems because it's both antiviral (for colds) and antibacterial (for strep throat). Try it in tea as a gargle.

❧❧ **Ginger (*Zingiber officinale*).** Here's another herb to gargle for a sore throat. Try adding ginger to lemon juice, vinegar and honey.

❧❧ **Marsh mallow (*Althaea officinalis*).** This herb has been used for thousands of years for treating sore throat and many other ailments. It contains a soothing water-soluble fiber (mucilage) that is quite effective at easing throat pain. Research shows that the plant also has anti-inflammatory action.

Commission E approves using marsh mallow root to soothe irritation of the mucous membranes of the mouth and throat and to help treat associated dry cough. I'd suggest a tea made from three teaspoons of crumbled root per cup of boiling water.

❧❧ **Wintergreen (*Gaultheria procumbens*).** Wintergreen has a cooling, soothing flavor, and it contains methyl salicylate, an herbal form of aspirin that can help treat sore throat pain. Try it as a gargle for fast cooling of inflamed throat tissue and as a tea for pain relief. I'd suggest putting 15 to 25 leaves in a cup of boiling water for both a gargle and a tea.

Don't give either aspirin or its natural herbal alternatives to children with sore throats. When children take aspirin-like drugs for viral infections (especially colds, flu and chicken pox), there's a chance that they might get Reye's syndrome, a potentially fatal condition that damages the liver and brain. Also, if you

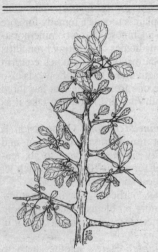

Myrrh

Ancient Egyptians added a gum resin from myrrh to perfumes and insect repellents.

are allergic to aspirin, you probably shouldn't take aspirin-like herbs, either.

☙ **Agrimony (*Agrimonia eupatoria*).** Commission E endorses using agrimony to soothe inflamed mucous membranes of the mouth and throat. Try a tea made with two to three teaspoons of dried herb per cup of boiling water.

☙ **Anise (*Pimpinella anisum*).** Anise tastes like licorice and is used as the flavoring agent in many "licorice" items. It's not as throat-soothing as real licorice, but Commission E suggests using it for respiratory problems, especially if you have a productive cough that produces phlegm. Anise helps break up bronchial congestion. You could make a tea by pouring a cup of boiling water over one to two teaspoons of crushed aniseed and steeping for 10 to 15 minutes. Strain the tea before drinking. The suggested dose is up to two cups a day.

☙ **Knotgrass (*Polygonum aviculare*).** Commission E approves using a tea made with two to three teaspoons of dried herb per cup of boiling water for treating sore throat and mild respiratory complaints. Knotgrass is astringent.

☙ **Myrrh (*Commiphora*, various species).** Here's another herb approved by Commission E as a treatment for sore throat. In Europe the tincture is added to water and used as a mouthwash and gargle.

☙ **Plantain (*Plantago*, various species).** Plantain is widely used as an external soother for skin problems. Commission E also endorses it for sore throat and inflammation of the mucous membranes of the mouth and throat. The plant has bactericidal activity, much of which may be lost if it's heated, so you could try three to four teaspoons of plantain in juice or cold water. Plantain also contains allantoin, a chemical that promotes the healing of injured skin cells and, I believe, the cells of the throat.

Sties

When you consider how common sties are, it's amazing how thoroughly the herb world has ignored them. I checked my top 20 herbals, and not one of them indexed sties. So I guess I'll be breaking some new ground here. It's about time somebody did, as there are several good herbs for sties.

A sty is a bacterial infection (typically staphylococcal) of an eyelash follicle. The infection causes a pus-filled bump to form on either the inside or outside of the eyelid. The bump grows for a week or so and then usually subsides, possibly rupturing spontaneously as it heals.

Sties should not be squeezed like pimples, as squeezing can spread the infection. Some people never get sties. Among those who do, they tend to recur.

Doctors often recommend holding a warm, moist cloth against the affected eye to hasten drainage. They also frequently prescribe antibiotics that attack the bacteria.

Green Pharmacy for Sties

Herbalists also have two approaches to treatment—antibiotic herbs plus herbs that boost the immune system so that the body can fight the infection more effectively.

✷✷✷ **Echinacea (*Echinacea*, various species).** This is one of my favorite immune stimulants. It was widely used to treat infections back in the days before antibiotics, and no wonder: Research clearly demonstrates its immunostimulant properties.

But in addition, this herb of our Great Plains, which is also known as coneflower, has antibacterial properties. Just six milligrams of the active constituents (echinacosides) in echinacea is the antibiotic equivalent of one unit of penicillin, according to herbal pharmacologist Daniel Mowrey, Ph.D., author of *The*

Scientific Validation of Herbal Medicine and *Herbal Tonic Therapies*. (A standard dose of penicillin is around 180 units.)

You take this herb orally, either in a tea or in capsules, rather than using it in a compress. (Although echinacea can cause your tongue to tingle or go numb temporarily, this effect is harmless.)

🌿🌿🌿 **Goldenseal (*Hydrastis canadensis*).** Like echinacea, goldenseal is both an immune booster and an antibiotic. In one study, berberine, an active constituent in this herb, was shown to be more active against staph infections, the kind that cause sties, than chloramphenicol (Chloromycetin), a powerful pharmaceutical antibiotic.

And berberine is only one of the medicinal compounds in goldenseal and its herb-medicinal relatives, barberry, goldthread, Oregon grape and yellowroot. You can take goldenseal orally, in either tea or capsules, but it also can be helpful when used in a compress.

🌿🌿🌿 **Potato (*Solanum tuberosum*).** I always like to quote herb conservative Varro Tyler, Ph.D., dean and professor emeritus of pharmacognosy (natural product pharmacy) at Purdue University in West Lafayette, Indiana: "To treat a sty, take fresh scrapings from the inside of a potato, put them on a piece of clean cloth and place on the sty. Replace once or twice with fresh scrapings. . . . It was amazingly effective. Within a couple of hours, the swelling was down, and the sty was significantly improved. By that evening it was almost gone."

If it's good enough for Dr. Tyler, it's good enough for me.

🌿🌿🌿 **Thyme (*Thymus vulgaris*).** If I had a sty, in addition to taking echinacea and goldenseal, I think I'd apply concentrated thyme tea directly to the sty with a cotton swab or in a compress.

Thyme is rich in thymol, a potent antiseptic, and contains more than a dozen other antiseptic compounds.

🌿 **Camomile (*Matricaria recutita*).** Camomile has eyelike flowers resembling miniature oxeye daisies, so it's not surprising that traditional herbalists suggested eye baths with camomile for sties. Ancient herbalists used to base many of their treatments on the physical resemblance that plants bore to parts of the body.

But—surprise—modern scientific herbalists have found that camomile really helps heal sties. Rudolf Fritz Weiss, M.D., the dean of German medical herbalists and author of *Herbal*

Medicine, suggests using hot compresses made with camomile tea.

❦ **Garlic (*Allium sativum*).** Naturopaths seem to recommend garlic for almost any infection, and I have to agree, because garlic is a potent antibiotic. I suggest taking a dozen chopped cloves. Even if you just can't get this much down, use more garlic when you have a sty.

❦ **Fruits and vegetables.** Naturopaths suggest eating more fruits and vegetables to combat infections. They are rich in vitamins, particularly beta-carotene (the vitamin A precursor) and vitamins C and E. You might also take a multivitamin supplement, if you don't already. One study of elderly people showed that a daily multivitamin significantly improved their immune function.

Stroke

Here's a quote from one of the thousands of letters I have received over the years, written by people disillusioned enough with their physicians to seek an alternative: "My husband, age 57, suffered a stroke a year ago. The doctors believe he still has a blood clot somewhere in his brain, though they can't seem to dissolve it. He is currently taking many, many drugs, but they don't seem to be doing much to help him. Can you suggest anything herbal he might take?"

That's the usual loaded question, the one that always prompts me to remind everyone that I'm a botanist, not a doctor. Strokes are very serious—the nation's third leading cause of death—and anyone who has had one should certainly be under a physician's care and follow their doctor's advice.

With that said, however, there are, indeed, quite a few herbal approaches to preventing stroke and stroke recurrence, at least the type caused by blood clots in the brain (ischemic strokes).

Brain "Attack"

Approximately 500,000 Americans have strokes annually. Eighty percent of those strokes are ischemic: A blood clot lodges in a brain artery, cutting off the supply of oxygen and nourishment to part of that essential organ. Wherever the blood clot forms, the area around it dies or becomes damaged, and the body function controlled by that area becomes impaired. While such a stroke often causes death, it might lead instead to severe disability, such as loss of the ability to speak or paralysis of part of the body.

Ischemic strokes are often preceded by mini-strokes known as transient ischemic attacks (TIAs). TIAs last anywhere from a few seconds to several hours and cause stroke symptoms that eventually resolve on their own. Those who suffer TIAs typically make full or almost full recoveries. But TIAs indicate a real risk of future catastrophic stroke and often signal the start of aggressive preventive treatment.

The other 20 percent of strokes are hemorrhagic. In this kind of stroke, a cerebral blood vessel bursts, and the result is the same as in ischemic stroke—impairment of the part of the body that the damaged area controls.

Whether you're talking about mainstream or herbal medicine, stroke prevention and treatment are tricky, because many of the approaches that help prevent ischemic stroke may actually increase the risk of the less common but equally disabling or deadly hemorrhagic stroke.

To prevent the more common ischemic stroke, physicians try to prevent arterial blood clots by prescribing anticoagulant (blood-thinning) medication. But when that is done, the risk increases that any bleeding in the brain won't stop, thus increasing the risk of hemorrhagic stroke. So stroke prevention involves a complicated balancing act.

Green Pharmacy for Stroke

Because the vast majority of strokes are ischemic, most of the suggestions in this chapter relate to preventing cerebral blood clotting. But I reiterate that hemorrhagic strokes are also a possibility, especially for those with a personal or family history of hemorrhagic stroke or aneurysm (a dangerously dilated blood vessel).

If you have high blood pressure, which is the major risk factor for stroke, see a doctor and have it treated. (You can also enlist the help of the herbal alternatives suggested in the chapter on high blood pressure on page 308.)

Please remember: It's important to follow any stroke-preventive medical advice that comes from your doctor. In fact, if you've had a stroke or know that you are at risk, it would be a really good idea to discuss any stroke-preventing herbs that you'd like to try with your doctor.

That said, here are a number of good herbal approaches to stroke prevention and treatment that you should be aware of.

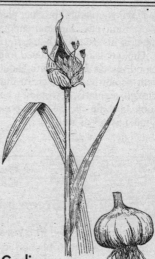

Garlic

A powerful healing herb, garlic was used to treat infected wounds and amebic dysentery during World War I.

❧❧❧ **Garlic** (*Allium sativum*). Garlic is the best anti-clotting herb. According to my database, it contains more anticoagulant compounds than any other herb—nine, to be exact. It is a major herb for heart attack prevention because of its blood-thinning effect and its ability to help control high blood pressure. These same effects also help prevent ischemic stroke.

If I were at risk for stroke, I'd increase my use of garlic in cooking and also take garlic capsules, which are available at health food stores and many drugstores. Garlic's close relatives, onions, scallions, leeks, chives and shallots, have similar benefits.

On the other hand, if I had reason to be concerned about hemorrhagic stroke, I'd steer clear of garlic and its other anti-clotting herbal relatives. (If you're not absolutely sure which category you fall into, ask your doctor to help you make this decision.)

❧❧❧ **Ginkgo** (*Ginkgo biloba*). Ginkgo is widely used in Europe to treat complications of stroke, including memory and balance problems, vertigo and disturbed thought processes. Many studies show that this herb increases blood flow to the brain. Varro Tyler, Ph.D., dean and professor emeritus of pharmacognosy (natural product pharmacy) at Purdue University in West Lafayette, Indiana, endorses this herb as a stroke treatment in his excellent book, *Herbs of Choice.*

Ginkgo also helps reduce fragility of the capillaries, the tiny blood vessels that fan throughout your body, which can help prevent hemorrhagic stroke. In Europe, many elderly people take ginkgo regularly. I wouldn't be surprised if this herb doesn't soon become increasingly popular with elderly folks in the United States as well.

The Green Insurance Plan

Are you interested in a sure-fire method for preventing stroke? A report published in the *Journal of the American Medical Association* suggests that stroke risk might be reduced 22 percent simply by eating more than three servings of fresh fruits and vegetables a day.

You should be eating at least that much anyway, since the National Cancer Institute recommends at least five servings a day to help prevent cancer. And if you follow those guidelines, you're helping to ward off two major threats, since fruits and vegetables contain many vitamins and minerals that are helpful in preventing stroke. One British study, for example, suggested that eating the amount of vitamin C in just half an orange, somewhere between 100 and 300 milligrams, every day significantly decreased the incidence of stroke.

To take this herb, you'll need to buy a standardized extract. Ginkgo extracts are widely available in health food stores and drugstores. You can try 60 to 240 milligrams a day, but don't go any higher than that. In large amounts, ginkgo may cause diarrhea, irritability and restlessness.

🍂🍂🍂 **Pigweed (*Amaranthus*, various species) and other foods containing calcium.** A six-year Harvard study of more than 40,000 health professionals showed that compared with those who consumed the least calcium, those who got the most had just one-third the risk of succumbing to heart attack. Personally, I believe these results also apply to ischemic strokes, because they are biologically so similar to heart attack.

Pigweed is an excellent plant source of calcium, with 5.3 percent on a dry-weight basis. According to my calculations, about one-third of an ounce of fresh pigweed leaves would provide 500 milligrams of calcium. (The Daily Value is 1,000 milligrams.)

You can use the young leaves in salads or steam the more mature leaves like spinach. You might also try pigweed pesto. To make the sauce, prepare your favorite pesto recipe, but use pigweed instead of basil.

Pigweed is not the only good herbal source of calcium. Here are some others, in descending order of potency (on a dry-weight basis): lamb's-quarters, stinging nettle, broadbeans, watercress, licorice, marjoram, savory, red clover shoots, thyme, Chinese cabbage (bok choy), basil, celery seed, dandelion and purslane.

🍂🍂🍂 **Willow (*Salix*, various species).** Willow bark is herbal aspirin, and low-dose aspirin—half of a standard tablet to a whole tablet a day—has been shown in several studies to reduce the risk of ischemic stroke by about 18 percent. (Low-dose aspirin also cuts heart attack risk by about 40 percent in men and 25 percent in women.)

You can take the little white aspirin pills, if you like. I personally prefer the herbal route: teas made from willow bark, meadowsweet or wintergreen. I add a teaspoon or two of any of these dried herbs to either hot herbal teas or cold lemonade and drink two to three cups a day. (I must confess, though, that I tend to be lazy and often take my own low-dose aspirin in pills.)

Again, willow bark and the other aspirin-like herbs should only be used to prevent and treat ischemic stroke. They are powerfully anticoagulant and may increase risk of hemorrhage, including hemorrhagic stroke. In fact, the Physicians Health Study, the large scientific study that showed aspirin's ability to prevent heart attack, showed a slight increase in risk of hemor-rhagic stroke from taking aspirin daily. The increase was small and not statistically significant, but if you're at risk for this type of stroke, consult your doctor before taking aspirin or any aspirin-like herbs. (You probably also should avoid them if you're allergic to aspirin.)

&-& Carrot (*Daucus carota*). In a Harvard study of 87,245 female nurses, consumption of carrots (and to a lesser extent, spinach) significantly reduced stroke risk. Women who ate five servings of carrots a week suffered 68 percent fewer strokes than those who ate carrots less than twice a month.

Carrots are rich in beta-carotene and other carotenoids, all members of the vitamin A family. Other studies show that peo-ple can reduce their risk of stroke by as much as 54 percent if they eat lots of fruits and veggies that are rich in beta-carotene and vitamins C and E.

The message is clear: Eat more carrots. I munch them as snacks, include them in my vegetable soups and juice them, too, sometimes with garlic.

&-& English pea (*Pisum sativum*). It turns out that nearly all legumes contain genistein, which appears to be a cancer-preventive nutrient. Scientists now believe that a diet high in genistein-rich tofu, a soy product, is an important reason that Asian women have such a low rate of breast cancer.

In addition to guarding against cancer, genistein also appears to have a significant anti-clotting effect, meaning that it may also help prevent ischemic stroke and heart attack. I like English peas more than I like soybeans, so this relatively new information was welcome news to me. I also eat lots of other beans and legumes. I suggest that you do, too.

&-& Pineapple (*Ananas comosus*). Pineapple contains a com-pound known as bromelain that is best known for its ability to break down proteins. It's a key ingredient in meat tenderizers. But bromelain also has an anti-clotting action that might help prevent ischemic stroke and heart attack. The bottom line: Eat more fresh pineapple.

&-& Scurfy pea (*Psoralea corylifolia*). These peas also con-tain genistein. After four long years of searching and research-ing, I finally have data to show that scurfy peas, consumed as a food (and reputed to be an aphrodisiac) in Asia, contain much more genistein than soybeans. I thank my colleague, Peter Kaufman, Ph.D., at the University of Michigan in Ann Arbor, for helping me to determine the genistein content of scurfy peas.

❧ Bilberry (*Vaccinium myrtillus*). Bilberries and their close relatives, blueberries and huckleberries, contain compounds known as anthocyanidins. Good European studies show that these compounds help prevent blood clots and also break down plaque deposits lining the arteries. In addition, some evidence suggests that bilberries help to maintain capillaries.

For all of these reasons, bilberries and their relatives might help prevent ischemic stroke without increasing the risk of hemorrhagic stroke. Medical anthropologist John Heinerman, Ph.D., author of *Heinerman's Encyclopedia of Fruits, Vegetables and Herbs*, says that one glass of huckleberry juice taken twice a week can help prevent stroke. I'm not as convinced as he seems to be, but these berries are delicious, and if they do help prevent stroke, so much the better.

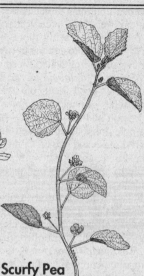

Scurfy Pea

Scurfy peas have a high concentration of a compound that may help protect a woman's body from harmful estrogens.

❧ Evening primrose (*Oenothera biennis*). The oil of this herb is rich in gamma-linolenic acid (GLA), which has potent anti-clotting and blood pressure–lowering actions. I think it's probably quite useful in the prevention of stroke and heart disease. Borage oil is also rich in GLA. You can purchase both of these oils at health food stores. To use them, follow the package directions.

❧ Ginger (*Zingiber officinale*). This is another herb with proven anti-clotting ability. In one Indian study, taking about two teaspoons of ginger a day for a week neutralized the blood-clotting effect of 100 grams of butter. (But please don't think you can continue to eat butter if you up your ginger intake. Butter is very high in cholesterol, which contributes to strokes.)

You might try using more ginger in cooking, or you could brew ginger tea using one to two teaspoons of fresh grated root per cup of boiling water. Steep until cool.

❧ **Spinach (*Spinacia oleracea*) and other foods containing folate.** A good deal of evidence shows that nutritional approaches can help prevent stroke. Studies at Tufts University in Boston and the University of Alabama in Birmingham, for example, have demonstrated that folate can help prevent both heart disease and stroke. Compared with people who consumed little folate, those who ingested the most were only half as likely to show narrowing of the carotid artery, the artery that leads to the brain.

Folate is not plentiful in plants, but according to my database, spinach, cabbage, endive, asparagus, parsley, okra and pigweed all have this important nutrient, so the more of these veggies you get in your diet, the better.

❧ **Turmeric (*Cucurma longa*).** Many studies show that the compound curcumin, which is found in this herb, helps prevent the formation of blood clots.

Turmeric is a key ingredient in most curry spice blends. You might consider eating more curry dishes or even making your own turmeric capsules. Many health food stores sell empty gelatin capsules.

Sunburn

From grade school through high school, I lounged around by the swimming pool all summer, soaking up the sun. In college, I played the bass fiddle and guitar at several beaches during the summers. That meant more days lying around in the sun at prime spots such as Grand Haven, Michigan, and Atlantic Beach, Ocean Drive and Myrtle Beach in the Carolinas.

All that sun exposure placed me at considerable risk for skin cancer, and I've lived with the consequences. I have already had a patch of cancer removed, and other blemishes have appeared that will soon need attention.

I've learned my lesson. Now, whenever I'm on a boat in the tropics, I use sunscreen and wear long-sleeved shirts, and sometimes even lightweight gloves and a broad-brimmed hat. All this sun protection goes against my upbringing, but given the places I travel, it's essential. And although I do what I can to keep the sun off, in Amazonia I seem to get sunburned even when I'm all covered.

Green Pharmacy for Sunburn

As burns go, most sunburns are comparatively mild. But sunburns cover a lot more of the body than most other everyday burns. And in addition to increasing cancer risk, they can be quite painful. Fortunately, Nature has provided us with several good remedies.

✿✿✿ Tea (*Camellia sinensis*). The Chinese recommend applying cooled black tea to the skin to soothe sunburn. That sounds good to me because of several beneficial chemical compounds that tea contains.

One researcher I know says that the tannic acid and theobromine in tea help remove heat from sunburn. Other compounds in tea called catechins help prevent and repair skin damage and may even help prevent chemical- and radiation-induced skin cancers. The latest studies show that green tea is also high in chemicals called polyphenols. When ingested, these chemicals help protect the skin against damage from the ultraviolet radiation that causes sunburn.

There's no doubt that it's better to avoid sunburn than endure the after-effects. But if you do spend too much time in the sun with not enough sunscreen, soothe the burn by sipping iced green tea. Then apply cool compresses of the tea to any areas of skin that have been overexposed.

✿✿ Aloe (*Aloe vera*). The inner gel of the aloe vera leaf has been shown to speed the healing of radiation-induced burns. You can scoop the gel directly from split leaves or buy commercially prepared gel at a health food store or herb shop.

Apply aloe gel after showering, then reapply it a few more times each day until the pain has subsided, suggests cardiac surgeon and sports medicine specialist Robert D. Willix, M.D., of Boca Raton, Florida. Usually, he says, the redness disappears in a day or two, and the skin does not peel.

✿✿ Black nightshade (*Solanum nigrum*). Some Indiana folk herbalists crush nightshade leaves, stir them into heavy cream and pat the mixture on sunburn, notes Varro Tyler, Ph.D., dean and professor emeritus of pharmacognosy (natural product pharmacy) at Purdue University in West Lafayette, Indiana.

I've witnessed a similar practice in the Amazon. A Peruvian shamanistic healer I know uses an Amazonian species of nightshade to treat all manner of burns, not just sunburn. He chops the leaves to express a greenish juice, which he applies to a burn as soon as possible, swearing that it prevents scarring.

If you have access to a black nightshade plant, you might want to give this one a try. Compounds in other species of *Solanum* have proved useful in helping to prevent skin cancer.

✷✷ Calendula (*Calendula officinalis*). Research shows that calendula flowers speed the healing of burns by closing wounds, reducing inflammation and stimulating the growth of new skin cells. You can buy commercial skin creams containing calendula at many health food stores.

✷✷ Cucumber (*Cucumis sativus*). The cool cucumber is often used for soothing burns, notes pharmacognosist Albert Leung, Ph.D. Simply slice open a cucumber and wipe it directly on your skin.

✷✷ Eggplant (*Solanum melongena*). Like black nightshade and its Amazonian cousin, which are also in the nightshade family, eggplant has a folk reputation as a sunburn treatment. It actually contains compounds used in sunny Australia for the treatment of skin cancers.

Of course, you're better off using sunscreen to protect yourself from the sun. But if you do get a sunburn, there's probably no reason why you shouldn't try applying some mashed eggplant to your skin to see if it will help soothe the burn.

✷✷ Plantain (*Plantago*, various species). The late Alabama folk herbalist Tommie Bass used plantain for sunburn, stings, poison ivy and poison oak. And he was right, since plantain contains allantoin, a proven healer of injured skin cells.

✷✷ Witch hazel (*Hamamelis virginiana*). In one study, researchers compared three sunburn treatments: witch hazel, 1 percent hydrocortisone, and camomile cream. The hydrocortisone beat the witch hazel, which in turn beat the camomile. Still, the witch hazel worked pretty well, and it's free where I come from.

You can buy a commercial solution and apply it straight from the bottle in a compress. Or try one teaspoon of witch hazel combined with one teaspoon of honey and a beaten egg white. You can also mix one tablespoon each of witch hazel, olive oil and glycerin and give that a try.

❧ Vitamins and minerals. In my database, vitamin E (tocopherol) is the nutrient most cited for anti-sunburn activity. You might want to try a cream containing vitamin E to soothe sunburned skin.

In addition, one study showed that l-selenomethionine, a natural amino acid, reduces the skin damage caused by sunburn. The study was done by Karen E. Burke, M.D., of Cabrini Medical Center in New York City. Selenomethionine is effective both applied to the skin and taken orally. Dr. Burke recommends taking 100 micrograms a day during the summer months, and she suggests 200 micrograms a day for anyone with a family history of any kind of cancer. (Brazil nuts are particularly rich in this nutrient.)

Swelling

An editor called me with a plea for help. She sounded like an upwardly mobile young woman working for one of those upwardly mobile women's health magazines. But she was stumped and in a hurry. With a deadline looming, her boss had challenged a statement that cucumber is good for swollen areas, especially swollen eyelids. She wanted me to find out if it was really true—in an hour. Where's the proof? her boss wanted to know.

Swelling is an enlargement of a localized area caused by abnormal fluid accumulation between cells. It is usually the result of infection, injury or retention or shifting of body fluids. In medical jargon, the word for swelling is *edema*, which is the Greek word for it. And any medicine or poultice that reduces swelling is called an anti-edemic.

Now I knew that cucumber had enjoyed a long folk reputation as an anti-edemic, but that information wasn't good enough for this editor. She needed scientific proof. So I laboriously plowed through my database and discovered that yes, indeed, cucumber contains at least two anti-edemic compounds: ascorbic acid and caffeic acid. It also contains a chemical relative of vitamin A, which may help as well.

Of course, once I got going, I became fascinated by all the anti-edemics I turned up, and I offered her the list—notably ginger, pineapple and turmeric. But all she wanted was verification of cucumber, which I gave her, although as anti-edemics go, it's on the weak side.

Still, as a result of that database search, I can now offer this tip: If you ever develop swollen eyelids, cut two circular sections of cool cucumber, lie down and place the slices on your closed eyelids. It just might help.

Green Pharmacy for Swelling

Besides cucumber slices, there are a number of other herbs that can also help reduce swelling.

❧❧❧ Ginger (*Zingiber officinale*). For centuries, India's traditional Ayurvedic physicians have recommended ginger, especially for swelling caused by arthritis. More recently, several researchers have shown that enzymes that help digest protein, known as proteolytic enzymes, also have anti-inflammatory action.

According to one report, the compound zingibain, which is one of the most active constituents in ginger, is also one of Nature's most potent proteolytic enzymes. Just one gram of zingibain can tenderize as much as 20 pounds of meat.

A Danish researcher reported one case of a woman with rheumatoid arthritis who found no relief from taking corticosteroids, which are commonly prescribed to treat the pain and swelling associated with this condition. She began taking 50 grams of ginger a day (that's almost two ounces, or 25 teaspoons) and within 30 days reported considerable reduction of swelling, as well as some pain relief. "Ginger," the researcher wrote, "produced better relief of swelling, pain and stiffness than nonsteroidal anti-inflammatory drugs."

Of course, 50 grams of ginger a day is a tall order (and you should definitely not take this much if you are pregnant). But given ginger's traditional use for treating arthritic swelling and the herb's proteolytic action, I'm inclined to believe this report.

I have, on occasion, enjoyed 50 grams of candied ginger. It's a hot, spicy candy that's available in many shops that sell gourmet items. It would be a fairly easy way to get this much ginger if you want to give this treatment a try, but ginger is also available in capsules.

❦❦ Pineapple (*Ananas comosus*). This fruit contains the proteolytic enzyme bromelain. Naturopath Michael Murray, N.D., co-author of the *Encyclopedia of Natural Medicine* and several other scholarly books on nutritional and naturopathic healing, recommends taking the pure compound, which is available in health food stores, to reduce swelling, particularly the kind caused by surgical incisions and traumatic injuries. Bromelain blocks the production of kinins, the compounds produced during inflammation that increase swelling and induce pain.

Dr. Murray's suggested dose is 400 to 500 milligrams taken three times a day on an empty stomach. Personally, I love pineapple, and my own recommendation is to simply eat more of this delicious fruit.

❦❦ Turmeric (*Curcuma longa*). India's traditional Ayurvedic physicians apply two parts turmeric and one part salt to swollen areas. Some also include ginger in this mixture. Science confirms this ancient wisdom. When researchers gave turmeric oil to experimental animals, they found that it had anti-inflammatory, anti-edemic and anti-arthritic activity.

Dr. Murray hails curcumin, the most active constituent in turmeric, as one of Nature's most potent anti-edemic and anti-inflammatory agents. He recommends taking 400 milligrams of the pure compound curcumin three times a day. Again, I prefer the whole-herb approach. I suggest simply eating more curries, heavy on the turmeric.

❦ Aloe (*Aloe vera*). People in the West Indies apply the gel of aloe to treat the swelling that comes from water retention. Bahamians even drink aloe juice for this purpose. West Indians also heat the split leaves and apply the warm interior of the leaf to bruises and swollen areas.

Aloe contains an enzyme (bradykininase) that helps decrease swelling and relieve pain. It also contains magnesium lactate, which is an antihistamine, so the herb may also help relieve the itching associated with some swelling.

❦ Arnica (*Arnica montana*). Arnica, also known as mountain daisy, is a favorite among homeopathic physicians for treating the swelling caused by sports injuries.

In larger doses—more than homeopathic doctors would recommend—this herb gets a thumbs-up from Commission E, the German government's group of herbal medicine experts. This group endorses external applications of arnica flowers as a quick fix for water retention, bruises, dislocations, sprains and rheumatic muscle and joint complaints. The commission suggests using two teaspoons of dried herb per cup of boiling water to make a tea to use as a wash. You can also dilute a tincture (one part tincture and three to ten parts water) to use in a compress.

❧ **Cat's claw (*Uncaria*, various species).** Also known as *uña de gato*, cat's claw is an Amazonian herb that's becoming quite popular in the United States, and with good reason. Two researchers sent me a report in which they discuss several compounds (quinovic acid glycosides) that show systemic anti-inflammatory activity. They suggested that cat's claw extract was better at relieving swelling than indomethacin (Indocin), a standard nonsteroidal anti-inflammatory drug that is often prescribed for that purpose.

My own experiments with cat's claw haven't been that positive, but you can try it and see if it works for you.

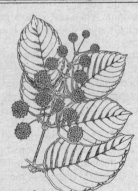

Cat's Claw

A newcomer from the Amazon, cat's claw contains substances that can help relieve swelling and inflammation.

❧ **Corn (*Zea mays*).** The Chinese have used cornsilk successfully to treat swelling caused by kidney disease, according to pharmacognosist (natural product pharmacist) Albert Leung, Ph.D. In one small three-month study of 12 people with kidney disease, water retention disappeared in 9 people and mostly disappeared in 2 others. The people were given about two ounces of dry cornsilk twice a day. Cornsilk is an effective diuretic and is thus useful for getting rid of excess water.

❧ **Dandelion (*Taraxacum officinale*).** Also a potent diuretic, dandelion can remove some of the excess fluid that causes swelling. You can eat the fresh roots, flowers and leaves or use them to make tea. You can also buy capsules.

✽ **Multiflora rose (*Rosa multiflora*).** Now a serious weed in the eastern part of the United States, multiflora rose is listed in Chinese pharmacy reference books as a good treatment for swelling. You can try a tea made with two to three teaspoons of dried herb per cup of boiling water.

✽ **Spanish needles (*Bidens pilosa*).** This is a plant that belongs to the same botanical family as feverfew. It is a popular folk medicine in Taiwan for all sorts of illnesses, from influenza to hepatitis. In one study with laboratory animals, Taiwanese scientists showed that this herb has significant anti-edemic and anti-inflammatory activity. More research is needed here, but I'm intrigued, and I'm on the lookout for further reports of its effectiveness.

Tinnitus

My sister-in-law, Barb, who lives in Hawaii, has tinnitus, or ringing in the ears. She asked me if there are any herbs that can be used to treat it. Yes, indeed, I replied—ginkgo. She tried this marvelous herb, and the ringing went away.

But Barb no longer takes ginkgo. When I last spoke with her, she was back on prescription drugs to treat this condition. Why? It seems that Barb gets her synthetic drugs free from her HMO and Medicare, but she can't get ginkgo free. And ginkgo tends to be pretty expensive.

Of course, Barb's drugs are not really free. She pays for them through her HMO membership and her taxes that support Medicare.

Barb's drug was approved by the Food and Drug Administration (FDA) without having been tested against ginkgo. The FDA really should have tested ginkgo, too. It's cheaper than the drug—if you have to pay for the drug out of your own pocket, that is. It's also more natural, at least as effective and perhaps safer.

Green Pharmacy for Tinnitus

Tinnitus is chronic ringing in the ears, although sometimes the sound is more like a roaring or whooshing. Doctors don't really know what causes tinnitus and often have very little success in alleviating it. Fortunately, natural approaches can help.

✺✺✺ Ginkgo (*Ginkgo biloba*). Hundreds of European studies have confirmed the use of standardized ginkgo extract for a wide variety of conditions associated with aging, including tinnitus, vertigo, memory loss and poor circulation. Ginkgo does not work in every case of tinnitus, but it is the herb I'd try first.

The active constituents in ginkgo leaf, ginkgolides, occur in concentrations too dilute to allow the use of teas or tinctures. The way to take ginkgo is as a 50:1 standardized extract, meaning that 50 pounds of ginkgo leaves are processed into 1 pound of extract. You'll have to buy this extract in a pharmacy or health food store; look for 50:1 on the label. Most experts recommend taking 40 milligrams of ginkgo extract three times a day to treat tinnitus.

✺✺ Sesame (*Sesamum indicum*). Chinese herbalists recommend sesame seeds for the treatment of tinnitus, blurred vision and dizziness. If you'd like to give sesame seeds a try, there's probably no harm in adding it to foods. Or try tahini, the peanut-butter-like spread made from sesame seeds, or halvah, which is sesame candy.

✺ Black cohosh (*Cimicifuga racemosa*). In her interesting feminist herbal, *The Roots of Healing*, Deb Soule, distinguished Maine herbalist and founder of Avena Botanicals, spins the tale of a professional flutist neighbor of hers who had been troubled for years by tinnitus. This neighbor took black cohosh tincture for a few weeks, and his tinnitus almost disappeared. He became a disciple of herbalism. Deb adds that black cohosh and ginkgo are a good combination.

✺ Goldenseal (*Hydrastis canadensis*). British herbalist David Hoffmann, author of *The Herbal Handbook* and one of my favorite practitioners, suggests that goldenseal may help some cases of tinnitus. It seems as if it might be worth a try.

✺ Lesser periwinkle (*Vinca minor*). This evergreen groundcover adorns some of my sunny and sandy slopes, but I'd never heard of using it medicinally until I checked a reference from Rudolph Fritz Weiss, M.D., Germany's leading herbal doctor and author of *Herbal Medicine*. Dr. Weiss reports that lesser periwinkle contains vincamine, a chemical compound that reportedly gives good results with tinnitus and Meniéré's syndrome. He suggests taking 20 milligrams of dried herb three times a day. Since there are some safety issues with this herb, however, you should follow a physician's advice if you want to try it.

❧ **Spinach (*Spinacia oleracea*) and other foods containing zinc.** Noting that zinc deficiency seems to be associated with tinnitus and certain kinds of hearing loss (sensorineural), Melvyn Werbach, M.D., assistant clinical professor of psychiatry at the University of California, Los Angeles, School of Medicine and author of *Nutritional Influences on Illness*, suggests taking 60 to 120 milligrams of zinc a day. This is a lot of zinc (the Daily Value is 15 milligrams), so you should not try this therapy without discussing it with your doctor.

My preference would be to simply increase the amount of zinc you get from food. According to my database, good sources of zinc include spinach (the best), parsley, collards, brussels sprouts, cucumbers, string beans, endive, cowpeas, prunes and asparagus.I doubt that anyone could get 60 milligrams of zinc a day from diet alone, but you could certainly make a point of taking in more zinc from your food while trying other herbal treatments for tinnitus. I can also recommend whipping up a tasty Zincophile Soup. Toss any or all of the vegetables listed (except the prunes) into a good vegetable soup.

Herbs to avoid. If tinnitus bothers you, don't take aspirin or aspirin-like herbs—willow bark, meadowsweet and wintergreen. High doses of aspirin may cause ringing in the ears. I've also seen reports that a few other herbs may aggravate tinnitus, among them cinchona, black haw and uva ursi.

Tonsillitis

A lthough I frequently had trouble with my tonsils when I was a kid, my mother never had them taken out, in spite of pressure from the M.D.'s she consulted. But when my younger brother came along, she followed the doctors' advice.

Brother Dan's tonsils came out. He then faced a constant

round of allergies and infections. Were these problems caused by his genes? I doubt it. Could it have had something to with his tonsillectomy? I'll never know for sure, but I suspect that it may have beeen a factor. Doctors now know that tonsils do help fight off infections. And medical opinion now holds that far too many tonsils were removed back in the days when my brother had his taken out.

I still get infections in my tonsils. Would I be better off without them? I can't say for sure, but I do thank my mom for leaving them where they belong.

Tonsillitis is an inflammation of the tonsils, the small round lymph glands sitting on the sides of the throat. It occurs most frequently in children under nine. Usually the tonsils become inflamed because they have been exposed to infection-causing microorganisms, frequently streptococcal bacteria or a virus. If you have tonsillitis, you should see a doctor for treatment. It's especially important to treat a strep infection with antibiotics because this kind of infection can lead to a heart-damaging bout of rheumatic fever.

Green Pharmacy for Tonsillitis

Tonsillitis—and inflammation of the related glands, the adenoids—shows that the body is defending itself from infection. Here are the herbs that can help fight off the infection and soothe the inflammation.

❧-❧-❧ Echinacea (*Echinacea*, various species). Herbs that enhance immunity are useful in almost all infections. Echinacea, also known as coneflower, is a fine one, according to many European studies. Echinacea stimulates phagocytosis, the devouring of bacteria and viruses by certain types of white blood cells. As with so many mouth and throat infections, I'd recommend going with a double whammy by taking echinacea along with goldenseal, another potent antiseptic, antibiotic and immune stimulant.

❧-❧ Garlic (*Allium sativum*). Garlic is useful in treating any kind of throat infection, including tonsillitis. James Balch, M.D., a urologist, and his wife, Phyllis, a certified nutritional consultant, recommend taking two garlic capsules a day for either sore throat or tonsillitis. (They also suggest eating more of garlic's close relative, onions.)

Capsules are a convenient way to take garlic, but not all

experts give them top billing. Jane Guiltinan, N.D., chief medical officer at Bastyr University in Seattle, for example, prefers whole garlic cloves to capsules or extracts. I agree.

May I suggest that my Tonsil Soup is also good for treating tonsillitis? To make it, use any favorite recipe for an onion/garlic soup. Then be very generous with any or all of the hot spices that contain vitamin C and other good sore-throat fighters, including chili pepper, ginger, horseradish, mustard seed and pepper.

❦❦ Honeysuckle (*Lonicera japonica*). Honeysuckle flowers are used in China to treat tonsillitis, bronchitis, colds, flu and pneumonia. Extracts made from these flowers act strongly against a broad spectrum of bacteria. It's small wonder, since the flowers contain more than a dozen antiseptic compounds.

In one study, researchers looked at 425 Chinese students with strep throat. This is not tonsillitis, admittedly, but it is a related throat infection. In this study, researchers spurred rapid healing by introducing an herbal preparation that included powdered dried honeysuckle flowers into the backs of the students' throats.

I would not hesitate to use honeysuckle, by itself or combined with forsythia, to treat tonsillitis. In fact, I do use the leaves of both plants to treat many midwinter respiratory infections.

❦❦ Sage (*Salvia officinalis*). In Germany, where herbal medicine is more mainstream than it is in the United States, physicians recommend a hot sage gargle for tonsillitis. The reason appears to be that sage has fairly high levels of tannins, substances that have a soothing, astringent action and an antimicrobial effect. Sage is loaded with other antiseptics, too.

❦❦ Citrus fruits and other foods containing vitamin C. There is some evidence that the vitamin C in citrus fruit is effective in treating the strep bacteria that often cause tonsillitis. Vitamin C also stimulates the immune system to produce more macrophages, scavenger cells that literally gobble up strep bacteria.

Besides citrus fruits, good plant sources of vitamin C include bitter melon, rosehips, bell peppers, red pepper, pokeweed shoots, guavas and watercress.

❦ Blackberry (*Rubus*, various species) and persimmon (*Diospyros virginiana*). Blackberry root and persimmon, either alone or in combination, were early American folk remedies for tonsillitis. Since both are rich in tannins, this is a rational formula.

❧ **Dandelion (*Taraxacum officinale*).** The Chinese suggest simmering about an ounce of dandelion root in two to three cups of boiling water until only half of the liquid remains. The resulting syrup is recommended for tonsillitis.

❧ **Elderberry (*Sambucus nigra*).** Many cultures use elderberry juice to treat tonsillitis, according to medical anthropologist John Heinerman, Ph.D., author of *Heinerman's Encyclopedia of Fruits, Vegetables and Herbs*. This makes sense to me in view of medical research showing that this herb has antiviral action and helps treat influenza.

❧ **Redroot (*Ceanothus americanus*).** The late Alabama herbalist Tommie Bass, whom I respected, used redroot, also known as New Jersey tea, for tonsillitis, sore throat, cough and thrush, a type of throat infection. The active constituent seems to be the tannins. Redroot can be as much as 10 percent tannins.

❧ **Assorted fruits.** Elsewhere around the world, blackberry's close relative, raspberry, is used to treat inflamed tonsils. One recipe involves adding sugar to boiled raspberry juice, and after it has cooled, gargling and swallowing it. Now that's one medicine I could enjoy.

Healing claims have been made for sugary syrups of blackberries, blueberries, papaya, red grapes and strawberries. In fact, this approach could be easily worked into what I call Tonsilade: Start with one cup of the juice of any or all of the above fruits. Then add a little juice from one of the citrus fruits—lemon, lime or orange—plus a bit of sage tea and sugar to taste.

❧ **Herbal formulas.** British herbalist David Hoffmann, author of *The Herbal Handbook*, suggests a treatment for tonsillitis that I might try myself: a tea brewed from two parts echinacea, two parts garden or red sage and one part balm of gilead. If you like sweet teas, you may add licorice, which is soothing.

Toothache

The Choco Indians have lived for probably thousands of years in eastern Panama and adjacent Colombia. Today, unfortunately, they are disappearing, victims of "development." I've worked more closely with them than with any other Indian group.

As early as 1960, my Choco confidants told me about a plant of the genus *Piper*, a close relative of black pepper, which they used as a remedy for toothache. They handed me a twig, and when I bit into it, my mouth went numb.

You certainly won't have access to the Chocos' plant. But another tropical toothache herb is probably sitting in your spice rack right now. It's clove, the flower buds of a tropical tree. Oil of clove contains a great deal of the anesthetic, antiseptic chemical eugenol. Cloves are 5 to 20 times richer in eugenol than other eugenol sources listed in my database. In fact, many dentists use it as a dental anesthetic and pain reliever, especially when doing root canals.

There's no need to define toothache. I've suffered quite a few over the years, and to this day, I stupidly procrastinate about going to the dentist. It turns out that I'm not alone. An estimated 98 percent of Americans have dental cavities, according to the National Institute of Dental Research.

All this adds up to millions of toothaches a year. Any persistent toothache should be checked by a dentist, but fortunately, you don't have to suffer on your way there, thanks to some good herbs.

Green Pharmacy for Toothache

The use of herbal oils for toothache is not new to scientific dentistry. As early as 1946, M. A. Lesser published a review in the journal *Drug and Cosmetic Industry* entitled "Preparations for Toothache." He noted that essential herbal oils "are the chief active ingredients of toothache preparations. Of these, oil of clove and eugenol are undoubtedly most important . . . "

✿✿✿ **Clove (*Syzygium aromaticum*).** Germany's Commission E, the body of natural medicine experts that makes herbal recommendations to that country's counterpart of the Food and Drug Administration (FDA), endorses oil of clove as a local anesthetic and antiseptic for toothache. Even a scientific committee reporting to our FDA commented that oil of clove was the only one of 12 ingredients commonly found in toothache preparations that was "safe and effective for temporary use on a tooth with throbbing pain."

❦

Jungle Wisdom

At the beginning of this chapter, I mentioned a pepper plant that the Choco Indians use to numb the pain of toothache.

I encountered this plant again years later, on my first ecotour to Iquitos, Peru. My Indian guide pointed to the plant and reiterated that it relieves toothache. He pulled it up by the root, scraped off the dirt and invited me to bite into it. As before, it immediately anesthetized my mouth.

Fruits and roots of some species of pepper plants are known to contain anesthetic compounds. Even black pepper contains some.

People who have lived for thousands of years in the world's jungles have toothache remedies that really work. And that's the main reason I wrote this book—to show that traditional medicine has legitimate scientific value.

Scientific critics counter that "old folk tales" are no match for Western-style scientific experimentation. But the basis of science is careful observation, and that's what traditional peoples have been doing since time immemorial—observing and experimenting with the world around them.

In general, traditional people have managed to select the good medicines and have rejected the bad, leading to what we today call folk medicine. Most of these folk medicines have thousands of years of experimental selection behind them, and few are associated with adverse reactions.

That's something that you really can't say about our modern pharmaceuticals, only a few of which have been on this earth for more than a hundred years. All too often, synthetic drugs turn out to be hazardous. This is evidenced by the number of pharmaceuticals that the Food and Drug Administration orders withdrawn because of adverse reactions.

❦

You can buy over-the-counter preparations of clove oil to use yourself to numb toothache. The oil is placed directly on the tooth, not ingested.

❧❧ **Ginger** (*Zingiber officinale*). A compress made with this hot spice seems to help alleviate toothache pain. I'd add more heat to such a compress myself, in the form of red pepper. Both ginger and red pepper seem to work like the old mustard plasters. They act as counterirritants, meaning that the surface irritation of the ginger or red pepper helps to diminish the deeper toothache pain.

To make a compress for your tooth, mix the powdered spice or spices in enough water to form a gooey paste. Then dip in a small cotton ball and wring it out. Apply the cotton directly to the tooth without letting it touch your gum. If you can't stand the heat, rinse your mouth and try some other remedy.

❧❧ **Red pepper** (*Capsicum*, **various species**). In 1992, while the world celebrated Columbus's voyage, I celebrated the introduction of red pepper outside America. Columbus was introduced to the spice by the Caribbean Indians.

When applied to the skin, capsaicin, the hot ingredient in red pepper, burns for a while, but it depletes the action of substance P, the chemical in the body responsible for transmitting pain. In addition, red pepper is fairly well endowed with salicylates, aspirin-like chemicals that can relieve pain. It's no wonder that this herb is an old folk remedy for toothache. To use red pepper on a toothache, use the cotton compress technique described for ginger.

✺✺ Toothache tree (*Zanthoxylum americanum*). This tree got its name because it's an old folk remedy for toothache. The late Alabama folk herbalist Tommie Bass recommended it right up until he died in 1996. He suggested chewing the bark or making a tea out of the bark or berries. I know from chewing on the twigs that it has anesthetic properties. This one may be a little hard to locate, but you may be able to find the dried herb in a shop that specializes in herbs.

✺✺ Willow (*Salix*, various species). For my toothaches, I have on occasion resorted to chewing a wad of willow bark and then tamping it into the painful tooth to temporarily alleviate the pain. Willow bark contains salicin, a chemical relative of aspirin that has considerable pain-relieving power. You can also drink a tea made from the herb or take a tincture to help banish the pain. (If you are allergic to aspirin, however, you probably shouldn't use aspirin-like herbs, either.)

✺ Rhubarb (*Rheum officinale*). Rhubarb root is used for toothache in China, where they call it *da-huang*. They prepare a toothache remedy by frying the root, then steeping it in alcohol to create a tincture. Then, using a cotton ball, they apply the tincture directly to the painful tooth for five minutes.

I'd try this if I couldn't find the better herbs mentioned earlier. Rhubarb contains at least six pain-relieving chemical compounds.

✺ Sesame (*Sesamum indicum*). Pharmacognosist (natural product pharmacist) Albert Leung, Ph.D., shares this fourth-century Chinese folk remedy for toothache: Boil one part sesame seed with two parts water until half the liquid remains. The resulting decoction, when applied directly to the tooth, was said to work wonders for toothache and gum disease. There's good reason to believe that this treatment might work, as sesame contains at least seven pain-relieving compounds.

Tooth Decay

An estimated 98 percent of Americans have cavities; most develop between the ages of 5 and 15. Researchers believe that cavity formation drops off by the midteens because the body develops immunity to decay-causing bacteria, primarily several types of streptococcus.

Green Pharmacy for Tooth Decay

Tooth decay was an even bigger problem before the fluoridation of water in this century. From ancient times until the nineteenth century, herbalists put a great deal of effort into studying plants that helped preserve teeth. They discovered quite a few that were very effective.

❧❧❧ **Tea (*Camellia sinensis*).** In addition to a generous endowment of several compounds that work together to prevent tooth decay, tea also contains a considerable amount of tooth-preserving fluoride.

Green tea may contain more fluoride than black tea. To get potent decay-preventive action from just the fluoride in tea, you'd have to drink three to ten cups a day. But you actually need less because of all the other anticavity compounds in tea. (There's also a good chance that the water you use for your tea already contains fluoride.) If you sweeten your tea, try using licorice instead of decay-promoting sugar. To do this, simply brew your regular tea with a little dried licorice root.

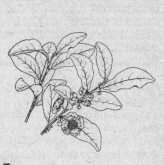

Tea

Tea, which is native to China, was originally used to flavor water that had been boiled for purification.

❧❧❧ **Bay (*Laurus nobilis*).** Bay's aromatic oil contains a powerful bacteria killing chemical (1,8-cineole) that is used in some dentifrices. Check the toothpaste label for bay if you'd like to take advantage of this herb's decay-preventing potential. If you don't find a toothpaste containing this ingredient in your pharmacy, you might have better luck at your local health food store.

❧❧ **Bloodroot (*Sanguinaria officinalis*).** Many studies have shown that dental-care products containing bloodroot help reduce the amount of dental plaque deposited on the teeth in as little as eight days. Bloodroot contains a compound known as sanguinarine, which seems to be responsible for the plaque-reducing effect.

Sanguinarine chemically binds to dental plaque and helps prevent it from adhering to the teeth. And since dental plaque is responsible for gum disease as well as tooth decay, bloodroot is also a good choice for adults who are fighting gum disease.

You can take advantage of bloodroot's plaque-fighting potential by looking for toothpastes and mouthwashes that contain this herb. One popular brand is Viadent.

❧❧ **Licorice (*Glycyrrhiza glabra*).** In addition to containing the bacteria-killing, nonsugar sweetener glycyrrhizin, licorice also contains indole, a powerful decay-preventive compound.

❧❧ **Peanut (*Arachis hypogaea*).** Before I retired as the U.S. Department of Agriculture's expert on medicinal plants, people always ribbed me about keeping peanuts as munchies in my office. I did it because I like peanuts. But I have learned that researchers at the Eastman Dental Center in Rochester, New York, have shown that peanuts are less likely to cause cavities than pretzels. Pretzels, in turn, are less likely to cause cavities than dried fruit, potato chips, saltines, graham crackers, fruit, chocolate and anything containing sugar.

I often mixed my decay-preventive peanuts with sugary, decay-promoting raisins. If I were more concerned about cavities, I guess I'd go with just the peanuts.

❧❧ **Stevia (*Stevia rebaudiana*).** This sweet herb from Paraguay is another tasty, nonsugar sweetener. Simply buy a box of tea and use a pinch whenever you want to sweeten a beverage. You'll find that it's extremely sweet. (Come to think of it, this is good advice for anyone who's trying to cut calories, too.)

❧❧ **Toothache tree (*Zanthoxylum americanum*).** This herb is best known for minimizing the horrible pain of toothache. It also contains a bacteria-killing chemical that can help prevent

tooth decay. The late Alabama herbalist Tommie Bass recommended chewing twigs. You could make a concentrated tea to
swish in your mouth. You'll probably find the herb only in some
specialty herb shops.

❧☙

Herbal Antiseptic
Mouthwash

Use this mouthwash after dinner by simply swizzling
some around in your mouth. Then, if you enjoy herbal
liqueurs, go ahead and swallow it; you'll find that it's delicious. This mixture contains more than 20 antiseptic
compounds and could help prevent tooth decay.

 1 pint vodka
 2 tablespoons eucalyptus
 2 tablespoons cardamom
 2 tablespoons rosemary or spearmint
 1 tablespoon cherry birch or wintergreen
 1 tablespoon horsemint
 1 tablespoon thyme
 1 tablespoon wild bergamot

In a glass jar, mix the herbs into the vodka. Close the jar
and put it away for one month.

❧☙

❧❧ **Wild bergamot** (*Monarda fistulosa*). This herb can
contain up to 30,000 parts per million of the decay-preventive
compound geraniol. Bergamot has about 20 times more geraniol than tea has.

Wild bergamot also contains a great deal of thymol, another
powerful antiseptic that is the active ingredient in Listerine, the
popular mouthwash. But why stop at just thymol? My own

recipe for a potent mouthwash contains several oral antiseptics that can help prevent tooth decay.

❦ **Chaparral (*Larrea divaricata*).** One scientific study, initiated by researchers who knew that chaparral has been used as a folk remedy for toothache, showed that chaparral mouthwash reduced cavities by 75 percent. And scientists have learned that one compound in the plant, nordihydroguarietic acid, is a potent antiseptic. Just brew a tea with chaparral to use as a mouthwash, but be careful to spit it all out without swallowing any.

❦ **Myrrh (*Commiphora*, various species).** Myrrh's antiseptic uses go back to biblical times. Tincture of myrrh has both deodorant and disinfecting properties, and it can be used as a dental rinse, gargle and mouthwash.

Tuberculosis

In late 1995, I addressed a group of more than 100 physicians at Flower Hospital in Toledo, Ohio. After my talk on herbal medicine, one older doctor drew me aside and told me this story: Decades earlier, when he was much younger, he met a man who had been admitted to a sanatorium for tuberculosis (TB). That was during the time when sanatoriums were in vogue and people with TB were usually sent away to them for their remaining days. Once consigned to a sanatorium, few people ever went home again.

The man the doctor described, however, had somehow been given a reprieve. And this was the curious thing. According to the doctor, the patient with tuberculosis happened to find a discarded load of onions on the grounds of the sanatorium. Tired and depleted from TB, he began eating the onions, enjoying several a day. Within a month he was well enough to leave the institution.

Now there's a story to delight and intrigue a plant medicine enthusiast. It turns out that onions really do have antibacterial properties, so it's just possible that this man's multi-onion diet really had something to do with his cure.

An Old Scourge Makes a Comeback

Tuberculosis is a chronic, usually contagious bacterial infection that can spread through the body in the bloodstream and lymph nodes, but it usually focuses on the lungs. To become infected, most people need to be repeatedly exposed—by living or working at close quarters with a carrier of the disease, for example.

If you spend 8 hours a day for six months or 24 hours a day for two months with anyone with active TB, there's a 50 percent chance that you will get it. It's no wonder that the disease centers in poverty-stricken areas where people live crowded together without adequate medical care.

Fortunately, my own family had lots of living space in Panama 30 years ago when we learned that our live-in maid had tested positive for TB. My whole family immediately was checked for the disease. Luckily, the test results showed that we were all TB-negative.

TB is the most common cause of death from infection in developing countries, causing 26 percent of avoidable adult deaths and 6.7 percent of all deaths. In the United States, those at highest risk include health-care workers, long-term hospital patients, prison inmates and guards and people with HIV, the virus that causes AIDS.

The bacteria generally remain dormant after entering the body, and only about 10 percent of infected individuals actually come down with overt TB. The remaining 90 percent produce TB antibodies, signifying exposure, but they show no signs of infection and cannot spread the disease.

In most cases, antibiotics eradicate TB. But in recent years, as AIDS has triggered an upsurge in cases, the bacteria have become resistant to one or more of the standard antibiotics. Currently, about 1 percent of new TB cases in New York City are caused by bacteria resistant to one antibiotic, while up to 7 percent of recurrent cases are resistant to two or more antibiotics. People who have TB that is resistant to multiple drugs have only about a 50 percent chance of survival, about the same chance as people had before antibiotics were developed.

TB is very serious. If you test positive, by all means get evaluated by a physician. If your doctor recommends medication, take it, and take all of it.

Green Pharmacy for Tuberculosis

In addition to your medical treatment, there are a number of herbs that might prove helpful.

✿✿✿ **Echinacea (*Echinacea*, various species).** Confronted with any bacteria, including the type that causes TB, I'd take echinacea to boost my immune system even after I started on antibiotics. That's precisely what I did in 1996 when I may have contracted Lyme disease. I took two 450-milligram capsules of echinacea three times a day, hoping to spur my immune system to resist the bacteria. Alternatively, you might also consider trying up to 40 drops of tincture three times a day. (Although echinacea can cause your tongue to tingle or go numb temporarily, this effect is harmless.)

✿✿✿ **Forsythia (*Forsythia suspensa*).** The Chinese use forsythia as an antibacterial antiseptic. Strong teas are very active against several bacteria. The plant has been used clinically against TB, often combined with honeysuckle. To fight a variety of infections, I use forsythia twigs in a 1:2 ratio with honeysuckle in a tea or hot lemonade. I think this approach would be good for treating TB.

✿✿✿ **Garlic (*Allium sativum*).** If I suspected that I had TB, I'd take garlic until I could get to a physician, and maybe even afterward. The Chinese use garlic to treat TB, with decent results, I hear. If I feared that I'd been exposed to TB, I would take at least one garlic capsule a day, and I'd make sure the label said that each capsule was standardized to the equivalent of at least one gram of fresh garlic.

In their excellent new book, *Garlic: The Science and Therapeutic Application of Allium Sativum and Related Species*, Heinrich P. Koch, Ph.D., professor of pharmaceutical chemistry and biopharmaceutics at the University of Vienna, and Larry D. Lawson, Ph.D., a research scientist at Nature's Way, an herb company in Springville, Utah, suggest that garlic may help antibiotics do their job in fighting TB. Studies show that allicin, the antibacterial compound in garlic, enhances the action of such antibiotics as chloramphenicol (Chloromycetin) and streptomycin against TB bacteria.

✿✿✿ **Honeysuckle (*Lonicera japonica*).** Honeysuckle has been used for centuries in China to treat a variety of respiratory problems, including TB, bronchitis, colds, flu and pneumonia. Honeysuckle flower extracts are strongly active against several bacteria, including those that cause TB.

I would not hesitate to use this herb if I had TB. In summer I'd make a tea with a handful of flowers per cup of boiling water and drink up to three cups a day. In winter I'd boil twigs and dried leaves to make a bitter tea, which I would mask with lemon and honey, turning it into hot honeysuckle lemonade.

≈≈≈ Licorice (*Glycyrrhiza glabra*). Since, according to my database, licorice has up to 33 percent antibacterial compounds on a dry-weight basis, it's small wonder that the Chinese use licorice to treat TB. I often use licorice roots, which are also antiviral, to sweeten my herbal teas when I have colds, and I drank licorice tea when I was flirting with Lyme disease. I'd probably add licorice to any herbal preparation I took for TB if I were battling this disease.

≈≈ Eucalyptus (*Eucalyptus globulus*). This is another herb used in Asia to treat TB. Unless you live in tropical America or in the San Francisco Bay area, you may have trouble finding fresh eucalyptus leaves, but the essential oil is readily available at shops that sell aromatherapy supplies.

Try a drop or two added to water or tea. That's a rough equivalent of the Chinese dose. You cannot ingest many essential oils, but eucalyptus is an exception, as long as you don't get overly enthusiastic. Don't use more than a drop or two: This is powerful stuff.

≈≈ Onion (*Allium cepa*). Onions have almost as much antibacterial action as their close relative, garlic, so I wasn't surprised to hear that story about the TB sanatorium resident who cured himself by eating onions. If I had TB, I'd eat lots of garlic and onions.

Ulcers

Back in 1991, I had an injury that caused the most excruciating pain I've ever had. My doctor prescribed large doses of nonsteroidal anti-inflammatory drugs (NSAIDs), which are powerful pain relievers.

Unfortunately for me and for anyone who's ever taken NSAIDs, these drugs are also notorious for causing ulcers.

Luckily for me, however, I knew about licorice, and I still regularly sweeten some herb teas with it. Now I'd say that I may owe my freedom from ulcers to this habit.

I never got an ulcer from taking all those NSAIDs. And even more amazing, I never developed one during the 30 years that I was employed by the federal government in the U.S. Department of Agriculture.

I don't think this proves that I have a stomach of steel. Rather, I think I owe my freedom from ulcers to the fact that sweet licorice root contains compounds that have remarkable anti-ulcer effects. And perhaps I also benefited from eating many of the ulcer-preventing herbs and foods discussed in this chapter.

The Sore That Won't Heal

Technically, an ulcer is any sore. But when people say that they have an ulcer, they almost always mean an internal sore in the lining of the stomach or duodenum, the gateway to the small intestine just downstream from the stomach. These kinds of ulcers are also called peptic ulcers because they occur in areas that are exposed to the digestive enzyme pepsin.

An estimated 10 percent of Americans have an ulcer at some point in life, with about one million new diagnoses a year. Men are four times more susceptible than women, and risk rises with age. Allergies somehow make people more ulcer-prone: In one study, 98 percent of people with peptic ulcers also had respiratory allergies.

Not long ago, scientists thought that stress caused ulcers. It may well play a role, but now we know that the real culprit is often an infection caused by the bacteria *Helicobacter pylori*, sometimes known as *Campylobacter pylori*. Simply having *H. pylori* bacteria in your system doesn't mean that you will get an ulcer. However, more than 75 percent of people with ulcers show evidence of *H. pylori* infection, and that's straight from the pages of the *Journal of the American Medical Association*.

Green Pharmacy for Ulcers

These days, doctors generally treat ulcers caused by *H. pylori* with a combination of antibiotics plus bismuth (Pepto-

Bismol) or similar drugs. In addition, you might try a number of herbal anti-ulcer approaches.

❧❧❧ **Ginger (*Zingiber officinale*).** How about candied ginger as an herbal alternative to cimetidine (Tagamet), ranitidine (Zantac) and famotidine (Pepcid)? It would sure taste a lot better!

❧❧

Anti-ulcer Fruit Cocktail

Every one of the ingredients in this tasty, no-fat dessert contains significant amounts of stomach-soothing, anti-ulcer compounds. You'll probably have a hard time thinking of this scrumptious treat as potent medicine, but that's exactly what it is.

    Bananas
    Pineapple
    Blueberries
    Ground cinnamon
    Ground cloves
    Ground ginger
    Honey (optional)

Cut up the bananas and pineapple; the amount and proportions will vary depending on how many people you're serving and which fruits you like best. Place them in a serving bowl and add the blueberries. Season to taste with the cinnamon, cloves and ginger (try to be generous) and sweeten with the honey (if using).

If you like, you can also make a between-meal anti-ulcer drink by blending blueberry juice, pineapple juice, a banana and the spices listed above. Garnish each serving with a peppermint sprig.

❧❧

❧

Folk Wisdom Vindicated Again

Here's a story I'd like to share with you about herbal folk wisdom and modern science. An old herbalist whom I respected, the late A. L. "Tommie" Bass, who had a little herb farmette outside Leesburg, Alabama, became the subject of a book, *Herbal Medicine: Past and Present* by John K. Crellin and Jane Philpott, published by Duke University Press in 1989.

In this book Crellin and Philpott discussed some 300 herbs that Tommie recommended over the years. For each herb, the authors recounted what Tommie had to say about the herb and then interpreted his account in the light of pharmacological research.

One herb that Tommie recommended for ulcers was yellowroot, which contains some of the same chemicals as goldenseal. Here's what Tommie said about it: "More people are taking it now for ulcers than anything we know of. I've used yellowroot to help so many people with their ulcers. They come back to thank me and offer me money. But I'm not in the business for the money. I'm in it to help people. And yellowroot can help an ulcer, more than that Tagamet. They throw away their Tagamet once they try the yellowroot."

But Crellin and Philpott noted that "little physiological evidence exists to suggest any specific activity on ulcers" from yellowroot's known active compounds, most notably berberine.

Perhaps they were understating the case. When I checked my database, I saw that berberine had, in fact, been reported to have anti-ulcer effects. In addition, Crellin and Philpott's commentary was written before the discovery that most ulcers are caused by bacterial infections. Yellowroot is a potent antibiotic, and berberine is a compound that has antibacterial effects even at very low concentrations, meaning that a few spoonfuls of tincture a day might well cure an ulcer, just as Tommie claimed.

I'm including this story as yet another example of how often folk wisdom about plants turns out to be scientifically valid. It also serves as a reminder that sometimes scientists need to take a second look at something that they've initially rejected as unscientific, especially when new data accumulate. The wisdom gained by long experience may prevail.

❦

Ginger is well-known for its anti-inflammatory activity, but it's considerably less known as an herbal treatment for ulcers. In fact, ginger contains 11 compounds that have demonstrated anti-ulcer effects. These chemical compounds are a real mouthful, but I think that you might find it interesting to know just how much anti-ulcer chemistry can be concentrated in a single, humble spice. Here they are in order, from most to least abundant: 6-shogaol, 6-gingerol, 8-shogaol, 8-gingerol, 10-gingerol, ar-curcumene, beta-bisalene, 6-gingediol, betases-quiphellandrene, 6-gingerdione and 6-paradol.

Eating honey-candied ginger is a pleasant-tasting treatment for ulcers, according to Paul Schulick, New England herbalist and author of *Ginger: Common Spice and Wonder Drug*. The combination of honey and ginger is particularly effective, he notes. In addition to the antibacterial compounds that are available from ginger, honey has antibacterial action, and the two together seem to produce synergistic effects. Ginger is a key ingredient in my Anti-ulcer Fruit Cocktail.

❦❦❦ **Licorice (*Glycyrrhiza glabra*).** German physicians have always been more open to herbal medicine than doctors in the United States, and they have researched herbal alternatives extensively. Commission E, the body of scientists that advises the German counterpart of the Food and Drug Administration, approves licorice as an ulcer treatment. This recommendation is based on the medical traditions of Asia, the Middle East and Europe, plus literally dozens of scientific studies.

Licorice contains several anti-ulcer compounds, including glycyrrhizic acid. Licorice and its extracts are safe for normal use in moderate amounts, up to about three cups of tea a day. However, long-term use—daily use for longer than six weeks—or ingestion of excessive amounts can produce symptoms such as headache, lethargy, sodium and water retention, excessive loss of potassium and high blood pressure.

These side effects, however, can be largely eliminated by using a slightly processed form of the herb called deglycyrrhizinated licorice (DGL). In one good study, DGL was at least as effective in speeding ulcer healing as the newest class of pharmaceutical drugs, called histamine-blocking agents, that were designed to do this. DGL also seems to protect the digestive lining from aspirin's ulcer-promoting effects.

Commercial licorice preparations containing DGL are readily available in natural food stores that sell herbs. If you have an ulcer, this is the preferred form of licorice to take, but clearly some of the power of the herb is lost with the lost glycyrrhizin.

If you'd like to take licorice from time to time as an ulcer preventive, you can do what I do. When you're brewing some other herbal tea, add a little licorice. Licorice by itself makes a sweet, pleasant-tasting tea, and when added to other teas, it serves as a sweetener.

❧❧❧ **Yellowroot (*Xanthorrhiza simplicissima*).** If the late Alabama herbalist Tommie Bass's experience with yellowroot can be believed—and I'm inclined to believe it—this herb is worth a try. (For details, see "Folk Wisdom Vindicated Again" on page 528.) Yellowroot is an antibiotic that should work by helping to control *H. pylori* bacteria.

I personally would try a teaspoon of yellowroot tincture in juice or tea once or twice a day before moving on to the antibiotics my doctor might prescribe for ulcer. If you're already taking antibiotics, however, do not make this switch without first discussing it with your doctor. Be warned: Untreated *H. pylori* virus is linked to stomach cancer, so you must take this condition seriously.

❧❧ **Banana (*Musa paradisiaca*).** Bananas are an old folk remedy for many gastrointestinal problems because they soothe the digestive tract. And studies with experimental animals suggest that bananas do, in fact, have an anti-ulcer effect.

One researcher noted that "bananas may be another useful

addition to such well-established anti-ulcer foods as raw cabbage, green tea, garlic and legumes."

❧❧ **Cabbage (*Brassica oleracea*).** Raw cabbage juice is a hallowed folk remedy for ulcers. It turns out that cabbage and its juice contain considerable amounts of two compounds with anti-ulcer activity, glutamine and S-methyl-methionine.

Melvyn Werbach, M.D., assistant clinical professor of psychiatry at the University of California, Los Angeles, School of Medicine and author of the excellent *Nutritional Influences on Illness*, cites a study of people with ulcers who were given raw cabbage juice as a treatment. Ninety-two percent showed significant improvement within three weeks compared with 32 percent of those taking a lookalike treatment (a placebo) without cabbage juice.

In studies of just the active compound glutamine, daily doses of 1,600 milligrams proved as effective as conventional antacids in treating ulcers.

The folk recommendation for treating ulcers is to drink one quart of raw cabbage juice a day. That may be hard to swallow, so I offer a recipe that might help: Anti-ulcer Cabbage Soup.

❧❧ **Calendula (*Calendula officinalis*).** Calendula, sometimes known as pot marigold, has antibacterial, antiviral and immune-stimulating properties. Calendula has been shown to alleviate symptoms of chronic stomach inflammation, what doctors call hypersecretory gastritis, a condition that has been associated with ulcers. Clinical trials in Europe suggest that this herb may also be useful for treating ulcers.

You can make a tea with the dried herb or take a tincture. I personally enjoy a cup or two of tea made with about five teaspoons of fresh calendula flowers. It's especially good with lemon balm and lemon.

I've also enjoyed calendula liqueur (the petals impart their golden color to the beverage) but I can't recommend that for treating ulcers. In fact, it's a good idea to go easy on alcohol if you have an ulcer. Finnish researchers have discovered that alcohol abuse increases the risk of *H. pylori* infection by 500 percent. If you have hay fever, however, you might want to avoid taking this herb, because people who are allergic to ragweed might react to calendula as well. If you take it and have a reaction—itching or any other discomfort—discontinue use.

❧❧ **Camomile (*Matricaria recutita*).** Several herbalists I

❧

Anti-ulcer Cabbage Soup

Here's a basic cabbage soup that's chock-full of anti-ulcer compounds. You'll have to do a little experimenting to arrive at a flavor that pleases you. If you try the optional spices, use them sparingly. While they are delicious in cabbage soup, the flavor is rather exotic.

    3   cups water
    2   cups shreddded cabbage
    1   cup chopped celery
    1   cup diced potatoes
    ½   cup chopped okra
    ½   cup diced onions
    ½   cup chopped green pepper
         Ground red pepper
         Ground ginger
         Ground black pepper
         Ground cinnamon (optional)
         Ground cloves (optional)
         Dried licorice root (optional)

Place the water, cabbage, celery, potatoes, okra, onions and green peppers in a soup pot. Bring to a boil over high heat. Reduce the heat, cover and simmer until the vegetables are tender. Season to taste with the red pepper, ginger, black pepper, cinnamon (if using), cloves (if using) and licorice (if using).

❧

admire recommend camomile tea for ulcers, notably Rudolf Fritz Wiess, M.D., the dean of German medical herbalists and author of *Herbal Medicine*. He writes that for stomach ulcers, "the remedy of choice is camomile. . . . There can be no other remedy more tailor-made, including all synthetic products." Widely used as a digestive aid in Europe, camomile is uniquely suited to treating digestive ailments, including ulcers. This is because it combines anti-inflammatory, antiseptic, antispasmodic and stomach-soothing properties. If I had an ulcer, I'd take my camomile tea with licorice.

🌿🌿 **Garlic (*Allium sativum*).** Garlic is a potent, broad-spectrum antibiotic. Paul Bergner, editor of *Medical Herbalism*, suggests that those who are wary of pharmaceutical antibiotics for ulcer treatment might want to try a course of garlic therapy. This would involve eating nine raw cloves a day. You can chop the garlic and mix it with any food that makes it palatable, such as carrot juice. Try blending two raw cloves of garlic with one carrot, for instance. I tried it, and the combination tasted better than I thought it would. It's a painless way to take a couple of cloves of garlic. You can also try whipping up an anti-ulcer gazpacho, heavy on the garlic and red pepper.

🌿🌿 **Gentian (*Gentiana officinalis*).** This is one of several bitter herbs traditionally used to aid digestion. Commission E reports that the bitter compounds in gentian stimulate the flow of saliva and stomach secretions.

Studies with experimental animals suggest that gentian might also be useful in the treatment of ulcers. Herbal pharmacologist Daniel Mowrey, Ph.D., author of *The Scientific Validation of Herbal Medicine* and *Herbal Tonic Therapies*, whose opinions I respect, recommends using gentian along with ginger, goldenseal and licorice root to treat ulcers.

🌿🌿 **Pineapple (*Ananas comosus*).** Like cabbage, pineapple is fairly well endowed with glutamine, a compound with experimentally verified anti-ulcer effects. Pineapple also contains bromelain, a general digestive aid.

🌿🌿 **Red pepper (*Capsicum*, various species).** Many Americans believe that hot spices cause ulcers. The truth is, they don't. In fact, they may even protect the stomach and duodenal lining against them. Capsaicin, the compound that gives red pepper its heat, has been shown to prevent ulcers in experimental animals that were given high, ulcer-causing doses of aspirin.

🌿 **Bilberry and blueberry (*Vaccinium*, various species).** Both of these fruits contain compounds known as anthocyanosides. In studies with experimental animals, these compounds have been shown to offer significant protection against ulcers.

They help stimulate the production of mucus that protects the stomach lining from digestive acids.

❧ Meadowsweet (*Filipendula ulmaria*). Like willow bark, meadowsweet is a type of herbal aspirin. Aspirin in high doses causes ulcers, so it might seem strange to recommend it as an ulcer treatment. Many prominent herbalists do, however, among them British herbalist David Hoffmann, author of several good herbals, including *The Herbal Handbook*. The active compounds in meadowsweet are salicylates. Aspirin, on the other hand, is nothing but salicylates. Hoffmann says that while pure salicylates do indeed cause ulcers, whole meadowsweet helps prevent and treat them despite its salicylate content.

Other chemical compounds in whole meadowsweet, among them tannins, phenolic glycosides and the herb's essential oil, give it an anti-ulcer effect. Hoffmann unflinchingly maintains that meadowsweet is one of the best digestive herbs and recommends it for ulcers and heartburn. This makes sense to me. Several plants with proven anti-ulcer effects, including camomile, also contain salicylates.

❧ Rhubarb (*Rheum officinale*). In a Chinese study of 312 people with bleeding ulcers, rhubarb helped improve some 90 percent within a few days. I'd be careful when using this herb, as it's also a powerful laxative. If you experience diarrhea, cut back the amount you're taking or discontinue use altogether.

❧ Turmeric (*Curcuma longa*). This culinary herb, used in Indian and Asian curry dishes, might be called the poor person's ulcer treatment. In a good study by physicians in Thailand, turmeric (250-milligram capsules taken three times a day) relieved ulcer pain only about half as well as pharmaceutical antacids after six weeks. However, the antacid was eight times more expensive than the turmeric. If you're low on dough, this herb might be a good way to go.

Vaginitis

Up in the backwoods of Maine lives an herbalist whom I respect and admire. Deb Soule is the founder of Avena Botanicals and author of the feminist herbal *The Roots of Healing*.

Over the years, many women have asked her to treat their vaginal yeast infections. She often recommends carefully peeling a clove of garlic so that it does not suffer any nicks and then wrapping it in clean gauze with a clean, unbleached string attached, thus creating a small, tamponlike packet. She says to insert a freshly prepared packet into the vagina each night for up to six consecutive nights. In many cases, she says, this treatment cures the infection. I'm not surprised, as garlic has potent antifungal properties.

By some estimates, vaginitis, which is any inflammation of the mucosal lining of the vagina, accounts for about half of all gynecological visits. There are several different causes of vaginitis, but yeast infections are the most common. (For more information on yeast infections, see page 557.)

Until just a few years ago, the most common treatment for vaginitis was a prescription antifungal medication. Within the past few years, many of those medications have become available over the counter, allowing women to treat themselves if they know for sure that they are dealing with a yeast infection.

This is a good place to point out that doctors do not recommend self-treatment for vaginitis unless you know exactly what you're dealing with. If you've been diagnosed in the past and have a pretty good suspicion as to the cause, you can give self-treatment a try. But if the symptoms don't clear up within a few days, or if you experience recurring bouts of vaginitis, you should see your doctor.

Green Pharmacy for Vaginitis

There are a number of herbs that can help treat vaginitis.

✿✿✿ **Garlic (*Allium sativum*).** If inserting a gauze-wrapped garlic clove does not appeal to you as a vaginitis treatment, and I can understand that it might not, try adding a teaspoon of fresh garlic juice to a few tablespoons of yogurt, then either soak a tampon in it or use it as a douche twice a day while symptoms persist. This treatment may not win any awards in the odor department, but it can be very effective.

There's a great book out called *Garlic: The Science and Therapeutic Application of Allium Sativum and Related Species* by Heinrich P. Koch, Ph.D., professor of pharmaceutical chemistry and biopharmaceutics at the University of Vienna, and Larry D. Lawson, Ph.D., a research scientist at an herb company in Utah. Dr. Koch and Dr. Lawson praise the "extraordinary fungicidal activity of fresh-pressed garlic juice and dried garlic." And they identify allicin as the major compound in garlic that kills *Candida albicans*, the fungus that causes vaginal yeast infections.

❧❧❧ **Teatree (*Melaleuca*, various species).** Australian teatree oil has become prominent only in the past few years as an antiseptic, but as word of its considerable healing power has spread, annual production in Australia has increased from 20 tons of oil to more than 140.

Australian chemists have shown that teatree oil is particularly effective against candida. One compound in the oil, terpinen-4-ol, appears to be the key to this herb's anti-candida action. Studies have shown that creams and douches containing high amounts of this compound have been as effective against yeast infections as the pharmaceutical antifungals nystatin (Mycostatin) and clotrimazole (Gyne-Lotrimin).

For recurrent yeast infections, Soule suggests mixing two to three drops of teatree oil in a tablespoon of yogurt and then soaking a tampon in it. Insert the tampon at night for up to six nights. Just don't take teatree oil, or any essential oil, internally. They are extremely concentrated, and even small quantities of many of them can be poisonous.

❧❧ **Cardamom (*Elettaria cardamomum*).** Cardamom may have twice as much terpinen-4-ol as teatree. You can follow the instructions given for teatree oil, but instead use two to three drops of cardamom oil.

❧❧ **Goldenseal (*Hydrastis canadensis*).** Goldenseal is a broad-spectrum herbal antibiotic, thanks to two chemical compounds, berberine and hydrastine, that it contains. Several studies show that these compounds help treat trichomonal vaginitis, a type that is caused by an amoeba.

Goldenseal also has some immune-stimulating activity. I often combine it with echinacea, which is immune-stimulating and antibiotic. Both of these herbs are taken orally in the form of teas, tinctures or capsules.

🌿 **Comfrey (*Symphytum officinale*).** Most cases of vaginitis are caused by infection, but sometimes, particularly in post-menopausal women, vaginal dryness can lead to irritation and inflammation during or after intercourse. Rose recommends applying a moisturizing lotion or egg white mixed with the contents of a vitamin E capsule and a couple of drops of comfrey tincture just prior to intercourse.

🌿 **Lavender (*Lavandula*, various species).** My friend Jeanne Rose, California herbalist and author of several good herb books, suggests essential oils, notably lavender, for treatment of trichomonas and gardnerella vaginitis. She recommends adding a few drops to douches, sitz baths, creams, lotions and tampons. (Remember that essential oils are for external use only.) In addition to lavender, she is partial to teatree oil and occasionally clary sage and German camomile.

She wisely cautions against routine douching; you should douche only for treatment of vaginitis. Regular douching can kill off beneficial microorganisms and leave you open for invasion by the infection-causing variety. In fact, studies show that women who douche regularly are at increased risk for pelvic inflammatory disease.

🌿 **Yellowdock (*Rumex crispus*).** Rose often recommends using a combination of yellowdock and other herbs for most types of vaginitis. Her formula includes one ounce of yellowdock root, two ounces of echinacea root, one ounce of goldenseal root and

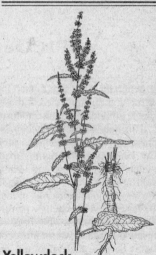

Yellowdock

Also known as curly dock, this herb has deep roots that are split and dried for use in tonics and ointments.

one ounce of ginseng root as a tonic for overall health.

You can use a mixture of dried herbs in the listed proportions to make a tea. You could also pulverize them and insert the mixture into empty gelatin capsules, which are available at many natural food stores that sell herbs. Admittedly, this is a lot of work, but women who face recurrent vaginitis are willing to make the extra effort if they find that the treatment works for them. You can try taking two or three capsules a day.

❧ **Apple cider vinegar.** Here's an old folk remedy, which many physicians also recommend, for several types of vaginitis: Add three cups of apple cider vinegar to a hot bath and soak in the tub for at least 20 minutes, spreading your legs to allow water to flow into the vagina. Rose suggests that vinegar baths and douches help restore normal vaginal acidity. Normal acidity helps banish candida, trichomonas and gardnerella.

Varicose Veins

I generally don't like to step into controversies, but here's one for you: I think there's reason to believe that eating violet flowers might help treat varicose veins.

This may sound far-fetched. None of the recent spate of "food pharmacy" books mentions violets for this common problem. But I have some intriguing evidence to support my claim that violets might prevent and treat some varicose veins and spider veins. But before we get to that, it's necessary to understand what we know about the causes of these problems.

Varicose veins occur when the valves in the veins that prevent blood from flowing backward don't work properly. Blood forms pools, and where this occurs, the veins and nearby capillaries become distended and swollen, leaking blood and fluid into surrounding tissue. This condition occurs most frequently in the legs; in areas where veins are near the surface, it causes unsightly bluish streaks, trails or spidery markings. But this condition can develop elsewhere as well. When they occur in and around the anus, these problem veins (varicosities) are known as hemorrhoids. When they occur in the scrotum, they are known as varicoceles.

Varicose veins affect about 15 percent of Americans, especially women, and the tendency to have this condition seems to run in families. When they occur in the legs, varicose veins are most common on the calves and along the inner thighs.

Green Pharmacy for Varicose Veins

A number of herbs, including violets, can help prevent or treat this problem.

🌿🌿🌿 **Horse chestnut (*Aesculus hippocastanum*).** In traditional herbal medicine, horse chestnut seeds were used to treat varicose veins and hemorrhoids. Eventually, botanists isolated the most active compound, aescin, and experiments with laboratory animals supported its traditional use as a remedy. Aescin helps strengthen capillary cells and reduce fluid leakage.

Commission E, the committee of scientific experts that advises the German counterpart of the Food and Drug Administration, endorses horse chestnut for treating varicose veins. On this side of the Atlantic, Varro Tyler, Ph.D., dean and professor emeritus of pharmacognosy (natural product pharmacy) at Purdue University in West Lafayette, Indiana, is also an advocate. In his excellent book for clinicians, *Herbs of Choice*, he singles out horse chestnut seed as by far the most effective plant drug for treating varicose veins.

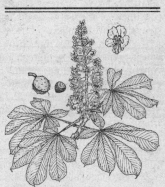

Horse Chestnut

The leaves, bark and seeds of horse chestnut are made into standardized extracts, widely available in Europe, that can help treat varicose veins.

In Europe, horse chestnut preparations are marketed as extracts of the leaves, bark and/or seeds, which are taken orally. Like most European plant medicines, horse chestnut extracts are standardized, and the dosage should be on the label. Unfortunately, these standardized extracts are not yet widely available in the United States.

You must obtain a standardized extract and follow package directions if you're going to use horse chestnut as a healing herb. It's simply not safe to use otherwise. If you can't find the extract, you'll have to rely on other herbs mentioned in this chapter.

❧❧❧ **Violet (*Viola*, various species).** Violet flowers contain generous amounts of a compound called rutin, which helps maintain the strength and integrity of capillary walls. Medical texts say that taking 20 to 100 milligrams of rutin daily can significantly strengthen the capillaries.

According to my database and some calculations, I estimate that a half-cup of fresh violet flowers would contain anywhere from 200 to 2,300 milligrams of rutin. You'd probably need only a few tablespoons to get 100 milligrams.

Are violets safe to eat? Yes. I've eaten 100 or so violet flowers on several different occasions, and I've never suffered any ill effects. Both violets and pansies, which also contain significant amounts of rutin, are usually cited in the books about edible flowers. As far as I can determine, they are safe when consumed at these low levels, and both flowers make impressive additions to salads.

If you'd rather not munch on flowers, you might try buckwheat, which is also high in rutin. A half-cup serving could contain about 6,000 milligrams of rutin, much more than necessary to curb capillary fragility. Eating a plate of buckwheat pancakes strikes me as a particularly nice way to take medicine. You might also investigate kasha, a cereal-like product made from buckwheat groats. Packaged kasha is widely available in supermarkets.

❧❧❧ **Witch hazel (*Hamamelis virginiana*).** Witch hazel comes in two commercial preparations, water extracts (witch hazel water) and alcohol extracts (tincture of witch hazel). Both are soothingly astringent, which makes witch hazel a popular external herbal treatment for various skin conditions from bruises to varicose veins.

Studies with laboratory animals have shown that this herb helps strengthen blood vessels. Commission E endorses using witch hazel extracts externally to treat both hemorrhoids and varicose veins. Simply wipe the affected area with a cotton ball that has been dipped in the extract.

Tincture of witch hazel can be taken internally for varicose veins, says the *Lawrence Review of Natural Products*, a respected newsletter. Or to make a tea, steep one to two teaspoons of dried witch hazel leaves in a cup of boiling water for ten minutes. You can drink two to three cups a day.

✷✷ Butcher's broom (*Ruscus aculeatus*). This herb has a long history of treating venous problems like hemorrhoids and varicose veins. It contains two anti-inflammatory compounds, ruscogenin and neoruscogenin, that constrict and strengthen veins.

✷✷ Lemon (*Citrus limon*). Lemon peel helps relieve varicose veins. It contains substances known as flavonoids, including rutin, that reduce the permeability of the blood vessels, especially the capillaries. I almost always add citrus peel to my fruit juices when I'm blending up a batch. It's worth a try.

✷✷ Onion (*Allium cepa*). Onion skin is one of our best sources of the compound quercetin. Like rutin, quercetin reportedly decreases capillary fragility. To get the full benefit of the quercetin, you should cook with whole, unpeeled onions whenever possible and discard the skin before serving.

✷ Bilberry (*Vaccinium myrtillus*). Bilberry helps circulation by stimulating new capillary formation, strengthening capillary walls and increasing the overall health of the circulatory system. Although capsules are available, I prefer whole bilberries whenever they are available. Related berries, which have the same benefits, include blackberries and blueberries.

✷ Ginkgo (*Ginkgo biloba*). Ginkgo is an all-around circulation booster. It's most widely known for its ability to increase blood flow through the brain, but it also improves circulation elsewhere in the body. German physicians use ginkgo preparations for treating varicose veins. However, large oral doses may be required, and that might prove expensive.

To use this herb, you need to buy a 50:1 extract, which will be specified on the label. No toxic side effects have ever been reported from using these standardized leaf extracts, although amounts higher than 240 milligrams daily may cause diarrhea, irritability and restlessness.

✷ Gotu kola (*Centella asiatica*). Several studies show that extracts of this Asian herb are useful in treating circulatory problems in the lower limbs, including venous insufficiency, water retention in the ankles, foot swelling and varicose veins. The plant has three active compounds, asiatic acid, asiaticoside and madecassic acid, that appear to work together. Although gotu kola is available in capsules, and it's fine to take it this way, I prefer to add the diced fresh leaves to juices and salads.

❧ **Spanish peanut (*Arachis hypogaea*).** The healing agent here is not the goobers themselves but rather their reddish, papery skins. Peanut skins are one of the better dietary sources of oligomeric procyanidins (OPCs), which are compounds that decrease capillary fragility and permeability, thus helping to prevent and treat varicose veins.

Pycnogenol, a major source of OPCs, is widely available in the United States as a rather expensive supplement, and if anything, it is overpromoted. Since it occurs naturally in most fruits and vegetables, I prefer to get my OPCs from food. Munching a few handfuls of Spanish peanuts—skins and all—is a particularly nice way to get a daily dose of OPCs.

❧ **Assorted essential oils.** Aromatherapists suggest massaging the affected area with the essential oils of cypress, juniper, lavender, lemon and marjoram. The oils should be diluted before they come in contact with the skin, so add a few drops of the oils of your choice to a couple of tablespoons of any vegetable oil. This massage treatment can't hurt, and it might help. Just don't ingest essential oils, as even a small amount can be toxic.

Viral Infections

Viruses are very strange. They are incredibly small—so tiny that while ordinary microscopes can see the body's cells and the bacteria that may infect them, you need much more powerful electron microscopes to see virus particles.

I use the word *particle* because by most definitions of life, viruses aren't really alive. They contain only genetic material (DNA or RNA) surrounded by a protein capsule. Viruses don't ingest food, breathe oxygen or eliminate wastes. All they do is reproduce after they've infected cells that are susceptible to them.

Antibiotics are generally useless against viruses; they work most actively against bacteria. Since the discovery of penicillin in 1928, mainstream medicine has come up with dozens of antibiotics. But today we still have only a handful of antiviral drugs, among them acyclovir for herpes, AZT for AIDS and interferon, the body's own virus fighter.

Green Pharmacy for Viral Infections

The good news is that several herbs used in traditional herbal medicine have scientifically documented antiviral effects. They're what I use when I have colds, flu and other viral infections. I discuss many of these herbs in the chapter on colds and flu (see page 164), but I want to devote one chapter to a look at herbs that can be tried as a treatment for any viral infection.

✿✿✿ **Echinacea (*Echinacea*, various species).** This is by far the most popular antiviral herb, and for good reason. Echinacea fights viruses in two ways. It contains three compounds with specific antiviral activity—caffeic acid, chicoric acid and echinacin. Root extracts of echinacea have also been shown to act like interferon, the body's own antiviral compound. In addition, echinacea is an immune stimulant that helps the body defend itself against viral infection more effectively.

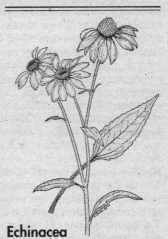

Herbalists are quick to tout echinacea as an immune booster, but the fact is, scientists still don't fully understand how it stimulates the immune system. Some suggest that it increases the body's levels of a compound known as properdin, which activates the specific part of the immune system, called the complementary pathway, that is responsible for sending disease-fighting white blood cells into infected areas to battle viruses and bacteria.

Other researchers maintain

Echinacea

Echinacea, the Plains Indians' primary medicine, today is the world's best-recognized herbal immunity booster.

that other compounds in the herb, lipophilic amides and polar caffeic acid derivatives, are at the root of its immunostimulant activity. One compound, chicoric acid, inhibits integrase, an enzyme that's important in viral reproduction.

I'm generally impressed with the way all the compounds in a plant have a way of working together harmoniously, so I'm inclined to believe that all of these immune-boosting properties work together.

Commission E, the German expert committee that judges the value of herbal medicines for the German government, has approved echinacea for treatment of influenza-like symptoms. That constitutes a significant scientific endorsement of this herb, which is native to America.

✸✸ Astragalus (*Astragalus*, various species). Also known as *huang qi*, this is an immune-boosting herb from China. In one small Chinese study, ten people whose heart muscles were infected by *Coxsackie B* virus, which causes the heart inflammation known as myocarditis, received injections of astragalus extract for three to four months. The activity of their natural killer cells, a component of the immune system, rose 11 to 45 percent. They also showed increased levels of alpha- and gamma-interferon, the body's own antiviral compounds. Not surprisingly, their symptoms improved. European studies suggest that, as with echinacea, many of the immune-stimulating compounds in astragalus are active when taken orally.

✸✸ Dragon's blood (*Croton lechleri*). This herb is also known as *sangregrado* or *sangre de drago*. There's a good reason why dragon's blood is on the back cover of the *Amazonian Ethnobotanical Dictionary*, which I co-authored in 1994 with Rodolfo Vasquez, botanist at the Missouri Botanical Garden. Several compounds in it, among them dimethylcedrusine and taspine, have antiviral and wound-healing properties that may be especially useful against the viral sores caused by herpes. The natural mixture of all three compounds heals wounds four times faster than the individual compounds alone.

I use dragon's blood when I get cuts or abrasions in tropical Peru. Unfortunately, this herb is not yet widely available in the United States, although I expect that it will be soon. It is applied externally.

✸✸ Garlic (*Allium sativum*). In addition to its well-known antibacterial action, garlic is also antiviral. Several of the sulfur compounds in garlic are active against the flu virus, according to Heinrich P. Koch, Ph.D., professor of pharmaceutical chemistry and biopharmaceutics at the University of Vienna, and Larry D. Lawson, Ph.D., a research scientist at an herb company in Utah, authors of *Garlic: The Science and Therapeutic Application of Allium Sativum and Related Species.*

Again, I'm reluctant to point to any specific compounds in garlic, because I suspect that they all somehow work together.

Some physicians who use herbs recommend taking two garlic capsules a day to treat colds, flu and other viral infections. But I prefer fresh garlic to capsules, and so does naturopath Jane Guiltinan, N.D., chief medical officer of Bastyr University in Seattle. She recommends consuming up to a dozen cloves a day. I'd have trouble with taking that many, except in salad dressing, garlic bread, soups and vegetable juice.

To avoid colds, I'd suggest you go ahead and eat a lot of garlic as a preventive. The other food to favor is onion, a close relative of garlic, which has similar though less potent antiviral action.

🌿🌿 **Goldenseal (*Hydrastis canadensis*).** Like echinacea, goldenseal is an immune stimulant, thanks to the berberine it contains. I often use it in combination with echinacea.

🌿🌿 **Juniper (*Juniperus*, various species).** Even among herbalists, it's not widely known that juniper contains a potent antiviral compound (deoxypodophyllotoxin). Juniper extracts appear to inhibit a number of different viruses, including those that cause flu and herpes. Sometimes when I feel a cold coming on, I make a juniper tea.

🌿🌿 **Lemon balm (*Melissa officinalis*).** Also known as melissa, this herb is highly recommended as an antiviral, especially against herpes. I would try lemon balm for treating any viral infection. It makes a very pleasant tea.

🌿🌿 **Licorice (*Glycyrrhiza glabra*).** Among its many other medicinal uses, licorice is active against many types of viral infections. One of its eight active antiviral compounds, glycyrrhizin, inhibits a number of processes involved in virus replication, among them penetration of the body's cells and replication of viral genetic material.

You could try a tea made by adding a few teaspoons of chopped dried root per cup of boiling water; steep for about ten minutes.

🌿🌿 **Shiitake (*Lentinus edodes*).** This tasty Asian mushroom contains a compound called lentinan that has antiviral,

immune-stimulating and anti-tumor properties, according to a
report published in the *Lawrence Review of Natural Products*,
a respected newsletter. Its antiviral action has been demonstrated in experiments with laboratory animals. Shiitake extract
helped protect mice against viral encephalitis.

Shiitake capsules are available, but I personally prefer to use
the whole mushroom as food.

❧ **Eucalyptus (*Eucalyptus globulus*).** Several compounds in
eucalyptus, hyperoside, quercitrin and tannic acid, have virus-
killing properties, according to pharmacognosist (natural product pharmacist) Albert Leung, Ph.D.

❧ **Forsythia (*Forsythia suspensa*) and honeysuckle
(*Lonicera japonica*).** Whenever I feel a cold or flu coming on,
I mix up a revered Chinese tea combo with honeysuckle and
forsythia. Sometimes I add a little antiviral lemon balm. Like
lemon balm, honeysuckle and forsythia contain compounds
that are proven virus killers. I find the combination of honeysuckle, forsythia and lemon balm especially nice in hot tea just
before bed.

❧ **Ginger (*Zingiber officinale*).** Good old ginger is good for
more than just motion sickness and upset stomach. According
to my database, it contains ten antiviral compounds. So if you
have a viral illness, you could try some ginger tea or add ginger
liberally to dishes you cook. Many of the antiviral compounds
in ginger also appear in turmeric.

Warts

The common wart is very common indeed. But sometimes it
seems as if folk treatments for warts are even more common. There's good reason for this: Not only do many folk treatments work, they often make physicians' treatments look
clumsy by comparison.

Warts are benign skin tumors that are caused by at least 35
different members of one family of viruses called papillo-
mavirus. The common wart typically appears on the hand, especially in older children, but warts can occur on other parts of the
body as well. (Plantar warts are the kind that show up only on

the feet.) Researchers have observed that individuals with suppressed immune systems are far more susceptible to warts than those with normal immunity.

Green Pharmacy for Warts

Here are the herbs you might want to consider if you're fighting this annoyingly persistent problem.

❧❧❧ **Birch (*Betula*, various species).** Birch bark has been used to treat warts in places as diverse as China, Scandinavia and Michigan. It contains two compounds, betulin and betulinic acid, that have antiviral activity. Birch bark also contains salicylates, which are approved by the Food and Drug Administration (FDA) for treatment of warts.

❧❧

Protect Your Skin

Some of the substances recommended in this chapter can be quite irritating to the skin. Everyone's skin is different, so if you try one of these remedies and it seems to make the skin around the wart red and irritated, rinse the area thoroughly and discontinue use of the herb.

❧❧

If you have access to fresh birch bark, you can tape a piece of moistened bark directly to the wart. You can also brew up some birch bark tea by adding a teaspoon or two of powdered bark to a cup of boiling water and steeping for ten minutes. You can drink the tea and also rub it directly on the warts.

❧❧ **Bloodroot (*Sanguinaria officinalis*).** This herb contains skin-irritant compounds (chelerythrine and sanguinarine) plus proteolytic enzymes, substances that help dissolve proteins such as wart-infected tissue. This may explain bloodroot's folk use as a wart remover. Look for an ointment containing this herb.

❧❧ **Castor (*Ricinus communis*).** Many people in many countries recommend castor bean oil for warts. They say you should massage the oil directly into the wart several times a day.

There are a number of ways that you might try to give the oil's anti-wart effects a little boost. I'd suggest putting a handful of willow bark into the oil and letting it steep for a couple of days. Willow contains aspirin-like compounds known as salicylates, which might prove helpful. Other herbalists drop in a few cloves of garlic, another folk remedy for warts, and allow the mixture to steep for a few days.

❧❧ **Celandine (*Chelidonium majus*).** Celandine contains some of the same compounds as bloodroot (chelerythrine, sanguinarine and proteolytic enzymes). Celandine juice can inhibit the wart virus or even kill it, according to Rudolph Fritz Weiss, M.D., dean of German medical herbalists and author of *Herbal Medicine*. If you have access to the fresh plant, you might apply the yellow juice directly to the wart once or twice a day for five to seven days. Otherwise, you can try applying a strong tea made from the dried herb.

❧❧ **Dandelion (*Taraxacum officinale*).** Several prominent herbalists recommend treating warts with milky dandelion latex, the substance that oozes out when you tear the leaves and stems. I suggest applying the white milk once a day for five to seven days. It didn't work for me, but you can give it a try if you like.

❧❧ **Fig (*Ficus carica*).** Figs contain a proteolytic enzyme known as ficin. In many cultures, people use several fig species for wart treatment. Using the white milk that oozes from the fruit and twigs, they claim, helps remove corns and warts. (This practice follows the lead of King Solomon, who used fig juice on his boils.) If you'd like to give this ancient treatment a try, I suggest applying the milk once a day for five to seven days.

❧❧ **Milkweed (*Asclepias*, various species).** Many people in many places recommend using the milky white fluid that oozes from milkweed to treat warts. I suggest massaging a little of the fresh fluid into a wart several times a day.

As an aside, I can't help but note that about half the folk remedies for warts involve milky white, green, orange, red or yellow plant resins. Many of these resins contain proteolytic enzymes. The active enzymes could help soften the warts and perhaps even inhibit the virus as well.

❧❧ **Pineapple (*Ananas comosus*).** Here's another plant rich in proteolytic enzymes. Medical anthropologist John Heinerman, Ph.D., author of *Heinerman's Encyclopedia of Fruits, Vegetables and Herbs*, suggests cutting a square of pineapple peel and taping the inner side to plantar warts overnight. The following morning, he says, remove the patch and soak the foot in hot water. Stubborn cases may require several applications.

❧❧ **Soybean (*Glycine max*).** Soybeans are an old Chinese medical treatment for warts, according to pharmacognosist (natural product pharmacist) Albert Leung, Ph.D. He cites a Chinese medical journal that published an intriguing study. Four people with warts were fed only plain, water-boiled yellow soybean sprouts, without seasoning or salt, three times a day for just three days. "All four patients treated were cured and their warts did not reappear," maintains Dr. Leung.

This is a treatment that I would try myself. There's good evidence to show that soybeans also help prevent cancer and heart disease.

❧❧ **Willow (*Salix*, various species).** The FDA has approved salicylic acid, which is found abundantly in willow, for wart removal, and it shows up in many over-the-counter preparations for removing warts, bunions and corns. You can buy one of these preparations if you wish and follow the package directions. My own preference would be to tape a piece of moistened inner bark from a willow tree to the wart and change it every day for five to seven days.

❧❧ **Yellow cedar (*Thuja occidentalis*).** Naturopaths suggest applying oil of yellow cedar to warts. It contains antiviral compounds, some of which are also found in mayapple. Dr. Weiss suggests painting a tincture on warts each morning and night for several weeks. This works well for smaller warts, he says, but not so well for large, solid warts. It sounds to me like it's worth a try.

❧ **Banana (*Musa paradisiaca*).** Some folk healers recommend scraping the inner white part of a banana peel and rubbing it onto a wart two to four times a day for five to seven days. There's even a report from the *Journal of Reconstructive Surgery* of a clinical trial that suggests that this treatment sometimes helps. I'd be willing to give it a try.

❧ **Basil (*Ocimum basilicum*).** This aromatic herb contains many antiviral compounds. One widely practiced folk remedy for warts involves rubbing crushed basil leaves on the growths. If I had a wart, I'd simply apply some fresh crushed basil leaves to the wart and cover it with a bandage, then reapply the leaves and change the dressing daily for five to seven days.

❧ **Papaya (*Carica papaya*).** I've tried this one and it didn't work for me, but many folk healers around the world recommend using papaya for removing warts. If you'd like to test it, apply juice from a fresh papaya twice a day for five to seven days. Maybe you'll have better luck than I did.

Worms

Here's a letter I received after one of my Amazon ecotours. It came from a tour participant who decided to put some of the herbal medicines he learned about on the tour to the test.

"I enjoyed finally meeting you and attending your lectures during the Pharmacy from the Rain Forest workshop last fall in Peru. I thought you might like to know that the field trip to the local *aguardiente* (rum) distillery proved to be unexpectedly educational.

"I believe that as a result of sampling the fermenting brew prior to pasteurization, I unwittingly ingested some intestinal parasite. An unpleasant experience followed, but my abdominal distress nevertheless afforded an opportunity to put to use some of the folk medicine of the region that you discussed.

"An infusion of wormseed in warm milk relieved all my symptoms for two days," my correspondent continued.

While I can't be sure from this letter that this fellow actually had worms, I felt glad that he learned something at the workshop and was able to treat his symptoms herbally.

The worms that we're concerned with in this chapter are tiny parasites that invade the human intestinal tract and occasionally other parts of the body. True worms include flukeworms, hookworms, pinworms, roundworms, tapeworms and whipworms.

More than one billion people worldwide are host to various intestinal worms. Don't make the mistake of thinking that this problem is confined to developing countries. The *New York*

Times estimates that 25 million Americans, mostly young children from all social classes, have worms.

Green Pharmacy for Worms

Mainstream medicine uses a variety of drugs to treat worms. They are generally effective, although some may cause severe side effects, including nausea, diarrhea, cramps and vertigo. If you suspect intestinal parasites, it's a good idea to get a diagnosis from a physician and follow his or her advice concerning treatment. Then discuss these herbal remedies with your doctor. If you try a natural approach, you might be able to deal with the problem without the side effects caused by many pharmaceuticals.

☙☙☙ Ginger (*Zingiber officinale*). New England herbalist Paul Schulick, author of *Ginger: Common Spice and Wonder Drug*, states that the tangy root is remarkably effective against some of the world's most dangerous parasites.

Among these is the anisakis worm, a Japanese worm that is carried in raw fish and is now increasingly common in the United States. No wonder the Japanese eat pickled ginger with their raw fish dishes: In one study, a ginger extract immobilized more than 90 percent of anisakis larvae within 4 hours and destroyed them in 16 hours.

If you're a big fan of sashimi, the Japanese raw-fish specialty, it probably wouldn't be a bad idea to adopt the Japanese custom of having some pickled ginger along with your meal or shortly afterward. This should offer a measure of protection. If it's not served in the restaurant where you have your sushi, you could enjoy a piece or two when you get home. Pickled ginger is available in Asian markets and many specialty food stores.

The same advice goes for eating ceviche, the Latin American dish made from marinated raw fish: Top off your meal with a piece of pickled ginger.

☙☙☙ Pumpkin (*Cucurbita pepo*). Pumpkin seeds and extracts have been shown to immobilize and aid in the expulsion of intestinal worms and other parasites. At least one patent has been granted for the use of a pumpkin extract in an intestinal worm treatment. Alternative practitioners often suggest that people with intestinal parasites eat one ounce of pumpkin seeds a day while the problem lasts. You could munch on pumpkin seeds and ginger for a double whammy.

❧·❧·❧ **Wormseed (*Chenopodium ambrosioides*).** Wormseed is not used as a dewormer only in the tropics. As a long-time resident of Maryland, I am proud to relate that wormseed was once produced commercially in my state's Carroll and Frederick counties for treatment of intestinal worms in American children and pets. I've also found that wormseed helps relieve gas, so I add it to bean soups. For worms, I'd try a concentrated tea. A word of caution: The concentrated wormseed oil is too potent to use.

You're far more likely to find this herb sold under the Spanish name *epazote*. Although wormseed is the correct English name, natural food stores tend to shy away from selling it under this name.

❧·❧ **Garlic (*Allium sativum*).** Naturopath Chris Deatheridge, N.D., a Missouri herbalist, uses garlic to treat pinworms, roundworms, giardia (an amoeba) and other parasitic infections. He suggests juicing three cloves with four to six ounces of carrot juice and taking it every two hours.

❧·❧ **Papaya (*Carica papaya*).** Here's another Panama-Peru connection: The Choco Indians that I studied more than three decades ago used to take the protein-digesting (proteolytic) latex of papaya to get rid of intestinal parasites. My new Peruvian Indian friends have gotten a mite more efficient and tidy: They swallow about a dozen of the pellet-size papaya seeds to accomplish the same end. I have chewed papaya seeds, and they are almost as hot as mustard seeds.

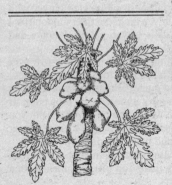

Papaya

The fruit of the papaya has plenty of vitamin C, which helps build immunity, and hot-flavored seeds that help repel intestinal worms.

❧·❧ **Pineapple (*Ananas comosus*).** Tapeworms may clear up after three days of eating nothing but pineapple. Pineapple contains the protein-digesting enzyme bromelain.

✨✨ **Turmeric (*Curcuma longa*).** Indian folk healers recommend this tasty spice for getting rid of worms, particularly nematodes. Turmeric contains four compounds with antiparasitic action. Individually, each of these compounds is ineffective, but when they're mixed together, they have strong worm-killing properties. The best way to take turmeric, as far as I'm concerned, is to enjoy curry dishes, in which it is a key ingredient. It is responsible for curries' yellow color.

✨ **Clove (*Syzygium aromaticum*).** Cloves have been demonstrated to be active against several parasites, including intestinal worms. I'd recommend taking a strong clove tea or adding powdered cloves to pineapple or papaya juices.

Finally, because proteolytic enzymes play such a major role in worm treatments, I'd recommend my Proteolade, a fruit smoothie made by blending the juice and pulp of fruits that are well-endowed with these enzymes. These include breadfruit, figs, papaya and pineapple. Spice the beverage to taste with cloves, ginger and turmeric. (Unless you live in the tropics, you probably won't be able to get the breadfruit. It's okay to leave it out.) You might also add a little prune juice as a laxative to help expel dislodged worms.

Wrinkles

When the tomb of King Tutankhamen, Egypt's boy pharaoh, was opened, archaeologists saw a treasure trove of artifacts. Researchers interested in the aging process found something else—a papyrus containing the king's anti-wrinkle formula: coconut oil and the herbs balsam and valerian mixed with animal fat.

The pharaoh's anti-wrinkle formula was not all that different from many others that have been touted through the centuries, including everything from bear grease and goose grease to tar and turpentine. The big question, of course, is, Do any of them really work?

Losing Elasticity

To answer that question we need to take a look at why skin develops wrinkles in the first place. Wrinkles result from changes in collagen, the protein that makes up the fibrous portion of your skin. Collagen is what holds you together. It makes up about one-third of your body's total protein and 70 percent of your connective tissue.

Young skin and connective tissue contain mostly elastic or soluble collagen, and as a result, it can absorb moisture and plump up. This ongoing process of moisturization and swelling keeps young, elastic skin looking sleek and smooth. But with sun exposure, cigarette smoking and normal aging comes oxidative damage to the skin. This damage is the same sort of thing that happens to iron when it rusts. In the body, this chemical process causes the formation of insoluble collagen, which is inelastic, is unable to absorb water well and does not plump up.

With loss of elasticity and moisture, lines and wrinkles form, especially in areas exposed to sunlight—the face, the neck and the backs of the hands.

Many commercial moisturizers are sold with the claim that they restore soluble collagen and rejuvenate the skin, allowing skin cells to absorb more fluid and banishing wrinkles. I honestly don't know whether or not these work. But before you spend a fortune on any of these products, I'd suggest trying some natural approaches.

Green Pharmacy for Wrinkles

Most natural anti-wrinkle treatments rely on antioxidants and emollients. Antioxidants are substances that mop up free radicals, the highly reactive oxygen molecules that are responsible for oxidative damage. Emollients help prevent dryness while moisturizing and softening the skin. Here are some natural treatments that might prove helpful.

🌿🌿🌿 **Horse chestnut (*Aesculus hippocastanum*) and witch hazel (*Hamamelis virginiana*).** Japanese scientists tested 65 plant extracts and found seven that showed sufficient antioxidant activity to have potential against wrinkles. The four that you probably can get your hands on are horse chestnut, witch hazel, rosemary and sage, but the researchers singled out horse chestnut and witch hazel as the best. Both of these are strong antioxidants. Soothing and astringent salves containing these herbs are available at health food stores, but I prefer to mix them myself.

Carrot (*Daucus carota*). Carrots are high in vitamin A, and deficiencies of this vitamin cause dry skin and wrinkling. Carrots also contain the antioxidant beta-carotene. I'd suggest munching a carrot or two a day, not only to prevent wrinkles but for all the cancer-preventive chemicals that this vegetable contains.

You might also consider topical application of carrot oil. Its high levels of vitamin A make it a good sunscreen, according to Aubrey Hampton, author of *Natural Organic Hair and Skin Care*. I confess I've never tried carrot oil, but on occasion, I've mashed carrots in a blender and experimentally applied the mash as a face mask. Someone once even called me a handsome old redneck. (Wash the mashed carrot off after 15 to 30 minutes.)

Cocoa (*Theobroma cacao*). A major emollient used in skin lotions and cosmetics, cocoa butter is the leading antiwrinkle suggestion of pharmacognosist (natural product pharmacist) Albert Leung, Ph.D. It melts at body temperature and remoisturizes dry skin, especially around the eyes (crow's-feet), the corners of the mouth and on the neck (turkey neck). I like it because it comes from the Amazon. Another similar tropical emollient is coconut oil.

Cucumber (*Cucumis sativus*). Cool, moist cucumber has a long history of use for soothing burns, including sunburn, and preventing wrinkles. Cucumbers are cheaper and probably as useful as many commercial moisturizers. You can cut thin, disk-shaped sections and wipe them on your skin. You can also whip them in your blender and apply the mash as a face mask. Rinse it off after 15 to 30 minutes.

Purslane (*Portulaca oleracea*). This plant is one of my favorite antioxidants. If you have access to fresh purslane, use it as a salad ingredient. Or try it in a soothing facial mask. Put the herb through a blender or juicer and dab it on your face, washing it off after 15 to 30 minutes.

Rosemary (*Rosmarinus officinalis*). Another potent antioxidant, rosemary was identified by Japanese researchers as a promising wrinkle preventive and treatment. Use it as a culinary spice or make a tea with a teaspoon or two of crushed, dried leaves per cup of boiling water. You could also blend it with your purslane.

✍✍ **Sage (*Salvia officinalis*).** Along with horse chestnut, witch hazel and rosemary, sage was the other common herb identified by the Japanese researchers, although it's somewhat less effective than the others. Use it as a culinary spice or try using a teaspoon or two of dried, crushed leaves per boiling water to make a tea. It's a good idea to be judicious, though, as sage contains a fair amount of thujone, a compound that in very high doses may cause convulsions.

✍✍ **Lac-Hydrin.** This drugstore item isn't exactly an herb, but it is a natural product. Lac-Hydrin is an alpha-hydroxy acid (AHA) found in fruits, sour milk and sugar cane. AHAs, often called fruit acids, help peel off dead skin cells by dissolving ceramides, which are substances that hold the cells together. Clearing dead cells off the surface of the skin reveals the plump, living cells underneath and contributes to a younger appearance. Dermatologists use strong concentrations of AHAs for face peels.

Lac-Hydrin also increases the thickness of the outermost layer of living skin cells (the epidermis), increasing the skin's ability to hold moisture and thus smoothing out fine lines and wrinkles.

Unlike some anti-aging treatments such as Retin-A, Lac-Hydrin does not cause sun sensitivity. In one study, Lac-Hydrin was applied twice a day for six months, and it diminished fine wrinkles noticeably in 90 percent of the people using it.

✍ **Almond (*Prunus dulcis*).** Almond oil, mentioned in the Bible and once used for anointing kings and priests, has increasingly worked its way into the cosmetic and perfume world. You can use it as an emollient and massage it into your skin to slow wrinkling.

✍ **Aloe (*Aloe vera*).** It's hard to separate aloe hype from fact. Cleopatra is said to have massaged aloe gel onto her face daily. Napoleon's wife, Josephine, added the gel to milk to make a face lotion. And aloe is an ingredient in many modern skin-care products. Does it help prevent wrinkles? It probably can't hurt to give it a try.

✍ **Avocado (*Persea americana*).** Pleasantly scented avocado oil is an emollient that's especially beneficial for people with dry skin. Just apply it directly to your face.

🌸 **Castor (*Ricinus communis*).** The oil of the castor bean has been used since biblical times as a facial oil and makeup ingredient. It's clearly an emollient, and I'd guess that if it didn't do some good, it would have been discarded generations ago.

🌸 **Grape (*Vitis vinifera*).** Grapes contain AHAs, the substances that help peel dead skin cells from the face. AHAs appear in dozens of over-the-counter (OTC) skin lotions, including those that claim to eliminate fine lines and wrinkles. But instead of opting for an OTC, why not go to a natural source? You can process grapes, even seeded varieties, in a juicer and apply the mash as a facial mask. Rinse it off after 15 to 30 minutes.

🌸 **Olive (*Olea europea*).** The prophet Hosea said, "Beauty shall be as the olive tree." He didn't say, "Wrinkles shall be removed with the olive oil." But since biblical times, olive oil has been used to soften and beautify the skin. Olive oil, as an emollient, just might help slow wrinkling. Many women steam their faces gently before applying it.

🌸 **Pineapple (*Ananas comosus*).** If the AHAs in pineapple husks can really remove bunions and corns, as I've read, I wouldn't hesitate to liquefy the peel and core from a whole pineapple in my blender and apply the mash to help remove the surface layer of dead skin cells. Rinse it off after 15 to 30 minutes. (As a corn remover, you would keep the pineapple on much longer.)

Yeast Infections

Most people think of yeast infections, also known as candidiasis, as a plague only upon women. But men can also develop candidiasis, especially those who are uncircumcised. A man with yeast typically shows no symptoms, but each time his partner is treated and gets rid of her infection, he reinfects her. So if you're a woman who's been having problems with yeast infections, be sure your partner is checked, too: Both of you might need some of these herbal remedies.

Yeast infection is caused by a group of yeastlike fungi called candida. *Candida albicans* is the most common culprit, but it's not the only one. Everyone has a certain amount of candida living on them and in them, but not everyone develops candidiasis.

❦

Candidicidal Soup

If you're dealing with the aggravation of recurring yeast infections, one of the best things you can do for yourself is to develop a taste for garlic and onions. Here's a tasty soup that might help.

     4   cups water
     2   onions, finely chopped
     4   cloves garlic, minced
         Sage
         Thyme
         Ground cloves
         Salt
         Gound black pepper
         Acidophilus yogurt

Place the water, garlic and onions in a medium saucepan. Bring to a boil over high heat, then reduce the heat, cover and simmer for 5 minutes, or until the vegetables are tender. Season to taste with the sage, thyme, cloves, salt and pepper, but use the spices somewhat sparingly. Top each serving with a dollop of yogurt.

Makes 4 servings

❦

Yeast live on moist areas of the body, such as the lining of the mouth and the vagina. They usually cause no problem, but sometimes they overgrow, causing infection. The vagina is the primary site. (See the chapter on vaginitis on page 535 for details about Green Pharmacy treatments for this problem.) But yeast infections can also develop in the mouth (thrush), in the respiratory tract (bronchocandidiasis) and on the skin (dermatocandidiasis).

Yeast has become more of problem than it was, say, 60 years ago, because several modern drugs spur yeast overgrowth. Among the leading culprits are antibiotics, steroids and birth control pills.

Mainstream medicine treats yeast infections with antifungal medications that used to be available only by prescription. But recently several, such as nystatin (Mycostatin) and miconazole (Monistat), have become available over the counter, and they are advertised extensively. It's too bad that herbalists can't afford to make TV commercials. If they could, people would understand that there's more than one way to treat a yeast infection.

Green Pharmacy for Yeast Infections

There are a number of herbs that can help fight yeast infections, but you'd better be sure of what you're dealing with before you self-medicate. If you have what you suspect is a yeast infection, please see your doctor for a diagnosis. Then, if you'd like to try an herbal alternative as your treatment of choice, you should discuss it with her. You might consider using these herbs in addition to whatever is prescribed for you.

✿✿✿ Echinacea (*Echinacea*, various species). This herb's immune-stimulating action seems to be particularly helpful for treating yeast infections. In studies using laboratory animals, treatment with the herb protected mice from *Candida albicans* infections. It works by stimulating the white blood cells to gobble up yeast organisms, a process known as phagocytosis.

In an impressive German study, women with recurrent vaginal yeast infections were given either standard antifungal medication or the antifungal plus an echinacea extract. Among those taking just the antifungal, 60 percent suffered recurrences. But among the women taking the drug plus echinacea, only about 10 percent experienced recurrences. That sounds to me like a good rationale for giving echinacea a try no matter what kind of yeast infection you're dealing with.

✿✿✿ Garlic (*Allium sativum*). Garlic is well-known as an antibacterial antibiotic, but it also inhibits fungi quite well and

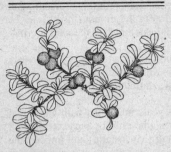

Cranberry

The tart berry that lends a distinctive taste to cranberry juice and sauce was used by nineteenth-century physicians to relieve inflammation.

can be used to treat both vaginal candidiasis and thrush. The typical oral dose may range up to a dozen raw, chopped cloves taken two or three times a day in juice. You have to like the taste of garlic pretty much to live with this particular treatment, but I think it's worth a try, as garlic does pack a powerful anti-yeast wallop. (Try blending it with carrots; it's surprisingly easy to take that way.) Onions have a similar but less potent effect.

❧❧ **Cranberry** (*Vaccinium macrocarpon*). Arbutin, a compound found in cranberries (and bearberries and blueberries), helps treat candida infections, according to naturopaths Joseph Pizzorno, N.D., president of Bastyr University in Seattle, and Michael Murray, N.D., authors of *A Textbook of Natural Medicine*. So if you're thinking of taking garlic, why not take it with cranberry juice? Or just eat some cranberry sauce plain. These colorful berries are not just for Thanksgiving.

❧❧ **Goldenseal** (*Hydrastis canadensis*). This is the best known among the "golden" herbs that contain the antibiotic berberine. Others include goldthread, yellowroot, barberry and Oregon grape. Berberine is effective against many microorganisms, including yeasts. At home, I take a tincture. In the field, I'd make a tea. You can use it either way.

❧❧ **Pau-d'arco** (*Tabebuia*, **various species**). Pau-d'arco contains the anti-yeast compounds lapachol and beta-lapachone, according to Dr. Murray, Dr. Pizzorno and other researchers. Lapachol is the weaker of the two, but its anti-yeast action is still comparable to that of the prescription anti-yeast medication ketaconazole (Nizoral). I have used a Latin American salve containing lapacho to clear up genital candida, and I would do so again if I had a flare-up. Flare-ups are frequent in the humid tropics. In the tropics, I'd boil up a concentrated decoction. At home, I'd empty a couple of capsules into a medicated salve.

❧·❧ Purslane (*Portulaca oleracea*). Vitamins A (and beta-carotene), C and E are my personal "ACE in the hole" for supporting the immune system. You definitely want to give the immune system help when it's fighting a yeast infection of any kind. Purslane is the best food source of all of these nutrients. I suggest enjoying young shoots of this tasty vegetable in a salad or steaming the leaves like spinach.

❧ Goldenrod (*Solidago virgaurea*). Commission E, the group of botanical medicine experts that advises the German government about herbs, approves using anti-inflammatory goldenrod for preventing and treating various urogenital disorders, including yeast infections. Compounds in goldenrod (ester saponins) are active against candida organisms. This herb can be used as an astringent beverage tea, and you can also use the tea as a douche.

❧ Ivy (*Hedera helix*). Ivy leaves are active against candida and quite a few bacteria. Commission E endorses using 0.3 gram (that's just a pinch of dried herb) for various chronic inflammatory conditions, and that seems like a reasonable dose for fighting yeast infections as well. You can steep the herb in hot water for about 10 to 15 minutes and drink the tea.

❧ Licorice (*Glycyrrhiza glabra*) and stevia (*Stevia rebaudiana*). Many specialists advise those with recurrent yeast problems against using alcohol, products that contain yeast and simple sugars. If you've had a yeast infection before and want to prevent a fresh outbreak, you should steer clear of honey and sugar. If you'd like to sweeten anti-candida teas, try using herbal sweeteners like licorice root or stevia.

❧ Sage (*Salvia officinalis*). Sage contains a mixture of anti-candida compounds. You could take sage tea as a beverage or use it as an astringent douche. If you're using it as a douche, you might add a drop or two of teatree oil, a potent anti-yeast herbal product.

❧ Spicebush (*Lindera benzoin*). Studying 54 plant species for antimicrobial effects, American scientists found that an extract of spicebush bark strongly inhibited *Candida albicans*. Throughout Appalachia, spicebush tea has long been a favorite, proving once again the wisdom of much folk medicine.

Author's Postscript

A Lifetime of Loving Plants

I've been interested in plants for at least 62 of my 67 years. My interest comes from my mother, who loved plants and raised me to love them as she did.

Much of my early botanical interest is shrouded in the mists of memory. I recall only snippets: playing with white cousins and black neighbors in the woods and pastures along the Koosa River outside Birmingham, Alabama, near my grandfather Truss's farm; visiting Uncle Bill's nursery and skinny-dipping in the Cahaba River. Even though I was born and lived in the East Lake suburb of Birmingham, we frequently got out to see the country cousins, where we played in the countryside forests and fields.

Even in Birmingham, the forests were close by. We had chickens, a small vegetable garden and arbors bearing magnificent scuppernong grapes. My grandmother made delicious scuppernong juice, and I've had a lifelong love affair with scuppernong fruit (*Vitis rotundifolia*). If by some fluke this sinner makes it to heaven, I imagine I will be greeted just the other side of the Pearly Gates by my grandmother, offering me a tall chilled glass of scuppernong juice.

Learning to Eat "Weeds"

In Birmingham, lonely old Mr. Brooks lived across the street. He had no close friends or family, and he spent most of his time talking to his rabbits in their hutch—and to me. He took me for walks in the nearby woods, and he introduced me to the world of edible wild plants such as chestnuts and watercress. Since that time, I have always had a keen interest in edible plants. And walking in the woods is still my number one therapy for personal rejuvenation.

But in addition to plants, another interest also crept in. Starting at around age five, I sold magazines at Howard University (now Samford University), just a few blocks from home. We were pretty poor in those days, and the guys in the dorm would buy the magazines, more out of pity for scraggly me than because they wanted them.

In one dorm, there was a group of bluegrass musicians. I loved what they played, and country music seemed to go quite well with all the country plants that my momma and Mr. Brooks were teaching me to love. Botany and country music— they may not go hand-in-hand for many people, but they always have for me.

Children's Garden of Delight

When I was seven, we were whisked away from the fields of Alabama to Durham, North Carolina, where my dad hoped to escape country poverty by getting into the insurance business. We were still poor, but I was happy, and so were my older brother, Ed, and my younger brother, Dan, just like poor children all around the world.

For a while we lived in a succession of low-rent apartments and bungalows. One apartment was a three-story tenement that bordered a vacant lot filled with honeysuckle. I have happy memories of my brothers and me tunneling through the honeysuckle vines and playing our games. One of the bungalows was close to the famous Duke Gardens of Duke University. Mother planted a small garden just outside our apartment, and I helped her tend the flowers. Jokingly, we called it Little Duke Gardens.

I should add that I am not related to the tobacco Dukes (Duke University was named for one member of this family) nor to the famous Doris Duke. I come from cotton-picking Dukes of Alabama, and I still have dozens of country cousins down there. Recently, one cousin told me that my great-great-grandfather Duke was an herbal doctor, so maybe herbs have always been in my blood.

From my mother's garden, I graduated to a part-time job

helping out in a florist's greenhouse nearby, where I added a great deal to what I already knew about ornamental flowers.

When I was about nine, Dad's insurance business picked up, so we moved to Raleigh, North Carolina, and purchased a large house with a big yard. Mom and Dad and I planted our first vegetable garden, and my botanical horizons expanded to vegetables. Mom also put in a big batch of four-o'clocks, introducing me to what later became a great interest of mine, floral clocks.

The Call of the Wild

There were thick woods nearby, and I explored them endlessly, sometimes alone and sometimes with my friends, a rather gentle gang of boys. We roved the woods, staking out campsites and defending them from imaginary enemies.

One friend's dad had a farm a few miles out in the country. We used to go camping out there, setting up tents in the cold, whistling pines (even in winter), fishing in the farm pond and challenging each other to name all the wildflowers.

The worst thing I ever did there still haunts me. We'd watch frogs by the pond and see their throats swell up like balloons as they croaked. We had BB guns, and with the unconscious cruelty of boys, I aimed at one frog's balloon-throat and pulled the trigger. I hit the mark, deflating his song-making balloon. I have regretted it ever since. I don't suppose it killed him, but he never sang again, and the forest was the quieter for it. Since then, I have killed a few frogs and other animals, but only for food in the field. From that time on, I abandoned mutilation or killing for sport.

I missed out on Cub Scouts, but I joined the Boy Scouts at the Tabernacle Baptist Church near my home. The rituals and uniform didn't do much for me, but I was very turned on by the camping trips and made as many as I could over the years, learning the forest and its plants even better. Mother made me a sleeping bag that was waterproofed by ironing on paraffin. It weighed a ton, but it kept me dry and warm. I also went on many non-Scout camping trips.

The Forest as Temple

By high school, music and puppy love started competing with the forest for my attention. Even as early as the sixth grade, I was singing country songs. My girlfriend, Greta Lewis, was involved in my Baptist church. Her parents didn't like me, but they tolerated me because of my church connection.

And then, all at once, I experienced a loss much greater than I had when I learned that there was no Santa Claus. Faced with the infinity of the universe, I lost faith in a theocratic God. That doomed Greta and me. But I believed deeply in the forest, in its infinite beauty and healing power. The forest became my temple, my theology. It's been my salvation ever since.

My older brother had a friend who was well-known around Raleigh as a wild mushroom hunter (mycologist), and we often went into the woods with him, trying to name all the plants. He and my brother both had part-time jobs at Crabtree (now Umstead) State Park, and I had become enamored of that wild place, with its miles of secret waterways. I spent seemingly endless hours canoeing through Umstead, silently observing the animals and birds; they apparently assumed that I was just another log—albeit oddly shaped—floating down the creeks.

Another neighbor was a forester who became impressed with my budding knowledge of field botany. Eventually, he got me my first summer job at Umstead Park, where they actually paid me to do all the things I loved to do: hike, camp, canoe and take stock of the plants and animals with the help of my trusty tree books, bird books and flower books. I got pretty good at living off the land.

Meanwhile, I started playing the guitar, and it wasn't long before the guitar became as close a friend as the forest. I never felt alone in the forest or with my guitar. I was always listening to country music and trying to play it. I had a pretty good ear and could pick up songs quickly. I knew where all the country music was on the radio and listened at all hours.

Tenth grade at Hugh Morson High found me in Miss Beddingfield's biology class. She was famous for making everyone in the class collect and identify 40 flowers. I collected over 100 and became legendary in my class as a result.

Music Beckons

Meanwhile, two beautiful brunettes arrived at school. They were part of the Saylor Sisters, a country vocal group that I'd heard on the radio. One of the sisters, Jeannie, offered to teach me to play the bass fiddle so that I could accompany them when they sang. Only I didn't have a bass. Of course, I would have done anything to spend time with her, so I leaned on my dad and he split the cost of a bass with me—$50 apiece, which was a lot of money in the 1940s. In fact, it was all I had. Buying my bass left me penniless but happy.

Jeannie taught me to play, and the next thing I knew, I was playing bass, but not for the Saylor Sisters. Instead I joined up with Homer A. Brierhopper and the Dixie Dudes, a local band I'd heard on the radio that played country schoolhouses throughout North Carolina. This was during World War II, and most of the good local musicians were in the Army, so old Homer turned to me.

I even cut a 78-rpm record with the band in Nashville. For a 16-year-old boy to make a record in Nashville, well, that was really something. I must admit that it gave me a swelled head, even if I was just a fill-in player for band members who were fighting the war. Then came gigs with the Woody Hayes orchestra for big money—$5 a night—and later other jobs at local nightclubs.

During my last two years of high school, I was just about making a living as a bass player, and even Dad had to admit that buying the bass had been a good investment.

Reluctant Academic

Dad wanted me to go to college, but I believed that music would support me well. So I kept playing nightclub gigs. But to appease my father, I enrolled at North Carolina State. The trouble was, with all of my time spent playing music and hiking in the woods, I didn't do much schoolwork. I dropped out right before I would have flunked out.

Dad was worried, but I wasn't. With my music money, I bought a motorbike and wheeled through the back roads of North Carolina, camping all over the place and putting together mental pictures of the ecosystems of the interesting state of North Carolina.

Then I got a phone call from Johnny Satterfield at the University of North Carolina (UNC) in Chapel Hill. He had a big band and had heard that I was pretty good on jazz bass. He wanted to add a second bass to his band. So off I went to Chapel Hill to audition. Johnny was a great admirer of Duke Ellington, and I think my name turned him on as much as my bass playing. He smiled broadly as my bassline danced around his piano fingering. He wanted me for the band and said he'd hire me, but only if I enrolled in UNC as a music major.

I didn't have much use for the music program at UNC, but one of my first electives was general botany. In short order, I switched my major to botany, making it my vocation and music my avocation. Dad was pleased. This time around, firmly entrenched in botany, I earned As and Bs. And when it came time to make a career choice, I enrolled in graduate school at UNC.

Getting Intimate with Plants

In graduate school, I soon teamed up with a professor, Al Radford, who specialized in aquatic plants. He knew that he and I were about the only people in the department who loved to wade waist-deep in blackwater swamps in search of rare aquatic plants. He took me under his wing, and I wound up writing my Master's thesis on a semi-aquatic plant, *Ludwigia*, that grew in roadside ditches.

I'll never forget the time that I was knee-deep in a roadside marsh looking for *Ludwigia* when some musicians I knew drove by. They stopped, amazed that I was wading in the muck, and asked if was all right. I told them that I was as happy as a clam. They drove off, probably convinced that I was crazy.

Another botany grad student was a petite, brown-eyed brunette who more than turned my head. I was interested in Peggy-Ann Wetmore Kessler from the moment I laid eyes on her. A graduate of Maryville College in the mountains of Tennessee, Peggy was working on her Master's at the time I met her.

Peggy earned her Master's degree, but she ended up spending more time as an illustrator than as a botanist. She worked part-time, illustrating several botany books produced by our professors, and to this day, she still illustrates. The illustrations that appear throughout this book are hers.

Together Peggy and I shared a love for botany, the outdoors and jazz. After we met, we spent many a weekend bouncing from botanizing around Carolina beaches and forests to jazz jam sessions and then back to the woods and beaches. It wasn't long before we were in love.

First Government Work: Germ Warfare

I completed my Master's degree in botany in 1955, and within a few days found myself drafted into the U.S. Army. At first the Army had no use for the fact that I was a botanist, but eventually, after a few hellish months under a sergeant who hated college graduates, especially those with Master's degrees, I wound up at Fort Dietrick, Maryland. There I joined many others with Master's and Ph.D.'s in the biological sciences who were hard at work trying to develop protection from biological warfare agents.

Germ warfare wasn't exactly a great love of mine, but otherwise, Fort Dietrick was terrific. My civilian boss was not very demanding. He had me culturing various fungi on different media to see how well they stood up in storage. He never told me why I was culturing fungi, but it didn't take long to figure out that we were reciprocating, looking for biological agents that could destroy enemy food crops.

When I was off duty, I hiked the nearby Catoctin Mountains, where I tried to draw the wildflowers as well as Peggy could—but I couldn't. (Ironically, my son, his Cherokee wife and my Cherokee grandchildren live there now.) I also went to town, nearby Frederick, where I played guitar and wound up teaching it. Before long, I put together a small jazz combo, the Dizzy Duke Group, that played at the NCO and Officers' clubs.

Peggy visited as often as we could work it out, and we spent some delightful times in a friend's cabin up on Yellow Creek, where she drew the flowers.

I wound up having such a fine time at Fort Dietrick that when my hitch ended, I was almost sorry to leave. But I wanted to get my Ph.D. in botany, and even though I never fought in Korea, I qualified for the Korean GI Bill. So I bought a big black Buick and returned to UNC, where I worked on my degree, had a teaching assistantship and rejoined my jazz-playing buddies.

Two of my professors were involved in a very ambitious project to obtain at least one specimen of every plant species in every county of the Carolinas in order to better map the distribution of those species. I signed on and so did Peggy, as the illustrator. So we two lovebirds spent a lot of time together at the university, in the field and at jazz jam sessions.

First Look at Latin America

I had a problem. By now I was academically inbred: I'd taken all my degrees at the same university with the same professors, which limited my education and my network for future employment.

As I completed my Ph.D. coursework, my adviser set me up with two projects that got me out of UNC. One was an expedition to collect botanical specimens in Mexico, Costa Rica and Guatemala, and the other was a 6- to 12-month job at the noted Missouri Botanical Garden in St. Louis, helping survey the medicinal plants of Panama and Peru.

It was hard leaving Peggy at UNC, but off I went with all sorts of camping gear and my best guitar. Our little group drove to Mexico in my adviser's station wagon; we were on a National Science Foundation Grant to study the chromosomes of the carrot family (*Umbelliferae*, or umbels for short).

We criss-crossed Mexico for two months, seeing all sorts of habitats and many umbels that were all but unknown outside Mexico. The itinerary was arranged so that we could catch as many species as possible when they were in bud. We collected the buds and popped them into chemicals that would preserve them until we got back to the lab to count their chromosomes.

We also collected many flowers, flattening them to preserve them. The Mexicans we met along the way were only too happy to tell us gringos the local lore about the plants we were collecting, including their medical uses. I didn't realize it at the time, but on that trip the seeds of medical botany were planted in my mind.

Unfortunately, my Spanish was too poor to catch most of

what our hosts said. But slowly it improved, and at night in our modest hotel courtyards, my guitar opened doors and made communication easier. The other thing I didn't realize at the time was that I was falling in love with Latin America.

After several fascinating months in Mexico, we flew into Guatemala for a few days to find rare umbels near Lake Atitlan. Then it was on to Costa Rica, where we ferreted out yet more umbels on the flanks of some volcanoes. At every stop, my love for the region deepened.

Learning about Medicinal Plants

Emerging from my Central American reverie, I found myself at the Missouri Botanical Garden for what turned out to be a postdoctoral appointment, long before I knew what a postdoc was. At UNC, I'd learned the plants of the Carolinas. In Missouri, I was introduced to plants of the world.

Half of my job was to identify specimens of medicinal plants collected in Peru or, if they'd never been previously identified, to name them. I'd pick up a dry, flattened Peruvian specimen with some Indian or Spanish colloquial name and maybe some notes about the color of the flowers and fruits, and I'd have to figure out what it was. Being trained in the difficult and tedious science of taxonomy, I knew how to identify plants by the placement and shape of their leaves and ancillary organs; the nature of the floral parts; the size, shape and number of floral parts and seeds; and the presence or absence of thorns, saps and peculiar aromas.

I wrestled intermittently with one medicinal plant my whole three years in Missouri before becoming convinced that the species had never before been named. The Peruvians called it *sanango*, which became its generic name. Twenty-five years later in the Peruvian Amazon, I saw a shamanistic healer use sanango in a healing ceremony.

Some plants I knew well, some didn't take much work to identify, and some took months to pin down. Still others I never identified for sure, although I could usually place them in the right plant family. Months or years later, a specialist in that family would see the specimen and identify it or name it. There are still many species unknown to science and unnamed (at least in Latin) in tropical America. More than a dozen were named after me. It was challenging, fascinating work.

But St. Louis was large and lonely. Then Peggy came out. She took an apartment close to the botanical garden and got a job as a lab technician. That improved the local scene considerably.

Becoming a Specialist

The other half of my job was to help the director of the botanical garden compile a catalog of the flora of Panama. Again I looked only at dried specimens that other scientists had collected. I had to make sure that they were named correctly and list their local uses, telling subsequent scientists how to identify them and the illustrator how to draw them. To check one specimen, I often had to look at hundreds to make sure that the same species didn't have different scientific names elsewhere in Central and South America.

As tedious as it could be, I loved the work, although such floristic endeavors are not considered as prestigious among botanists as monographic work, in which the scientist concentrates on a small group of related plants, digs in and learns more about them than anyone else. The next thing you know, you're the world authority on them. I wrote a monograph on the weedy tropical chickweed, *Drymaria*, and Peggy illustrated it. Today, more than 30 years later, I'm still the world's leading expert on *Drymaria*. But I can't recall the last time anyone called on that particular expertise.

Peggy and I married in 1960 at the St. Louis courthouse. We bought a beat-up house on the Loutre River 80 miles out of St. Louis, where we took long weekends. Our son, John, was born in St. Louis on Christmas Eve, 1961, about a year after we married.

In St. Louis, I also continued playing music at various clubs, some jazz combo gigs and some accompanying work with jazz, blues and country singers. Some botanists still looked askance at my avocation, but somehow, the deeper I delved into botanical medicine with its earthy folk roots, the more comfortably it "fit" with the music I played, which also had deep roots in the same earthy folk experience.

Loving the Jungle

In 1961, the U.S. military offered me a consulting job accompanying Swamp Fox I, an expedition to the remote Darien Province of Panama and the so-called Darien Gap, the only remaining hole in the Inter-American Highway linking Alaska and Chile. Military vehicles were trying to open a road through this muddy rain forest, with little success. My job was to describe the different types of vegetation and identify which were best suited to supporting vehicular traffic. I jumped at the chance.

My first night in a palm-thatched shack in Darien, a big iguana dropped from the rafters right onto me, almost scaring me to death. The second night the roar of a distant howler monkey was equally alarming. But as always, the local people were gracious, and they were happy to tell me all they knew about the area's plants, including their medicinal uses.

My Spanish was still only rudimentary, but I kept working on it, and little by little, it got better. Ethnobotany, the study of how native peoples use their local plants, was still in its infancy at the time. In fact, the word *ethnobotany* didn't become widely used until some years later, but I was already hip-deep into it, literally, there in the bush of Darien.

I made several Swamp Fox trips to Panama, and I loved working with tropical plants in the wild. Compared with the wonder and adventure of my Darien expeditions, my work at the Missouri Botanical Garden, studying dead, dry specimens of the same plants, began to look pretty dull. I began to put out feelers for another job.

I wound up at the U.S. Department of Agriculture Research Station, the research heart of the USDA, in Beltsville, Maryland. I spent most of the rest of my career there, from 1963 to 1995.

Right away, I got involved in a Latin American project, this time a study of succession—the natural changes in plant populations over time—in tropical Puerto Rico. I learned to identify tropical trees by their seeds and seedlings.

I was happy to learn to do this, but I wasn't happy with the reason behind the project, which was to check how herbicides (read "defoliants") might alter the normal succession of tree seedlings in tropical forests. I also spent some time as curator of the USDA seed collection.

Focusing on Medicinal Herbs

Two years into this USDA program, I got a call from the Battelle Memorial Institute, a research organization in Columbus, Ohio. Battelle had landed a big contract from the old Atomic Energy Commission for a feasibility study of a sea-level canal across Panama and Colombia. It may sound crazy now, but the idea was to use supposedly clean, low-power nuclear "devices" (bombs) to blast this canal through the rain forest to save ships the hassle of the locks in the Panama Canal.

Battelle needed a botanist on the team, and my future boss learned that I had a good deal of experience in Panama and with Panamanian flora. Once again, I jumped at the opportunity to go to Latin America.

I had no idea then, but the Battelle project changed my life. It marked my conversion from a botanist to an ethnobotanist focused on medicinal herbs.

The Battelle project was a dream come true for me, but it began as quite a nightmare for Peggy. We had a nearly four-year-old son and a six-month-old daughter, Celia, and here I wanted to pull up stakes and move us from Beltsville to Panama—in a howling snowstorm, no less. Somehow, though, we survived the trip, as well as six weeks in a fleabag hotel in the Panama Canal Zone.

We also survived gross culture shock and the six weeks and two lawyers it took to get through the formalities and free our earthly goods from customs and get them moved to our apartment in El Cangrejo, which was, by Panamanian standards, a well-to-do suburb of Panama City.

Living in Panama

At first I was unhappy that we were not allowed to live in the Canal Zone, which was very American. But as I was a private consultant not directly employed by the U.S. government, there was no housing for us in the zone. However, in short order, we changed our minds. The Canal Zone was like living in Florida. Where we were, we lived in Panama. When I'm in another country, I like to settle into the culture as much as possible, which is what we did.

Things in Panama were not easy for Peggy. She did not speak

Spanish and had to cope with the many challenges of living in a foreign country, always with two small children in tow and often without her husband around for weeks on end. But despite all the headaches, she enjoyed one wonderful, unexpected perk. For the only time in her life, she had a live-in maid, Edith Bristan, the sister of my most important Panamanian rain forest guide, Narciso Bristan.

Almost all of the apartments in our suburb had maid's quarters, and incredibly, we could afford live-in help. So we asked Edith to move in. She was great with the kids and great company for Peggy. Being of that culture, she taught us all the little details of Panamanian life that would have taken years for us to learn on our own.

By this time, after my Swamp Fox experiences, my Spanish was fairly decent, and one of my jobs was to talk with all the Panamanians, black, white and Indian, about what they ate from the local environment. Why? To put it crudely: If the United States dug that ditch using nuclear bombs, how long would we have to keep the locals from living their local lives— six days, six months, six years, six centuries or six millennia?

Of course, the Panamanians knew why we were there and were quick to ask how many canals the United States was planning to dig in the 50 states using nuclear weapons. They were always gracious, but their point was quite clear, and after my more than two-year stay in Panama, Uncle Sam decided that it was not feasible—biologically, geologically and politically—to build this canal with nuclear weapons.

Plants Yield Their Healing Secrets

The bomb business may have been the reason I was in Panama, but actually, it didn't intrude much on what I did from day to day. I spent most of my time traveling through the thick, lush rain forest of Darien, always by boat because there were no roads. Led by various Panamanian and Indian guides who became my friends, I visited the indigenous people of the forest. With camera and tape recorder, I documented how they lived and what they ate, always delving at length into the local medicinal herbs and how they were used. It was a fascinating two years, and I returned to the United States more convinced than ever that I would focus my career on herbal medicines.

Some experiences remain vivid in my memory, even after 30 years. On one trip into the bush, our group decided to climb Cerro Pirre, an enchanting 5,000-foot peak near the Colombian border. It was a slow, two-day, hand-over-hand climb through thick vegetation. Our Choco Indian porters handled the rigors much better than we gringos did.

We all wore high, thick boots to protect us from the many snakes, and I wished I had leather gloves as well because my hands got cut up something fierce by the vegetation, much of which I was collecting along the way. The first night, some of our guides went ahead to look for a good campsite, and when they found one, they built a fire whose smoke took us to them.

When we arrived at the little clearing they'd discovered, we saw not only the fire but also something right out of some Hollywood jungle movie—what looked like miniature human skulls on skewers. Our sharpshooting Choco porters had hunted up some meat, in this case white-faced monkeys.

After several days of little more than rice, beans and what the Choco and I could forage, I welcomed barbecued monkey, even though it felt a little cannibalistic to eat it. We got some rather grotesque pictures of the guides sucking the brains out of the monkey skulls.

A bigger surprise lay in store for us the next day. After climbing to the peak, we made it back down to the river, where some of our guides lived in a group of huts. It turned out that one of the monkeys we'd eaten had a baby, which our guide recovered on the way down. In the little village, one of the porters gave the baby monkey to his wife, who immediately offered her breast to the monkey to nurse. No one was surprised but me and my fellow gringos. I took a picture of that Choco mother nursing a monkey on one breast and her baby on the other. That picture was published in *Economic Botany*.

I thought about that scene years later, when Ebola virus was in the news and people were talking about how new viral diseases might move from monkeys to humans. The news media never mentioned nursing, but that's certainly one possible way.

Surviving in the Jungle

Being a botanist, I paid special attention to the unique plant spices of the tropics. In Panama, the culinary herb of choice in the bush was culantro, a close relative of coriander, which has the same chemistry and flavor. It really helped with some of those jungle meats.

One jungle meat, namely turtle, greatly increased my growing respect for herbal medicine. On one collecting trip, we camped on the banks of Rio Pirre, and our guides caught some turtles for stew. (They weren't considered endangered then.)

Soon after that meal, I developed a bad case of salmonella food poisoning. (Later I saw a scientific article documenting a high incidence of salmonella in turtle populations in Darien.) The diarrhea was violent and terrible, and I became so weak that I was unable to stand up, let alone work.

I invested several hundred dollars in mainstream Panamanian physicians and their U.S.-style pharmaceutical medicines. They helped a little, but I remained quite ill. Then a more herbally inclined Panamanian doctor gave me powdered carob, and it helped quite a bit. Thirty years later, in 1995, I read a study in the *Journal of Pediatric Gastroenterology and Nutrition* showing that carob powder is highly effective as a treatment for infant diarrhea. I can personally attest that it works.

Forming Friendships among the Indians

Since boyhood romps in the North Carolina forests, I'd been interested in living off the land, and those skills came in handy in Panama. Once a few of us gringos and my guide-buddy Narciso Bristan (our maid's brother) spent several days deep in the bush and ran low on rations. We subsisted on the remains of our rice, dry beans and flour, supplemented by local fruits and roots that I foraged, plus game skillfully shot by Narciso.

Little by little I became intimate with the forests and people of eastern Panama, who gave me some interesting Indian names. With the gregarious village-dwelling Kuna Indians, I was *tutu-sipu-nele-mergui* (gringo witch doctor white flower). The Choco Indians called me *jaibana borojo* (witch doctor borojo). (Borojo is a tree related to coffee but with grapefruit-size fruits that are used to make a fermented beverage called *chicha*.)

Everywhere I went, I always asked to be shown the local medicinal plants, and I talked with the local herbalists and shamanistic healers about how they used them.

In my 2½ years in Panama (with some time in northwestern Colombia as well), my team collected nearly 15,000 specimens, many rare and valuable finds from the wettest, most vegetation-rich area in the Western Hemisphere. Some are now at the New York Botanical Garden, and more are at the Missouri Botanical Garden. From a field botany perspective, the project was a major success, and I hope I had something to do with the decision not to set off nuclear bombs in that wonderful, fascinating, fragile region. Truth be told, I'd fallen madly in love with Latin America, particularly Panama, the Choco Indians, ethnobotany and herbal medicine. I'd become a "Panamaniac."

But all good things come to an end, and in 1968, the family and I returned to the United States, to Battelle's main office in Columbus, Ohio. What a transition. No rain forest, no extended expeditions into the bush, and no live-in maid at home for Peggy and the kids. But someone had to write up all our botanical data from the Panama project, and it fell to yours truly.

I wound up with a whole string of journal articles, including quite a few ethnobotanical papers about herbal medicine. I also published my first book, *The Isthmian Ethnobotanical Dictionary*.

Then funds ran low, and Battelle had no more money for the Panama project. The money was in a new project focusing on the ecology of Amchitka, an island off Pacific Alaska. With all due respect to the beauty and ecological importance of the northern latitudes, I was smitten by the tropics. When Battelle hinted that I might be sent to the North Slope of Alaska, I knew we had come to a parting of the ways.

Investigating a Different Kind of Drug

Once again, the USDA came to my rescue. I was invited back to Beltsville in 1971 to work on a program that involved herbal medicine, but not the kind I advocate using.

In looking to leave Battelle, I'd drafted a proposal on the feasibility of genetically subverting marijuana to make it unappealing to its users. The euphoria-producing compound in marijuana is tetra-hydrocannabinol (THC). The higher the THC level, the more potent the pot. I proposed to breed marijuana with next to no THC and then spread the seed Johnny Appleseed–style in areas where high-THC pot was being illegally grown. I argued that natural cross-breeding would eventually lower the potency of all the local marijuana. Frankly, I had no idea if my notion would work, but the USDA liked the proposal.

We bought a nice suburban house on a half-acre lot within walking distance of my office at Beltsville. But within a year, and with a loan from Momma, we bought a great six-acre farm with a brick ranch house.

I wanted to grow grapes organically, repelling insects and diseases with aromatic herbs, so I intercropped French grapes with old-fashioned aromatic herbs. After a while, the herbs took over from the grapes, but nonetheless, I called the farm Herbal Vineyard. Today we have hundreds of herb species, plus blueberries, blackberries, grapes, raspberries and wineberries, all pretty much untended.

Shortly after I returned to the USDA, there was a dramatic reorganization at Beltsville. I was made chief of what was called the Plant Taxonomy Laboratory, which dealt in part with narcotics. Before I knew it, I was sent back to my beloved Latin America to help the State Department help Bolivia, Peru and Ecuador clamp down on cultivation of coca, the plant source of cocaine.

I also visited Burma, Cambodia, Laos, Thailand and Vietnam to help limit cultivation of the opium poppy. My job was not to eradicate these crops, however. After all, they were being grown because they were a lucrative cash crop for very poor people. My challenging assignment was to develop a catalog of legal useful plants that might be grown as substitute cash crops. Can you guess what I suggested? Medicinal herbs.

Working with Medicinal Herbs

In 1977, I got a medicinal herbalist's dream job as chief of the USDA Medicinal Plant Laboratory, whose main function was to collect medicinal plants from around the world for the cancer screening program being run cooperatively by the USDA and the National Cancer Institute.

I inherited a team of scientists who had been involved in collecting potentially cancer-fighting plants for nearly two decades. (One was Judi duCellier, who became my career-long right-hand woman. She's still with me. She rode herd on this book through the entire editorial process.) The cancer screening program eventually analyzed 10 percent of the world's known plant species for anti-tumor activity and helped point the way to the development of several chemotherapeutic agents now in use, including Taxol from the yew tree, which is used for fighting advanced breast and ovarian cancer.

I dug right into the Medicinal Plant Lab, excited about my first formal job that was fully devoted to medicinal plants. I traveled the globe on collecting trips to China, Ecuador, Egypt, Panama, Chile, Honduras, Syria and the Dominican Republic. While in each of these countries, I also talked with local experts about all the other local medicinal plants that they used for purposes other than cancer treatment.

The cancer screening project was a huge effort, and my own interest in other medicinal plants made it even more ambitious. I needed a way to catalog and easily retrieve the information I was gathering from both folk medicinal and scientific sources. That led to my now-huge medicinal plant computer database, the source for much of the information in this book. If you have a computer, modem and World Wide Web browser, you can access it yourself at http://www.ars-grin.gov/~ngrlsb/.

I was becoming known as one of a small number of medicinal herb experts at the USDA, and that led to several side projects, such as my first trip to China in 1978 to study Asian ginseng (*Panax ginseng*) and the related plant, Siberian ginseng (*Eleutherococcus senticosus*). I had brought along a pound of American ginseng seed (*Panax quinquefolius*) as a gift, in hopes of receiving a pound of Asian ginseng seed in return. Although my hosts said that it was illegal for anyone to take the seed of either Asian or Siberian ginseng out of China, I managed to come home with a souvenir: several flattened twigs and leaves of Siberian ginseng. On a whim, I planted the twigs, and they sprouted, making me an inadvertent smuggler of ginseng.

Cancer Research Funding Dries Up

By 1981, my laboratory's annual budget for the cancer screening program was a half-million dollars, and I was doing such exciting work that I didn't notice the storm clouds gathering in the Reagan Administration.

Instead, I visited China with Dr. James Reveal of the

University of Maryland, with a goal of collecting as many medicinal plants as possible. But once again, the Chinese had a different idea. We only got to collect in one real forest in Kunming in southwest China. Otherwise, we spent our time in botanical gardens or herbal apothecaries or research facilities. Nevertheless, we visited Harbin, Beijing, Chunking, Kunming, Nanjing and Shanghai and returned with some 300 species for the cancer screening program.

Shortly after we got back, Ronald Reagan shut the program down and my laboratory along with it. (I continued to research botanical approaches to cancer treatment, but I did it at home on my own time.)

After a brief, unhappy stint working on trying to improve wheat's disease resistance by breeding domestic wheat with several wild species, in 1982 I returned to the narcotics program at the USDA. This move allowed me to return to my beloved tropics, looking again into alternative crops for cocaine, marijuana and opium poppy. The job took me to Hawaii, Puerto Rico and Thailand, and at every stop, I added material to my ever-expanding medicinal plant database.

Sharing the Rain Forest

Then, in 1991, a pivotal event occurred: I received my first invitation to teach a medicinal plant workshop to an ecotourist group in Amazonian Peru, about 200 miles downriver from the Upper Huallaga Valley, where I'd first looked into alternatives to coca farming years earlier during my first stint with the narcotics program. I was very excited about spending a week in the Amazon, but right before I was to go, I slipped a disk in my back while transporting a Christmas tree. (If you want the gory details, you can read the chapter on backache on page 87.)

I canceled the ecotour workshop but then reconsidered, figuring I'd be in pain either way. Why not at least be in the Amazon?

So I went, and I consider it among the best decisions I ever made. By the end of the week, my pain was much less intense, in part, I think, because I took control of my own medical care and in part because I used so many herbal medicines. In fact, I dedicated that workshop to the tropical papaya tree, the source of chymopapain, a drug used to treat slipped disks.

That first ecotour led to many others, in Belize, Costa Rica and Peru, and now Tanzania and Kenya. These trips helped Judi and me compile our book *The CRC Handbook of Alternative Cash Crops for the Tropics*. And my many trips to Peru led to my *Amazonian Ethnobotanical Dictionary*, co-authored with the excellent Peruvian botanist Rodolfo Vasquez Martinez, who patiently answered my incessant questions as we traveled along the Amazon and Napo rivers in Peru.

By 1997, I'd been involved in more than 30 week-long tropical ecotours, where I worked as a field instructor teaching about the medicinal plants of the rain forest. I even had a toll-free number so that people could call for information about pharmacy ecotours.

Retiring to Harder Work

Then by chance, Alice Feinstein, a book editor at Rodale Press, contacted me to say that she admired my work with herbal medicine and asked if I would like to write a book for Rodale. I said I'd love to. But I had to retire from the USDA to find the time to do it, and I did so in 1995. Those years with the USDA took me around the world many times, learning about the medicinal plants in *The Green Pharmacy*.

Retirement has allowed me to do more than just write this book. I've become deeply involved with The Amazon Center for Environmental Education and Research (ACEER), with its U.S. base in Helena, Alabama. I've become a consultant for the American Botanical Council in Austin, Texas, Herbalife in Los Angeles and Nature's Herbs in American Fork, Utah.

Today I'm as busy as I ever was, working to save the Amazonian rain forest while trying to persuade anyone who will listen that herbal alternatives often work as well as or better than pharmaceuticals. *The Green Pharmacy* furthers both of these objectives.

Join me in the Amazon, friends, and think green. If we all give herbal medicines the chance they deserve, botanical medicine will spread like kudzu, and the world will be the better for it.

—James A. Duke, Ph.D.
The Herbal Vineyard
Fulton, Maryland

Index

Boldface page references indicate primary discussions. Underscored references indicate boxed text. *Italic* references indicate illustrations. Prescription drug names are denoted with the symbol Rx.

TAKE YOUR HEALTH INTO YOUR OWN HANDS

ORDER TODAY:

THE ARTHRITIS CURE
Jason Theodosakis, M.D., M.S., M.P.H., Brenda Adderly, M.H.A.,
and Barry Fox, Ph.D.
___96453-6 $6.50 U.S./$8.50 Can.

SECRETS OF SEROTONIN
Carol Hart
___96087-5 $5.99 U.S./$7.99 Can.

FOODS TO HEAL BY
Barry Fox, Ph.D.
___95987-7 $6.99 U.S./$8.99 Can.

NATURAL HEALING FOR CHILDREN
Winifred Conkling
___96044-1 $6.99 U.S./$8.99 Can.

TAKE THIS BOOK TO THE HOSPITAL WITH YOU
Charles B. Inlander and Ed Weiner
___96326-2 $5.99 U.S./$7.99 Can.

HEADACHES: 47 WAYS TO STOP THE PAIN
Charles B. Inlander and Porter Shimer
___96263-0 $4.99 U.S./$6.50 Can.